Complementary and Integrative Medicine Part I: by Diagnosis

Editors

DEBORAH R. SIMKIN
L. EUGENE ARNOLD

CHILD AND ADOLESCENT PSYCHIATRIC CLINICS OF NORTH AMERICA

www.childpsych.theclinics.com

Consulting Editor
JUSTINE LARSON

April 2023 • Volume 32 • Number 2

ELSEVIER

1600 John F. Kennedy Boulevard • Suite 1800 • Philadelphia, Pennsylvania, 19103-2899

http://www.theclinics.com

CHILD AND ADOLESCENT PSYCHIATRIC CLINICS OF NORTH AMERICA Volume 32, Number 2
April 2023 ISSN 1056–4993, ISBN-13: 978-0-323-94027-6

Editor: Megan Ashdown
Developmental Editor: Arlene Campos

Child and Adolescent Psychiatric Clinics of North America (ISSN 1056-4993) is published quarterly by Elsevier Inc., 360 Park Avenue South, New York, NY 10010-1710. Months of issue are January, April, July, and October. Business and Editorial Offices: 1600 John F. Kennedy Boulevard, Suite 1800, Philadelphia, PA 19103-2899. Periodicals postage paid at New York, NY and additional mailing offices. Subscription prices are $369.00 per year (US individuals), $709.00 per year (US institutions), $100.00 per year (US & Canadian students), $411.00 per year (Canadian individuals), $862.00 per year (Canadian institutions), $473.00 per year (international individuals), $709.00 per year (international institutions), and $200.00 per year (international students). International air speed delivery is included in all *Clinics* subscription prices. All prices are subject to change without notice. **POSTMASTER:** Send address changes to *Child and Adolescent Psychiatric Clinics of North America*, Elsevier Health Sciences Division, Subscription Customer Service, 3251 Riverport Lane, Maryland Heights, MO 63043. **Customer Service: 1-800-654-2452 (U.S. and Canada); 314-447-8871 (outside U.S. and Canada). Fax:** 314-447-8029. **E-mail:** JournalsCustomer Service-usa@elsevier.com **(for print support) or** journalsonlinesupport-usa@elsevier.com **(for online support).**

Reprints. For copies of 100 or more of articles in this publication, please contact the Commercial Reprints Department, Elsevier Inc., 360 Park Avenue South, New York, New York 10010-1710 Tel.: 212-633-3874; Fax: 212-633-3820, E-mail: reprints@elsevier.com.

Child and Adolescent Psychiatric Clinics of North America is covered in *MEDLINE/PubMed (Index Medicus), ISI, SSCI, Research Alert, Social Search, Current Contents,* and *EMBASE/Excerpta Medica.*

Contributors

CONSULTING EDITOR

JUSTINE LARSON, MD, MPH, DFAACAP
Medical Director, Schools and Residential Treatment, Consulting Editor, Child and
Adolescent Psychiatric Clinics of North America, Sheppard Pratt, Rockville, Maryland

EDITORS

DEBORAH R. SIMKIN, MD, DFAACAP
Certified Functional Medicine, Diplomate, American Board of Integrative Holistic
Medicine, BCN, Adjunct Assistant Professor, Department of Psychiatry, Emory University
School of Medicine, Miramar Beach, Florida

L. EUGENE ARNOLD, MD, MEd
Professor Emeritus, Department of Psychiatry and Behavioral Health, The Ohio State
University College of Medicine, Columbus, Ohio

AUTHORS

L. EUGENE ARNOLD, MD, MEd
Professor Emeritus, Department of Psychiatry and Behavioral Health, The Ohio State
University College of Medicine, Columbus, Ohio

BETTINA BERNSTEIN, DO
Clinical Assistant Professor of Psychiatry, Philadelphia College of Osteopathic Medicine,
Clinical Affiliate, Department of Child and Adolescent Psychiatry, The Children's Hospital
of Philadelphia, Philadelphia, Pennsylvania

VINOD S. BHATARA, MD, MS, MSHS
Professor, Department of Psychiatry and Pediatrics, University of South Dakota, Sanford
School of Medicine, Sioux Falls, South Dakota

CHADI ALBERT CALARGE, MD
Associate Professor, Menninger Department of Psychiatry and Behavioral Sciences,
Department of Pediatrics, Baylor College of Medicine, Houston, Texas

VALENTINA CIMOLAI, MD
Child, Adolescent, Adult and Integrative Psychiatrist, Private Practice, REACH Faculty,
Bloom Psychiatry and Wellness and Mindful Healing Group, Clearwater, Florida

JEREMY DANIEL, PHARMD, BCPS, BCPP
Associate Professor, South Dakota State University, College of Pharmacy and Allied
Health Professions, Psychiatric Clinical Pharmacist, Avera Behavioral Health, Sioux Falls,
South Dakota

SWAPNA N. DESHPANDE, MD, DFAACAP
Clinical Associate Professor, Department of Psychiatry and Behavioral Sciences, Oklahoma State University, Tulsa, Oklahoma

SOLANGIA ENGLER, MS
Department of Psychological and Brain Sciences, Texas A&M University, College Station, Texas

SHEEBA FAZILI, MA
Clinical Instructor, University of South Dakota Sanford School of Medicine, Sioux Falls, South Dakota

DIMITRI FIANI, MD
Menninger Department of Psychiatry and Behavioral Sciences, Baylor College of Medicine, Houston, Texas

SHERECCE FIELDS, PhD
Department of Psychological and Brain Sciences, Texas A&M University, College Station, Texas

ROBERT L. HENDREN, DO
Professor of Psychiatry and Behavioral Sciences, University of California, San Francisco, San Francisco, California

REENA KUMAR, DO
Fellow, Andrew Weil Center for Integrative Medicine, University of Arizona, Tucson, Arizona

SHERIN KURIAN, MD
Department of Psychiatry, Psychiatry Research, Texas Children's Hospital, Baylor College of Medicine, Houston, Texas

NOSHENE RANJBAR, MD
Associate Clinical Professor of Psychiatry, University of Arizona College of Medicine, Tucson, Arizona

DOUGLAS RUSSELL, MD
Assistant Professor, Department of Psychiatry and Behavioral Sciences, University of Washington School of Medicine, Seattle, Washington

KIRTI SAXENA, MD
Chief of Child/Adolescent Psychiatry, Department of Psychiatry, Texas Children's Hospital, Associate Professor of Psychiatry, Baylor College of Medicine, Houston, Texas

DEBORAH R. SIMKIN, MD, DFAACAP
Certified Functional Medicine, Diplomate, American Board of Integrative Holistic Medicine, BCN, Adjunct Assistant Professor, Department of Psychiatry, Emory University School of Medicine, Miramar Beach, Florida

SHAYNA SWICK, MD
University of Arizona College of Medicine, Tucson, Arizona

KRISHNA S. TANEJA, MD, MBA
Psychiatry Resident, Southern Illinois University School of Medicine, Springfield, Illinois

PANKHUREE VANDANA, MD
Division of Child and Adolescent Psychiatry, Assistant Professor of Psychiatry, The Ohio State University, Nationwide Children's Hospital, Westerville, Ohio

SHIKHA VERMA, MD, FAPA
Medical Director of Northern California, Evolve-PC Residential Treatment Centers, California; Assistant Professor, Department of Psychiatry and Behavioral Health, Rosalind Franklin University of Medicine and Science, North Chicago, Illinois

TAMARA VIK, MD
Assistant Professor, Director of Child and Adolescent Residency Program, University of South Dakota Sanford School of Medicine, Sioux Falls, South Dakota

CAROL WHITMAN, MD
Clinical Instructor and Resident in Psychiatry, University of South Dakota Sanford School of Medicine, Sioux Falls, South Dakota

ALEEMA ZAKERS, MD
Staff Psychiatrist, MPH Georgia Institute of Technology, Adjunct Faculty, Moorhouse School of Medicine, Adjunct Faculty, Emory School of Medicine, Atlanta, Georgia

Contents

First-line psychopharmacologic and psychosocial treatments for
attention-deficit/hyperactivity disorder in children are effective but limited
by tolerability and accessibility problems. Many complementary and integrative strategies have been investigated as alternative or adjunctive treatments for the disorder, and the literature has progressed to meta-analyses
for several. Although heterogeneity of study methods and risk of bias pervades the literature, we conclude that Omega-3 supplementation, dietary
restriction of artificial food colorings, and physical activity can be considered evidence-based. Additionally, meditation, yoga, and sleep hygiene
are safe, partially effective, cost effective and sensible adjunctive treatment strategies.

An integrative approach to treating anxiety in children and adolescents
takes a biopsychosocial-spiritual approach. Early life stress may translate
into anxiety via epigenetic mechanisms, the adoption of maladaptive
coping tendencies (poor eating, sedentary lifestyle, substance use), and
dysregulation of central autonomic nervous system function. Each of these
mechanisms may increase inflammatory markers. This article will explore
the efficacy of CIM interventions that work on these mechanisms through
mind-body-medicine, acupuncture, nutrition, and supplements.

Substance use disorders are a growing concern for all ages, including adolescents. Even though there is an increase in recreational substance use
and a wider variety of drugs is available to this young population, treatment
options remain scarce. Most medications have limited evidence in this
population. Few specialists treat individuals struggling with addiction
along with mental health disorders. As the evidence grows, these treatments are usually included in complementary and integrative medicine.
This article discusses available evidence for many complementary and
integrative treatment approaches while briefly describing existing psycho-
therapeutic and psychotropic medications.

Sleep problems are very common in children and adolescents. Chronic insomnia is the leading cause of sleep disorders in children and adolescents. Adjunctive interventions that address low ferritin levels and vitamin D3 deficiency are helpful in children and adolescents. The addition of l-5-hydroxytryptophan, gabadone, l-theanine, Ashwagandha, omega 3 fatty acids, probiotics in bipolar disorder, and children with colic, meditation, and changing from a high-fat diet to a Mediterranean diet are also helpful adjunctive interventions. Actigraphy data should be collected in future sleep studies because subjective data may not indicate the true effect of the intervention.

The rationale for CIM treatments in youth psychoses is to optimize treatment by targeting symptoms not resolved by antipsychotics, such as negative symptoms (major drivers of disability). Adjunctive omega-3 fatty acids (ω-3 FA) or N-acetyl cystine (NAC usage for > 24-week) can potentially reduce negative symptoms and improve function. ω-3 FA or exercise may prevent progression to psychosis in youth (in prodromal stage). Weekly 90-minute moderate to vigorous physical activity or aerobic exercise can reduce positive and negative symptoms. Awaiting better research, CIM agents are also recommended because they are devoid of any serious side-effects.

Youth with emotional dysregulation (ED) and irritability/aggression, common in disruptive disorders (frequently comorbid with attention-deficit/hyperactivity disorder), are underserved by conventional treatments. Anger dysregulation is usually the core feature of ED. Complementary and integrative Medicine (CIM) treatments for youth with disruptive disorders and ED are reviewed. Broad-spectrum micronutrient supplementation has a medium effect and is supported by two double-blind randomized controlled trials using similar formulations. Other CIM treatments supported by controlled data but needing further research, include omega-3 fatty acid supplementation, music therapy, martial arts, restricting exposure to media violence, decreasing sleep deprivation, and increased exposure to green-blue spaces.

Response to PTSD treatments differ based on the age the abuse occurred, the type of abuse, and the chronicity of the abuse. Even when modifications to treatment are made based on the developmental age when the abuse occurred, therapies may be insufficient. In addition, when diagnostic criteria are modified to identify more children, some children continue to escape detection. Developmental Trauma Disorder, (akin to the RDoC), may be more suitable to identify epigenetic and inflammatory effects of early abuse that may be responsible for the nonresponsive to treatment. Complementary and Integrative Medicine interventions (meditation, EFT, EMDR, PUFAs, etc.) may reverse these effects.

Omega-3 polyunsaturated fatty acids, probiotics, vitamin C, vitamin D, folic acid and L-methyl folate, broad-spectrum micronutrients, N-acetylcysteine, physical activity, herbs, bright light therapy, melatonin, saffron, meditation, school-based interventions, and transcranial photobiomodulation are reviewed, with a focus on their use for treating mood disorders in children and adolescents. For each treatment, all published randomized controlled trials are summarized.

Childhood obesity is a significant global challenge with increasing prevalence. It is associated with long-term health risks. Interventions especially early on can be effective in the prevention and reducing the impact on health in children. In children, dysbiosis and inflammation are associated with obesity. Studies demonstrate that intensive lifestyle interventions in form of parent education, motivational interviewing to improve diet and exercise as well as mindfulness, and sleep improvement can help alleviate the risk. The article outlines the current research describing complementary and integrative approaches to the prevention and treatment of obesity in children.

Eating disorders (EDs) are a non-heterogeneous group of illnesses with significant physical and mental comorbidity and mortality associated with maladaptive coping. With the exception of lisdexamfetamine (Vyvanse) for binge eating disorder, no medications have been effective for the core symptoms of ED. ED requires a multimodal approach. Complementary and integrative medicine (CIM) can be helpful as an adjunct. The most promising CIM interventions are traditional yoga, virtual reality, eye movement desensitization and reprocessing, Music Therapy, and biofeedback/neurofeedback.

This article reviews the role of iron in brain development and function, with a focus on the association between iron deficiency (ID) and neuropsychiatric conditions. First, we describe how ID is defined and diagnosed. Second, the role of iron in brain development and function is summarized. Third, we review current findings implicating ID in a number of neuropsychiatric conditions in children and adolescents, including attention deficit hyperactivity disorder and other disruptive behavior disorders, depressive and anxiety disorders, autism spectrum disorder, movement disorders, and other situations relevant to mental health providers. Last, we discuss the impact of psychotropic medication on iron homeostasis.

Autism spectrum disorder (ASD) is a neurodevelopmental disorder that affects 0.6%-1.7% of children. The etiology of autism is hypothesized to include both biological and environmental factors (Watts, 2008). In addition to the core symptoms of social-communication delay and restricted, repetitive interests, co-occurring irritability/aggression, hyperactivity, and insomnia negatively impact adaptive functioning and quality of life of patients and families. Despite years of effort, no pharmacologic agent has been found that targets the core symptoms of ASD. The only FDA-approved agents are risperidone and aripiprazole for agitation and irritability in ASD, not for core symptoms. Though they effectively reduce irritability/violence, they do so at the expense of problematic side effects: metabolic syndrome, elevated liver enzymes, and extrapyramidal side effects. Thus, it is not surprising that many families of children with ASD turn to nonallopathic treatment, including dietary interventions, vitamins, and immunomodulatory agents subsumed under complementary-integrative medicine (CIM). Per recent studies, 27% to 88% of families report using a CIM treatment. In an extensive population-based survey of CIM, families of children with more severe ASD, comorbid irritability, GI symptoms, food allergies, seizures, and higher parental education tend to use CIM at higher rates. The perceived safety of CIM treatments as "natural treatment" over allopathic medication increases parental comfort in using these agents. The most frequently used CIM treatments include multivitamins, an elimination diet, and Methyl B12 injections. Those perceived most effective are sensory integration, melatonin, and antifungals. Practitioners working with these families should improve their knowledge about CIM as parents currently perceive little interest in and poor knowledge of CIM by physicians. This article reviews the most popular complementary treatments preferred by families with children with autism. With many of them having limited or poor quality data, clinical recommendations about the efficacy and safety of each treatment are discussed using the SECS versus RUDE criteria.

CHILD AND ADOLESCENT PSYCHIATRIC CLINICS

Preface

Complementary and Integrative Medicine/Functional Medicine in Child and Adolescent Psychiatric Disorders: Should It Be Taken Seriously?

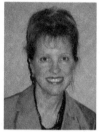 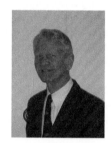

Deborah R. Simkin, MD, DFAACAP   L. Eugene Arnold, MD, Med
Editors

INTRODUCTION

According to the National Center for Complementary and Integrative Health (NCCIH) at the National Institute of Health, complementary interventions are non-mainstream approaches used together with conventional medicine and alternative interventions are the use of non-mainstream approaches used in place of conventional medicine. NCCIH states "Integrative health emphasizes multimodal interventions, which are two or more interventions such as conventional medicine approaches (like medication, physical rehabilitation, psychotherapy), and complementary health approaches (like acupuncture, yoga, and probiotics) in various combinations, with an emphasis on treating the whole person rather than, for example, one organ system". NCCIH defines whole person health as "helping individuals, families, communities, and populations improve and restore their health in multiple interconnected domains—biological, behavioral, social, environmental—rather than just treating disease. NCCIH also states that Functional Medicine (FM) may not fit neatly into CIM and sometimes refers to a concept similar to integrative health, but it may also refer to an approach that "more closely resembles naturopathy (a medical system that has evolved from a combination of traditional practices and health care approaches popular in Europe during the 19th century)" and includes such things as.

Child Adolesc Psychiatric Clin N Am 32 (2023) xiii–xxiv
https://doi.org/10.1016/j.chc.2022.09.001
1056-4993/23/© 2022 Published by Elsevier Inc.

childpsych.theclinics.com

- Dietary and lifestyle changes
- Stress reduction interventions like meditation
- Herbs and other dietary supplements
- Manipulative therapies
- Exercise therapy
- Practitioner-guided detoxification
- Psychotherapy and counseling

FM evaluations include antecedents (genetic risk and family history), triggers (environmental insults), and perpetuators (entities that cause the disease process to continue or worsen) (www.nccih.nih.gov/health/complementary-alternative-or-integrative-health-whats-in-a-name). Although FM and CIMED are not congruent, for simplicity we will here use the term CIM to refer to both overlapping types of treatment. Interest in pediatric integrative medicine has increased due to the desire to decrease prescription use, the need for more effective approaches to preventive health in children,[1,2] and the prevalence of use in children living with chronic illness.[3,4] Therefore, it is prudent that child psychiatrists familiarize themselves with empirical research on CIM/Functional Medicine (CIM) interventions summarized in this update. The American Academy of Child and Adolescent Psychiatry (AACAP) established the Committee on Integrative Medicine (CIMED) in 2010 to educate child psychiatrists in this field. This text continues in that mission as research has expanded. We assume familiarity with DSM-5 diagnoses, which are named without definition.

Overall, consumer interest in and use of complementary therapies in adults and children have outpaced training options in pediatric integrative medicine, leaving clinicians with a desire for more training and familiarity with resources. For example, a 2012 survey of academic pediatric training programs revealed that only 16 of 143 programs reported having an integrative medicine program.[5] Even fewer of these training opportunities exist in child psychiatry.

Data from the 2012 National Health Interview Survey (NHIS) showed that 12% of children (about 1 in 9) used complementary therapies in the prior year, similar to the prevalence documented in the 2007 NHIS survey. The 2012 NHIS showed an increase from 3.9% in 2007 to 4.9% of children using dietary supplements and a significant increase in the pediatric use of yoga, fish oil, and melatonin.[6] Prevalence jumps to approximately 50% in children living with a chronic illness (www.nccih.nih.gov/health/complementary-alternative-or-integrative-health-whats-in-a-name). Use was higher in children with more than one health condition and in children whose families could not afford conventional care. The percentage of children who used yoga in the past 12 months increased significantly from 3.1% in 2012 to 8.4% in 2017. However, lower-income families are at a disadvantage when it comes to services like massage therapy and yoga. Non-Hispanic white children were likelier to have used yoga and chiropractic care than non-Hispanic black or Hispanic children.[7] Lower-income families cannot afford the luxury of yoga and other mind-body classes, ranging from $12 to $20 per class. For low-income patients with little or no discretionary income, these fees are seen as unnecessary, and more basic needs, such as food, rent, heat, and clothing, take priority. Other difficulties in utilizing services involve time factors because lower-income individuals often work multiple jobs, lack transportation, and for those who recently migrated and have not had time to master the English language, difficulty following instructions.[8]

Both the 2007 and the 2012 NHIS results revealed that adolescents (ages 12–17 years) were more likely to use complementary therapies than younger children (ages 4–11 years).[6] Adolescents use supplements to enhance athletic performance, lose weight, increase energy, and improve their body image.[9] Adolescents, like children, are more likely to use complementary therapies if their parents do, but they also use them due to targeted marketing and advertising on television and the Internet.[10] Clinicians may disregard natural products merely because they originate "outside of conventional medicine" produced by large pharmaceutical companies and the lack of government oversight and regulation quality and safety of dietary supplements and natural products. Most families are unwilling to discuss this choice with their physicians because they expect disinterest, disapproval, or ignorance from physicians regarding complementary and integrative medicine (CIM) treatments.[11] However, without extensive training in critically appraising research literature, it can be challenging for the layperson to understand why the "evidence" they have heard or read for a particular treatment may not be meaningful or valuable. Engaging patients in the available evidence and the provider's experience can help them understand the compatibility and efficacy of using a broad and holistic approach to treatment.

Therefore, it is essential for child psychiatrists to be knowledgeable about what their patients may be using, the research for or against the use, and the side effects of supplements in order to provide informed consent, especially when the patient or the family refuses the standard treatment. In such situations, there is a risk to ignoring questions about a patient's use and/or using resources which cite the research validity for whether some CIM treatments may have benefit. This text should increase the knowledge of CIM empirically based interventions for clinicians who seek to improve the quality of care.

For the provider to maintain executive balance, it is essential to keep in mind that many current standardized treatments have limitations (e.g., selective serotonin reuptake inhibitors and antipsychotics). Many are expensive, and many CIM therapies have not or cannot be effectively studied in a well-controlled fashion.[12,13] In addition, it is essential to remember that research on CIM is limited because many of these treatments do not generate large profits. Therefore, even though some treatments appear valuable enough to validate the need for randomized, double-blind, placebo-controlled studies, funding is unavailable to support this.

Some treatments may derive most of their effect from placebo response (this is also true for some Food and Drug Administration [FDA] -approved medications). Increasing literature confirms the reality of placebo benefits, including EEG and brain-imaging changes.[14–16]

DEFINITIONS

The National Center for Complementary and Integrative Health (NCCIH) of the National Institutes of Health (NIH) defines complementary therapies as evidence-based health care approaches developed outside conventional Western Medicine that is used in conjunction with conventional care (www.nccih.nih.gov/health/complementary-alternative-or-integrative-health-whats-in-a-name). NCCIH defines integrative health as bringing conventional and complementary approaches together in a coordinated way. Integrative health also emphasizes multimodal interventions, which can be two or more interventions (such as conventional medicine, lifestyle changes, psychotherapy) in various combinations, with an emphasis on treating the whole person rather than, for example, one organ system. Functional medicine (FM) incorporates components of integrative medicine but goes a bit further by asking how and why illness began. NCCIH also states that Functional Medicine (FM) may not fit neatly into CIM and sometimes refers to a concept similar to integrative health, but it may also refer to an approach that "more closely resembles naturopathy (a medical system that has evolved from a combination of traditional practices and health care approaches popular in Europe during the 19th century)" and includes such things as: "Dietary and lifestyle changes, Stress reduction interventions like meditation, Herbs and other dietary supplements, Manipulative therapies, Exercise Therapy, practitioner-guided detoxification, Psychotherapy and counseling. It looks at the root cause of illness for each individual and the multiple systems that the illness may have affected. FM traces factors over a lifetime that act as antecedents, like family history or trauma that causes epigenetic changes, triggers, like infections or stress, and mediators, like obesity, lack of sleep, and diet, that may continue to influence the expression of genes or worsen the condition produced by gene expression. For instance, although a person may have an increased risk of developing Alzheimer, it does not have to be one's destiny. Many factors (including environmental toxins or trauma, lifestyle, diet, activity patterns, psycho-social-spiritual factors, and stress) can influence the progression of the disease and create other conditions, like diabetes, obesity, and heart disease (that also can influence the progression of the disease). Therefore, FM uses a biological systems approach to address the source of these conditions. FM will also seek to uncover acquired conditions, like Lyme disease or decreased hormone levels that occur in older individuals, that may contribute to the progression of Alzheimer.[17] By using this systems approach and addressing lifestyle, FM can, for instance, down-regulate or eradicate inflammation in multiple systems or sources. Inflammation may play a significant role in the progression of the disease.

FM ideally seeks to balance individuals' spiritual, mental, and emotional levels. Patients tend to be more satisfied with this approach. In a 2-year study following patients in an outpatient clinic versus those seen in a Center for Functional Medicine clinic at Cleveland Clinic, researchers evaluated continuous changes over time in the NIH validated Patient-Reported Outcome Measurement Information System (PROMIS). PROMIS measures patients' global physical and mental health over time, measuring factors like fatigue, physical function, pain, gastrointestinal issues, and emotional well-being. At both 6 and 12 months, patients in the FM clinic demonstrated improvements in PROMIS global physical health that were significantly larger compared with patients seen in a primary care setting.[17] Although this text will discuss empirically based interventions using CIM approaches, one must not forget that research usually addresses one intervention for one disease approach. Therefore, we do not want the reader to assume that using CIM interventions based on research equates to the multisystem approach of FM. Instead, we intend to provide a resource based on empirically proven research for CIM interventions that may be incorporated into the practice of child psychiatry if the practitioner chooses to do so.

DEFINITIONS OF AGE

Adolescence is defined by the World Health Organization as between 10 and 19 years, while youth are referred to as 15 to 24 years (http://undesadspd.org/Youth.aspx). Young people are defined as a combination of the ages of adolescents and youth (10- to 24-years-old). The Lancet commission designated definitions of age from a biological perspective.[18] In early adolescence (10–14 years) pubertal hormones come on board that activate the nucleus accumbens and the reward system. Without a mature prefrontal cortex to inhibit the reward system, this period is associated with risk-taking behavior. Late adolescence (15–19 years) brings continued development of executive and self-regulatory skills. Young adulthood (typically 20–24 years) is accompanied by the maturation of the prefrontal cortex and an increase in self-regulatory functions. It marks the end of a period of high brain plasticity whereby the final phase of the organization of the adult brain occurs. Based on the brain's neurodevelopment and because most studies refer to adults as 18 or older, we define children as up to 10 years of age, adolescents as ages 10 to 17 years, and young adults as ages 18 to 24 years.

LEGAL, REGULATORY, AND ETHICAL ISSUES
Informed Consent

There are two reasons parents are entrusted to give informed consent on behalf of their child. First, children are thought to lack the knowledge, experience, and maturity to make decisions. Second, it is assumed that with the assistance of a health provider, parents are expected to make decisions in the child's best interest. In CIM, risks and benefits, just as in conventional medicine, must be considered. Every element of informed consent or assent must be followed for both CIM and conventional treatments. Elements of informed consent include risks, benefits, alternative, conventional and CIM treatments, the degree to which the research supports the use of the CIM treatment, the absence of FDA approval, the parent/patient's understanding of known and unknown risks associated with CIM, and an explanation of why the CIM treatment is being used rather than a conventional treatment. No guarantees should be given. Having handouts available should a parent request one would be helpful.

Using Integrative/Functional Medicine- Liability

CIM is not always the standard of care found in conventional medicine, and by departing from conventional medicine, a clinician may increase the risk of a medical malpractice suit. However, it is now being recognized, and research is increasing. For example, the American Psychiatric Association now has a caucus on Complementary and Alternative Medicine (CAM). Research is beginning to find many avenues for using CIM as an adjunct to conventional medicine. In malpractice suits, battery claims are the most common occurrence secondary to not obtaining informed consent. Medical malpractice occurs when a clinician does not follow a standard of care and causes harm to the patient.[19] Therefore, in the latter example, it would be necessary for a clinician to know the risks and benefits, including drug interactions and side effects. Using the SECS criteria helps support CIM treatments with few side effects, such as meditation. Stabilizing a patient (for instance, that may be suicidal) must be done before using CIM treatments or referring a patient to a CIM treatment provider.

If a psychiatrist is working with a patient receiving a CIM treatment from a CIM provider, the psychiatrist should continue to follow the patient to ensure the integrative treatments are not interfering with a conventional treatment plan, harming the patient, or delaying necessary conventional treatment. Reaching out to the CIM provider after obtaining consent is wise. Not doing the above suggestions can be considered a liability. Documentation of any discussion with the parents, the child, and the CIM provider should be delineated in the chart. If a parent insists on using a treatment that is against medical advice, clear documentation should denote the parent's or young adult's refusal of medical advice.

Considering the hierarchy of published evidence of safety and efficacy is advisable when choosing the first intervention, whether conventional or CIM.

Some conventional and CIM treatments are used when there is no FDA quality control. However, the reasons the treatment is used must be documented. For instance, even though there may be no FDA recommendation for a conventional medicine within a specific age group, if research is available that validates the use, this must be explained to the parents and documented. Many supplements are marketed in CIM that have no FDA monitoring. Therefore, a clinician should be aware of the research that supports the use. For instance, omega-3 fatty acids have been shown to reduce the symptoms of depression in youth. Some authors suggest a 2/1 ratio of eicosapentaenoic acid (EPA) to docosahexaenoic acid (DHA) is best.[20] Clinicians should know the research on dosage and the best products to use. Much of this can be found in published research. Clinicians can also ask a supplement manufacturer if they allow the FDA to inspect their facility.

Introducing CIM treatments into practice is somewhat similar to introducing any new treatment. However, as CIM treatments and research continue to evolve, clinicians may need to change their practice to provide the best possible care to their patients and remain in compliance with the law.

Purity of Substances

Concerns exist about the purity and potency of herbal products and other dietary supplements sold in the United States, partly because of regulations that differ from those governing the use of pharmaceuticals.

Under the Dietary Supplements Health and Education Act of 1994,[19] a dietary supplement is considered the following.

  A product (other than tobacco) intended to supplement the diet that bears or contains one or more of the following ingredients: a vitamin, a mineral, an herb or other botanical, or an amino acid;
  Intended for ingestion in pill, capsule, tablet, or liquid form;
  Not used as a conventional food or as the sole item of a meal or diet; and
  Labeled as a dietary supplement.

The FDA can demonstrate that a supplement is unsafe only after it reaches the market and must prove that the product is unsafe before it can restrict a product's use or take other legal action. The FDA relies mainly on the MedWatch voluntary reporting system to collect safety data on dietary supplements.[21]

In contrast, dietary supplements in Canada are regulated through Health Canada's Natural and Non-Prescription Health Products Directorate, formerly known as the Natural Health Products Directorate. In addition, products manufactured or distributed in Canada must have a product license by Health Canada, certifying premarket safety, efficacy, and quality (https://health-products.Canada.ca/lnhpd-bdpsnh/index-eng.jsp. Accessed July 16, 2017).

Training and Licensure

Despite the high demand for integrative care, a lack of education about the safety and effectiveness of complementary and integrative therapies in pediatrics and child psychiatry still exists.

As of 2015, 50% of US medical school Web sites (n = 130) listed at least one course or clerkship offering in CAM.[22]

The Committee on the Use of Complementary and Alternative Medicine by the American Public recommends that the national professional organizations for all CAM disciplines ensure the presence of training standards and develop practice guidelines. Ideally, health care professional licensing boards and accrediting and certifying agencies (for both complementary and conventional medicine) should set competency standards in the appropriate use of both conventional medicine and complementary therapies, consistent with practitioners' scope of practice and referral standards across health professions.[23]

In 2020, the Academic Consortium for Integrative Medicine and Health assumed the role of recognizing integrative medicine fellowship programs. As of 2020, there were 19 fellowships approved by the American Board of Integrative Medicine (www.abpsus.org/integrative-medicine-fellowships/). Certification by the American Board of Integrative Medicine is recognized by the American Board of Physician Specialties, Inc (www.abpsus.org/integrative-medicine-who/).

The Institute of Functional Medicine offers certification in FM after completion of the Functional Medicine in Clinical Practice course and six advanced individual modules in Gastrointestinal, Environmental Health, Immune, Hormone Cardiometabolic, and Bioenergetics. Then the applicant must submit and pass the criteria required in a case report and a written exam. Recertification must be obtained every 10 years (www.ifm.org/certification-membership/certification-program/certification-process-and-requirements/).

For clinicians who have no training or certification and who partner with another clinician who practices CIM, it is best to know whether the CIM/FM clinician is certified in the area he/she claims to be.

HISTORY AND WHERE DO WE GO FROM HERE

The Flexner Report of 1910 transformed the nature and process of medical education in America with a resulting elimination of proprietary schools (chiropractors, physical therapy, naturopathic medicine, and so forth) and the establishment of the biomedical model as the gold standard of medical training.[24] A group of men, known as the Hopkins Circle, joined in a project that altered the course of medical education. Members included William Welch, the founding dean at Hopkins; William Osler, the Canadian son of a frontier minister and chief of medicine at Hopkins; Frederick Gates, a Baptist minister and trusted adviser to John D. Rockefeller; and Abraham Flexner, a former schoolteacher and expert on educational practices. At that moment in the history of American medicine, things changed. In order to be accredited, schools had to be more consistent in teaching medicine based more on scientific principles. However, William Osler was one of the critics of this report. While he noted the importance of scientific knowledge, he felt that the focus would become so narrow and that medical schools, students, and clinicians would see other interventions as less worthwhile. He also felt the practice of medicine would become more sterile. By focusing on the science of diseases in medicine and less on the emotional connection of the doctor-patient relationship and the mentoring in the teacher-student relationship (the art of medicine), a critical priority to Osler would be lost.

The Flexner Report led to the closure of 75% of medical and psychiatric facilities, five of the seven black medical schools, and a reduction of CAM-related educational programs at the existing medical schools.[25] However, unlike the effects of the Flexner Report (which was based on German medical education), the acceptance of CAM in Europe allowed aspects of CAM to continue to exist, enriching the teaching of medicine.[26] The medical schools and American medicine made substantial scientific gains after the Flexner Report emerged but the balance of art and science was lost. Naturopathic medicine declined after the Flexner report. Although the discovery of penicillin greatly advanced medicine and the need for the further development of surgery after World War II helped thousands, many people sought a pill as a fix. A review of medical care in the last century documents that the trust and respect that were extended to the profession 50 years ago have been substantially eroded.[27]

Two things seemed to have been lost. First, American medicine was isolated from other fields that focused on healing traditions and natural approaches, such as

Ayurveda, Yoga, and traditional Chinese Medicine (which had been used for thousands of years). In 1955 by Professor Roger Williams, a biochemist, in '*Biochemical Individuality*', argued that bad genes did not necessarily cause disease by themselves and that nutrition and environment can influence the outcome. He first discussed this in an article outlining the effect of nutrition and craving in alcoholism and called it the genetotrophic (geneto = genes, trophic = nutrition) effect. He also felt that many diseases were influenced by nutrition and other environmental insults that interacted with genes and played a role in allergies, mental diseases, cardiovascular diseases, arthritis, multiple sclerosis and cancer.[28] The effect of nutrition and environment upon genes has now been proven (epigenetics). The focus of preventative medicine, the doctor-patient relationship and the emotional and spiritual well-being of the patient as a human being, was lost. To address these issues, in 1977, the American Holistic Medical Association (AHMA) was formed and together with the American Board of Integrative Holistic Medicine (ABIHM) began developing certification. In 2013, leaders from AHMA and ABIHM came together with other leaders in integrative health to form the Academy of Integrative Health & Medicine (www.aihm.org/vision). Meanwhile, in 1991, Dr Linus Pauling appointed Dr Jeffrey Bland as the director of nutritional research at his Institute. Dr Bland recognized that today's most prevalent health issues are caused mainly by the interactions between genetics, lifestyle choices, and environmental exposures and that treating them requires understanding these interactions and subsequently using that understanding to design appropriate treatments that are personalized to each individual.[29] He founded the Institute of Functional Medicine (www.ifm.org/about/history). Using this model, the focus is on the spiritual, mental, and emotional health of the individual and a deep commitment to the doctor-patient relationship while still using interventions based on scientific research. Recent research has allowed clinicians the opportunity to utilize CIM/FM interventions. Child psychiatrists have an enormous opportunity to prevent the development of disease by utilizing conventional medicine alongside CIM/FM empirically based treatments.

METHODOLOGY

Much of the initial work for this text began as a Clinical Update for the American Academy of Child and Adolescent Psychiatry by the Committee on Complementary and Integrative Medicine while Dr Simkin and Dr Arnold served as co-chairs. In this text, each commonly seen child and adolescent psychiatric disorder is addressed from a CIM/FM perspective.

To update current published evidence (or lack thereof) for child/adolescent complementary-integrative interventions, we searched PubMed first, then PsychInfo for additional references and, then supplemented with additional reference found by following major journals after that.

Retrieval was limited to publication dates January 2000 to November 2022, English language, peer reviewed, human research, and the age ranges of children and adolescents.

Search terms were in the format established by Pubmed and PsychInfo respectively, and included the following: mental health, mental disorders, behavior disorders, emotional problems, autism, depression, anxiety, PTSD, bipolar, ADHD, traumatic brain injury AND complementary integrative medicine, alternative therapies, functional medicine alternative therapy complementary treatment, meditation, nutrition, sickness behavior, gut-brain axis, folate cycle, hypothalamic pituitary axis, methylation cycle, oxidative stress, micronutrients, bright light therapy, transcendental meditation, proinflammatory cytokines, IDO pathway, microglia, omega 3 fatty acids, N-acetylcysteine, SAM-E, vitamin D, microbiome, probiotics, antioxidants, gluta-thione, St. John's Wort, elimination diet, processed foods, pesticides, inflammation, mind-body therapies.

The strategy was to use meta-analyses and systematic reviews when available, and when there were none for a given treatment, substitute randomized controlled trials (RCTs). A search of the literature from 2000 was conducted on Medline initially in October 2020, yielding 4,434 English-language citations. Filtering for meta-analyses or systematic reviews reduced these to 175. Rerunning with filter of RCT yielded 474. Repeating the procedure in Psychinfo yield 25 additional nonduplicative refer-ences. These citations were supplemented by references suggested by section au-thors from Embase and web searches, including new publications after 2020. Final winnowing (eg, not using an individual RCT if included in a meta-analysis or systematic review) resulted in 357 total citations.

Tables rate treatments by an adapted version of the US Preventative Services Task Force principles (US Preventive Services|Grade Definitions; uspreventiveservicestaskforce.org) and the World Federation of Societies of Biological Psychiatry and the Canadian Network for Mood and Anxiety Treatments Taskforce (https://doi.org/10.1080/15622975.2021.2013041). The tables summarize the quality of the research and the benefit and safety. The tables also state a prac-tical conclusion/recommendation in the last column.

While awaiting better evidence, the best a clinician can do in many situations is to weigh what is known about possible benefits and risks and apply clinical common sense. For this text, the clinician can be guided by the safe, easy, cheap, and sensible (SECS) versus risky, unrealistic, difficult, or expensive (RUDE) criterion.[30] A treatment that is SECS does not require as much evidence of effectiveness to justify clinical application as one that is RUDE. Note that to qualify as SECS, a treatment must meet all four benchmarks, whereas to qualify as RUDE, treatment needs to meet only one of the benchmarks. Thus, over-the-counter RDA/RDI multivitamin/mineral supplements for a child with a poor diet induced by stimulants or meditation for a child with anxiety qualifies as SECS, not requiring much evidence for implementation.

On the other hand, although safe and sensible, neurofeedback is expensive and complicated, thus requiring good evidence of effectiveness. Oral chelation, although easy and not too expensive, is risky, thus also requiring good evidence of effective-ness for a different reason. Note that passing the SECS criterion does not make a treatment evidence-based; it just provides a clinical decision tool to make the best of the immediate situation.

In addition, each article focusing on child and adolescent psychiatric disorders will summarize the Strength of Recommendations based on benefit and safety, the level of certainty based on the quality of the research, the specific level of research used to rate the quality and the benefits of the research, whether the intervention fits the

---

Box 1
Ranking of Strength of Recommendations based on benefit and safety and Level of Certainty regarding quality and SECS criteria

Strength of recommendations based on benefit and safety

A = Recommend strongly. There is a high certainty that the net benefit is substantial **and safe.**

B = Recommend. There is a high certainty that the net benefit is moderate or there is moderate certainty that the net benefit is moderate to substantial **and safe.**

C = Neutral (offer or provide this service for selected patients depending on individual circumstances, based on professional judgment and patient preferences). There is at least moderate certainty that the net benefit is small.

D = Discourage. There is moderate or high certainty that the service has no net benefit or that the harms outweigh the benefits.

I = Insufficient (if the service is offered, patients should understand the uncertainty about the balance of benefits and harms). Current evidence is insufficient to assess the balance of benefits and harms of the service. Evidence is lacking, of poor quality, or conflicting, and the balance of benefits cannot be determined.

Level of certainty regarding quality

HIGH: Level of Evidence with robust positive data meta-analyses or metareviews involving 2 or more randomized controlled clinical trials (RCTs) of excellent, robust quality. The available evidence usually includes consistent results from well-designed, well-conducted RCTs in representative child, adolescent, or young adult (18–24-years-old) populations, assessing the effects on mental health outcomes.

MODERATE: Level of Evidence with robust positive data involving 2 or more RCTs of excellent, robust quality. The available evidence usually includes consistent results from well-designed, well-conducted RCTs in representative child, adolescent, or young adult (18–24-years-old) populations, assessing the effects on mental health outcomes, but confidence in the estimate is constrained by such factors as:

- The number, size, or quality of individual studies.
- Inconsistency of findings across individual studies.
- Limited generalizability of findings to child psychiatry/adolescent/young adult practice.
- Lack of coherence in the chain of evidence.

   As more information becomes available, the magnitude or direction of the observed effect could change, and this change may be large enough to alter the conclusion.

LOW: Level of evidence with less than 2 RCTs with good or average quality. The available evidence is insufficient to assess the effects on mental health outcomes. Evidence is insufficient because of:

- The limited number or size of studies.
- Important flaws in study design or methods.
- Inconsistency of findings across individual studies.
- Gaps in the chain of evidence.
- Findings are not generalizable to routine child/adolescent/young adult practice.
- Lack of information on important mental health outcomes.

   More information may allow estimation of effects on mental health outcomes.

SECS Criteria

A guide to clinical decisions is that Interventions that are Safe, Easy, Cheap, **and** Sensible (SECS) require less evidence to justify individual trials than those that are Risky, Unrealistic, Difficult, **or** Expensive (RUDE). Because some of the treatments do not have much solid, compelling evidence but would be reasonable to try with a lower bar of evidence, this criterion is also taken into account. Being risky, unrealistic, difficult, **or** expensive (RUDE) disqualifies from SECS. The bolded conjunctions are essential in applying this guide.

SECS model, and the personal recommendations of the authors of each article (**Box 1**).

Deborah R. Simkin, MD, DFAACAP
Department of Psychiatry
Emory University School of Medicine
8955 Highway 98 West, Suite 204
Miramar Beach, Florida 32550, USA

L. Eugene Arnold, MEd, MD
Department of Psychiatry
Ohio State University
McCampbell 395E
1581 Dodd Drive
Columbus, OH 43210, USA

E-mail addresses:
deb62288@aol.com (D.R. Simkin)
L.Arnold@osumc.edu (L.E. Arnold)

REFERENCES

1. McClafferty H, Vohra S, Bailey M, et al. Pediatric integrative medicine. Pediatrics 2017;140(3):e20171961.
2. Birdee GS, Phillips RS, Davis RB, et al. Factors associated with pediatric use of complementary and alternative medicine. Pediatrics 2010;125(2):249–56.
3. McClafferty H. Integrative pediatrics: looking forward. Children (Basel) 2015;2(1): 63–65 8.
4. Adams D, Dagenais S, Clifford T, et al. Complementary and alternative medicine use by pediatric specialty outpatients. Pediatrics 2013;131(2):225–32.
5. Surette S, Vohra S. Complementary, holistic, and integrative medicine: utilization surveys of the pediatric literature. Pediatr Rev 2014;35(3):114–27 [quiz: 128].
6. Vohra S, Surette S, Mittra D, et al. Pediatric integrative medicine: pediatrics' newest subspecialty? BMC Pediatr 2012;12:123.
7. Black LI, Clarke TC, Barnes PM, et al. Use of complementary health approaches among children aged 4–17 years in the United States: national Health Interview Survey, 2007–2012. Natl Health Stat Rep 2015;78:1–19.
8. Black LI, Barnes PM, Clarke TC, et al. Use of yoga, meditation, and chiropractors among U.S. children aged 4-17 years. NCHS Data Brief 2018;(324):1–8.
9. Saper R. Integrative medicine and health disparities. Glob Adv Health Med 2016; 5(1):5–8.
10. Wilson KM, Klein JD, Sesselberg TS, et al. Use of complementary medicine and dietary supplements among U.S. adolescents. J Adolesc Health 2006;38(4): 385–94.
11. Musaiger AO, Abahussain NA. Attitudes and practices of complementary and alternative medicine among adolescents in Saudi Arabia. Glob J Health Sci 2014;7(1):173–9.
12. Adler SR, Fosket JR. Disclosing CAM use in the medical encounter. J Fam Pract 1999;48(6):453–8.
13. Ioannidis JP. Effectiveness of antidepressants: an evidence myth constructed from a thousand randomized trials? Philos Ethics Humanit Med 2008;3:14.

14. Gollub RL, Kirsch I, Maleki N, et al. A functional neuroimaging study of expectancy effects on pain response in patients with knee osteoarthritis. J Pain 2018; 19(5):515–27.

15. Zhang W, Luo J. The transferable placebo effect from pain to emotion: changes in behavior and EEG activity. Psychophysiology 2009;46(3):626–34.

16. Zhang W, Qin S, Guo J, et al. A follow-up fMRI study of a transferable placebo anxiolytic effect. Psychophysiology 2011;48(8):1119–28.

17. Beidelschies M, Alejandro-Rodriguez M, Ji X, et al. Association of the functional medicine model of care with patient-reported health-related quality-of-life outcomes. JAMA Netw Open 2019;2(10):e1914017.

18. Patton C, Sawyer S, Santelli J, et al. Our future: a Lancet commission on adolescent health and wellbeing. Lancet 2016;387(10036):2423–78.

19. Cohen MH, Natbony SR, Abbot RB. Complementary and alternative medicine in child and adolescent psychiatry: legal considerations. In: Simkin D, Popper C, editors. Alternative and complementary therapies for child and adolescent psychiatric disorders, 1. Child Adol Clin N Amer Part; 2013. p. 493–507.

20. Guu TW, Mischoulon D, Sarris J, et al. International society for nutritional psychiatry research practice guidelines for omega-3 fatty acids in the treatment of major depressive disorder. Psychother Psychosom 2019;88(5):263–73.

21. Adams D, Cheng F, Jou H, et al. The safety of pediatric acupuncture: a systematic review. Pediatrics 2011;128(6). Available at: www.pediatrics.org/cgi/content/full/128/6/e1575. Accessed July 2022.

22. Cowen VS, Cyr V. Complementary and alternative medicine in US medical schools. Adv Med Educ Pract 2015;6:113–7.

23. Institute of medicine committee on the use of complementary and alternative medicine by the American public and board on health promotion and disease prevention, complementary and alternative that follow these standard medicine in the United States. Washington, DC: National Academies Press; 2005.

24. Duffy TP. The flexner report—100 years later. Yale J Biol Med 2011;84(3):269–76.

25. Miller L, Weiss R. Revisiting black medical school extinctions in the Flexner era. J Hist Med Allied Sci 2012;67(2):217–43.

26. Stahnisch FW, Verhoef M. The Flexner report of 1910 and its impact on complementary and alternative medicine and psychiatry in North America in the 20th century. Evid Based Complement Alternat Med 2012;2012:647896.

27. Rothman DJ. Medical professionalism—focusing on the real issues. N Engl J Med 2000;342:1284–6.

28. Williams RJ, Berry LJ, Beerstecher E. Individual metabolic patterns, alcoholism, genetotrophic diseases. Proc Natl Acad Sci U S A 1949;35(6):265–71.

29. Bland J. Defining function in the functional medicine model. Integr Med 2017; 16(1):22–5.

30. Hurt EA, Arnold LE. An integrated dietary/nutritional approach to ADHD. Child Adolesc Psychiatr Clin N Am 2014;23(4):955–64.

Complementary and Integrative Treatments for Attention-Deficit/Hyperactivity Disorder in Youth

Douglas Russell, MD[a],*, L. Eugene Arnold, MD, MEd[b]

KEYWORDS

- ADHD • Complementary • Integrative • Diet • Meditation • Neurofeedback
- Omega-3 • Physical activity

KEY POINTS

- Many complementary and integrative strategies have been extensively studied as a treatment for attention-deficit/hyperactivity disorder (ADHD) in youth.
- Effect sizes for Complementary and Integrative Medicine interventions in ADHD are generally small-to-moderate.
- Heterogeneity of study method and risk of bias pervades much of the available literature.
- Omega-3 supplementation, dietary restriction of artificial food coloring, meditation, yoga, physical activity, and sleep hygiene can be considered reasonable adjunctive treatments.
- If used as the sole treatment, most of these risk delaying more effective treatment.

INTRODUCTION

Attention-deficit/hyperactivity disorder (ADHD) affects an estimated 8.4% of children aged 2 to 17 in the United States and approximately 5% of children and adolescents worldwide.[1,2] First-line treatments for school-aged youth and older include psychostimulant medication, parent training, and school consultation.[3] Despite strong evidence supporting the efficacy of these treatments, in the United States only 62% report being treated with psychostimulants during the past year, and only 47% with behavioral treatment.[1] Tolerability problems and social stigma have long hindered efforts to increase medication adherence, whereas lack of access has limited evidence-based psychosocial interventions.[4–6] These troublesome barriers have led clinicians,

[a] Department of Psychiatry and Behavioral Sciences, University of Washington School of Medicine, c/o Seattle Children's Hospital, OA.5.154 PO Box 5371, Seattle, WA 98145-5005, USA; [b] Department of Psychiatry and Behavioral Health, The Ohio State University College of Medicine, 395E McCampbell Hall, 1581 Dodd Drive, Columbus, OH 43210, USA
* Corresponding author.
E-mail address: drusse@uw.edu

Child Adolesc Psychiatric Clin N Am 32 (2023) 173–192
https://doi.org/10.1016/j.chc.2022.08.005
1056-4993/23/© 2022 Elsevier Inc. All rights reserved.

researchers, patients, and families alike to seek alternative treatments for ADHD symptoms.

Complementary and Integrative Medicine (CIM) has been part of the treatment landscape for ADHD since before the modern definition of this neurodevelopmental disorder was codified. There have been multiple randomized controlled trials (RCTs) investigating a wide variety of complementary and integrative treatments for ADHD, and the evidence has progressed to meta-analyses for several of these modalities. This article reviews some of the most studied treatments, including restriction/elimination diets, single- and multiple-nutrient supplementation, neurofeedback, mind–body activities, physical activity, and traditional Chinese medicine (TCM). It will also consider emerging alternative treatment modalities.

Restriction/Elimination Diets

Restriction/elimination diets for what was then called the hyperkinetic reaction of childhood first came to national prominence with the 1974 publication of *Why Your Child Is Hyperactive* by Ben F. Feingold, MD.[7] Feingold, a pediatric allergist, argued that artificial food additives and naturally occurring salicylates in the diet were the etiology behind the behavioral and learning problems in these children, and argued that eliminating these foods resulted in symptom improvement in over 50%. Pressure from parent advocates of this dietary intervention encouraged the US Food and Drug Administration (FDA) to commission controlled studies, which failed to confirm Dr Feingold's claims. A 1983 meta-analysis by Kavale and Forness[8] found a negligible effect, essentially putting the matter to rest for the next 20 years.

Interest in restriction/elimination diets was renewed in 2004 with the first of the Southhampton studies, where Batemen and colleagues[9] investigated the effect of artificial food coloring and sodium benzoate in preschool children living in the Isle of Wight in the United Kingdom. This 4-week crossover study found a moderate effect based on parent ratings (effect size = 0.51) independent of preexisting hyperactive or atopic status. A follow-up study by McCann and colleagues[10] added a second comparison group of 8 to 9 year-olds in Southhampton, UK and a second formulation of artificial food coloring plus sodium benzoate. Results were largely confirmatory but much less robust (effect sizes 0.06–0.20). Based on strength of evidence from these studies, the United Kingdom's Food Standards Agency instituted mandatory warning labels for foods containing sodium benzoate and six artificial colors: sunset yellow FCF, quinoline yellow, carmoisine, allura red, tartrazine, and ponceau yellow.[11] The third Southhampton study in 2010 related the adverse effect of food additives on ADHD symptoms to histamine degradation gene polymorphisms.[12] One year later, Pelsser and colleagues[13] investigated the effect of individually tailored elimination diets on serum immunoglobulin G (IgG) and hyperactivity in a sample of 100 children and found a large response rate (64%) but no correlation to serum IgG levels. Nigg and colleagues[14] performed a detailed meta-analysis including this and other studies of restriction diets and synthetic food color additives in ADHD and found a small effect size of 0.29.

Nutritional Optimization

Nutritional supplementation for ADHD has also been extensively studied. Single-nutrient studies are most common, being more amenable to randomized, controlled designs than more complex dietary or lifestyle interventions. Owing to the generally small sample sizes and heterogeneity in dosing and design, it is typically difficult to draw generalized conclusions from any one of these individual studies. However, the number of studies has supported metanalyses with important implications for clinical practice. The most notable of these have focused on omega-3 polyunsaturated fatty-acid (PUFA) supplementation. Animal models have suggested a role for PUFAs in monoamine transmission, and an association with omega-3 PUFA deficiency in the frontal cortex of hyperactive rats.[15,16] Human studies have suggested that omega-3 PUFA composition in red blood cell membranes is decreased in adolescents with ADHD, and that ADHD is associated with the omega-6 heavy "western diet" that includes foods high in saturated fats, refined sugar, and sodium.[17–19] Relevant to the inflammation often found in ADHD, we should note that the omega-3 PUFA eicosaentaenoic acid (EPA) is the precursor for anti-inflammatory eicosanoids and the omega-6 PUFA arachidonic acid is precursor of pro-inflammatory eicosanoids. The rationale for supplementation is to rebalance PUFA composition away from omega-6 PUFAs, overexpressed in western diets, and toward omega-3 PUFAs prominent in the "Mediterranean" diet and other diets that emphasize consumption of seafood.

Bloch and Qawasmi's[20] meta-analysis in *Journal of the American Academy of Child and Adolescent Psychiatry* (JAACAP) included 10 RCTs investigating the effects of omega-3 PUFA supplementation on ADHD symptoms and discovered a standardized mean difference of 0.31. A secondary finding was a "dose effect" of EPA but not docohexaenoic acid (DHA). Specifically, the three studies with the strongest effect used formulations with EPA greater than 550 mg (DHA >150 mg). A second meta-analysis by Gillies and colleagues[21] included 13 studies looking at any combination of omega-3 and omega-6s, and reported a higher likelihood of improvement compared with placebo or no significant difference in parent or teacher ratings. Sonuga-Barke and colleagues[22] included 11 studies (seven overlapping with Bloch and Qawasmi and two of omega-6 PUFA supplementation) and found a standardized mean difference of .21 that was reduced to 0.16 when only "probably blinded" trials were included. Gillies' and Sonuga-Barke's methods have been criticized for including trials of omega-6 PUFA supplementation, which may explain their less robust findings. Hawkey and Nigg[23] analyzed 16 studies and concluded a standardized mean difference of 0.26, higher than Gillies and Sonuga-Barke but slightly lower than Bloch and Qawasmi. Cooper and colleagues[24] analyzed 10 studies looking specifically for effect on externalizing symptoms and saw no effect. Most recently Chang[25] separately analyzed seven RCTs of omega-3 supplementation as a clinical treatment of ADHD, three RCTs investigating effect on cognitive measures associated with attention, and seven studies looking at blood levels of omega-3 PUFAs in ADHD-affected youth. Effect sizes were 0.38, 1.09, and −0.58 for each analysis, respectively. A systematic review by Abdullah and colleagues,[26] which limited inclusion to RCTs that used the Conners Rating Scale as a primary measure, found a nonsignificant trend toward benefit. The field continues to debate the merit of recommending omega-3 supplementation for ADHD, but many consider the evidence base strong enough to suggest a role as an adjunctive treatment.

We should note that all the RCTs included in these meta-analyses mentioned above employed supplement formulations for ease of study. However, dietary intake of fish leads to up to nine times higher plasma concentrations than supplementation.[27] This suggests a potential further role for dietary counseling in ADHD treatment planning. According to the USDA's FoodData Central,[28] animal sources highest in EPA content include mackerel, herring, anchovy, barracuda, and salmon (generally cold-water wild ocean fish). In plants, omega-3s exist primarily in the form of alpha-linolenic acid (ALA), a precursor to EPA and DHA. Plant sources highest in ALA include flaxseed, chia seed, and hemp seed. Conversion of the 18-carbon omega-3 ALA in foods like flaxseed to the 20-carbon EPA and 22-carbon DHA requires enzymes such as fatty-acid desaturase that may be deficient in some patients or may be preempted by omega-6 fatty acids competing for the same enzymes in an omega-6-rich diet.

Other dietary and nutritional interventions studied in ADHD have included sugar restriction, high-protein breakfasts, amino acid supplementation, glyconutritional supplementation, single vitamin/mineral supplementation, broad-spectrum micronutrient supplementation, metabolites (melatonin, dimethlaminoethanol, L-carnitine, thyroid hormone), and several herbal preparations (pycnogenol, ginkgo biloba, St. John's Wort). However, in most cases small sample sizes and heterogeneity in dosing and design make it difficult to generalize conclusions. Broad-spectrum vitamins/minerals is one possible exception; two recent RCTs demonstrated improvement by CGI-I (not parent rating), and reduced inattention and emotion dysregulation (not hyperactivity).[29,30] Both of these studies used a formula with all known vitamins and essential minerals in doses above recommended daily allowance/recommended daily intake (RDA/RDI) but below upper tolerable limits. Notably, the micronutrient group grew significantly more than the placebo group, in contrast to the common side effect of stimulants. Because the formula can interact with medication and because the response rate of 54% is only slightly less than for a stimulant, one might argue that it should be tried first. Another evolving area of research in diet and ADHD involves the microbiota–gut–brain axis. Some evidence suggests differences in gut microbiome composition in youth with ADHD, a possible bidirectional effect between omega-3 PUFAs and the gut microbiome, and potential role of the microbiome in regulating circadian rhythm.[31] Probiotics may eventually play a therapeutic or preventative role, but studies to date have been mixed.[32]

Other than omega-3 PUFAs or nutrient repletion in the setting of known deficiency, there is little rationale to support single nutrient interventions for ADHD at this time. Similarly, other than the restriction of artificial color or elimination of foods or additives when there is known sensitivity, there is little evidence supporting other dietary interventions for ADHD. Of those interventions with evidentiary support, effect sizes are small to moderate, suggesting that they should be deployed as adjunctive as opposed to primary treatment strategies. When considering adjunctive omega-3 PUFA treatment, guiding parents toward naturally occurring foods that are rich in this nutrient may be preferable to supplementation.[27] Furthermore, even in a setting of limited clinical benefit in ADHD, interventions such as limiting consumption of foods with refined sugars and artificial additives, and increasing intake of foods containing omega-3 PUFAs may have additional general health benefits.

Neurofeedback

Neurofeedback is another complementary approach studied in ADHD. The procedure involves isolating electroencephalographic bands associated with the cortical activity of interest in ADHD, translating these into sensory outputs (visual and/or auditory) which are perceived by the subject in real time, and then modulating these signals using principles of operant conditioning. Theoretically, this self-regulation of brain activity leads to improved cognitive and behavioral control. There has been increasing interest in neurofeedback at a therapeutic intervention as we learn more about the Default Mode Network and its potential role in ADHD symptomatology through functional imaging research. The Default Mode Network (DMN) is comprised of brain regions that are typically more activated during rest than task. These include the medial prefrontal cortex (mPFC), posterior cingulate cortex (PCC), and angular gyrus (AG). Anti-correlation between the DMN and dorsolateral prefrontal cortex (DLPFC) is associated with better executive functioning and working memory. Mattfeld and colleagues[33] showed that adults with persistent ADHD symptoms show reduced anticorrelation between the PCC and mPFC. In a 4-year longitudinal study comparing attentional problems with functional connectivity in children, Whitfield-Gabrieli and colleagues[34] found that reduced anticorrelation between the DLPFC and mPFC at age 7 predicted worsening attention symptoms at age 11. There is emerging evidence to suggest that neurofeedback increases anti-correlation between the right inferior frontal cortex and posterior DMN regions in adolescents with ADHD, which in turn correlates with clinical improvement.[35] There is also evidence of sustained positive effects on longitudinal follow-up.[36]

The two most common variations of neurofeedback studied in ADHD are frequency band training and slow cortical potential training. Electroencephalogram (EEG) is typically used as the biomarker for neurofeedback, but functional magnetic resonance imaging (fMRI) has been proposed as an alternative.[35] Despite the strong theoretic rationale for neurofeedback as an intervention in ADHD, to date the evidence for its effectiveness has been mixed. Bussalb A and colleagues[37] suggest that this lack of consensus is related to a high degree of technical and methodological heterogeneity that pervades the existing research, and identify informant (parent vs teacher), treatment intensity (as opposed to duration), and quality of EEG equipment as specific factors that impact reported treatment efficacy. Micoulaud-Franchi's[38] meta-analysis of neurofeedback treatment in children with ADHD included five RCTs between 2021 and 2014. Results were moderate but significant for inattention (standardized mean difference [SMD] $= -0.46$) and hyperactivity/impulsivity (SMD $= -0.34$) parent report, but only teacher reports of inattention reached significance (SMD $= -0.30$). Hodgson's 2014 meta-analysis comparing seven psychological interventions in ADHD included 14 studies that found that neurofeedback showed the greatest efficacy when weighted across the 20 outcome measures, albeit with a very small effect overall (ES $d = 0.21$).[39] Cortese and colleagues's[40] meta-analysis in JAACAP included 13 RCTs published from 2004 to 2015 in children aged 3 to 18. Results included a combined effect size of 0.35, which diminished to non-significance when the analysis was limited to probably blinded studies. Catala-Lopez's[41] meta-analysis of comparing multiple pharmacologic and non-pharmacological interventions in ADHD concluded no significant effects for neurofeedback over placebo.

Neurofeedback is an important non-pharmacologic treatment option for ADHD with a rationale increasingly supported by emerging EEG and fMRI studies and a growing evidence base that shows moderate effectiveness for ADHD symptoms by parent report. The evidence is considerably less strong when teacher ratings, thought to be more effectively blinded, are considered. This has led to discussions about the role of placebo effects. The field would benefit from further research using more uniform treatment methodology and study designs. A recent well-designed double-blind RCT found very large pre–post improvement (ES $d = 1.5$) in both active NF and control groups but no significant difference between them.[42] The control treatment differed from neurofeedback only in having the operant conditioning based on another child's prerecorded EEG. The controls enjoyed pre–post improvement as great or greater than neurofeedback improvements in unblinded studies that reported significant superiority of neurofeedback over control treatment, suggesting that those improvements were due to nonspecific effects, not neurofeedback itself. In addition, when parents were blind to treatment assignment, they detected no greater advantage of neurofeedback than did teachers. These findings highlight the importance of a control condition that is both fundamentally distinct from the primary intervention while remaining similar enough to preserve effective blinding, which had not been done up to this point. This problem is relevant to many other complementary and integrative treatments that involve interventions or lifestyle modifications for which it is nearly impossible to effectively blind study participants.

Mind–body Activities

Meditation practices, including mindfulness and mantra meditation, as well as related mind–body activities (yoga, tai-chi, and chi gong), are also of interest for ADHD. Mindfulness refers to practices adapted from spiritual tradition to enhance attentional and emotional self-regulation by focusing on present-moment experience without judgment. Researchers have been investigating the effects of mindfulness and to a smaller extent other meditation on brain structure and function for over a decade. However, small sample sizes, significant heterogeneity of practice technique and study design, and lack of replication have made it challenging to conclude specific effects on the brain. There is general consensus that meditation engages multiple brain areas involved in attentional processing/regulation, emotional processing/regulation as well as self-awareness, including the frontoparietal network, sensory-motor network, and default mode network, with evidence of longitudinal alteration of brain structure and function.[43]

Five meta-analyses have attempted to estimate the efficacy of meditation and other mind–body activities on ADHD symptoms.[44–48] Krisanaprakornkit's[46] analysis included only four RCTs, two involving mantra meditation and two involving yoga. Design limitations and risk of bias in the included studies left the authors unable to draw any conclusions about the effectiveness of either treatment. A systematic review by Evans and colleagues[49] from 2017 included 16 studies and determined that it was impossible to come to any conclusions about efficacy due to pervasive risk of bias throughout the literature. Chimiklis and colleagues[45] analysis comprised 11 studies involving yoga, mindfulness, and other meditation practice and reports significant effects on hyperactivity, inattention, parent–child relationship, executive functioning, on-task behavior, parent stress, and parent trait-mindfulness, with effect sizes ranging from small to large. However, the authors caution that small samples size and bias limit the ability to draw definitive conclusions. Zhang and colleagues's[48] meta-analysis included 13 RCTs for a total 270 children and adolescents and 339 adults. Highlighting the difficulty of studying complex practices like meditation, only one of the included studies was double-blind. Results imply mild to moderate benefit for ADHD core symptoms, with effect sizes of $d = -0.44$ for children/adolescents and -0.66 for adults. There were no effects found on neuropsychological measures of inattention and inhibition in children and adolescents, but the authors found significant effects on working memory and inhibition in adults. Zue J and colleagues's[47] analysis included 11 studies, of which only 2 involved children, and conclude overall effect sizes of -0.83 for inattentiveness and -0.68 for hyperactivity/impulsivity, with no sub-analyses by age. Finally, Cairncross and Miller analyzed 10 studies and concluded an overall effect of -0.66 for inattention and -0.53 for hyperactivity/impulsivity. Subgroup analysis by age revealed effect sizes in the youth of $-0.66/-0.47$ versus $-0.91/-0.68$ in adults.[44]

Meditative practice, much like neurofeedback, has a strong rationale but lacks strong, unbiased evidence to support its effects on ADHD. The plethora of approaches, heterogeneity of study designs, and high potential for bias makes it difficult to derive definitive conclusions about meditation's effectiveness. Despite these significant limitations, the available literature to date does suggest a relatively consistent small-to-moderate effect in children and adolescents. This has been enough to convince some school districts to formally incorporate meditative practice into school curricula, with some evidence suggesting benefit for reducing stress and promoting self-regulation in children and adolescents.[50,51] This modality is also increasingly touted in popular culture and commercial enterprise as a way to center oneself in a world where reliance on digital technology has created unsustainable demands on our attention. The relative absence of adverse effects lowers the threshold for recommending mindfulness as part of an ADHD treatment plan, particularly for individuals with comorbid internalizing disorders.

Physical Activity

The rationale for physical activity in ADHD is based on observations that it exerts effects on the same catecholaminergic systems that stimulant medications target, increasing dopamine and norepinephrine in the PFC, hippocampus and striatum.[52,53] Cerrillo-Urbina and colleagues's[54] meta-analysis incorporates findings from eight RCTs grouped into either aerobic exercise (seven studies) or yoga therapies (one study), with a combined total of 249 children with ADHD. Compared to control conditions, results showed improved attention, (SMD = 0.84) and social functioning (SMD = 0.59), and reduced hyperactivity (SMD = 0.56), impulsivity (SMD = 0.56) and anxiety (SMD = 0.66).

A related meta-analysis by Watson and colleagues[55] looked at the effects of in-classroom physical activity and found a moderate effect on improving on-task and reducing off-task behavior (SMD = 0.33), as well as strong improvements in academic achievement when using a progress monitoring tool (SMD = 1.03). Zang's[56] meta-analysis examined the effects of physical exercise on executive functioning in children and included 14 studies (8 randomized, 6 observational) with a combined total of 574 participants. The author found the strongest effects on reducing anxious and depressive symptoms (weighted MD = −1.84), thought problems (weighted mean difference [WMD] = −3.49), social problems (WMD = −5.78), and aggression (WMD = −0.39). However, effects on hyperactivity, inattention, and oppositional behaviors were nonsignificant. A newly published meta-analysis by Seiffer and colleagues[57] restricted inclusion to only randomized, controlled trials of regular (at least two sessions per week) moderate to vigorous physical activity for children and adolescents with ADHD, and selected differences in core ADHD symptoms between control intervention groups post-intervention as its primary outcome measure. 11 studies were included in the analysis, totaling 448 participants. The authors concluded that physical activity had a small but significant effect on core symptoms (Hedges' g = −0.33).

Little is known about which type, intensity, or setting is optimal for children with ADHD. However, we do know that popular sports, cycling, and aerobic/gym exercise are associated with a greater reduction in overall mental health burden in adults compared with other activities, and that team sports seem to afford the most benefit for anxious youth.[58,59] Thygesen and colleagues[60] cohort study of individuals born in Denmark between 1992 and 2007 found an association between decreased access to green space and risk for developing ADHD. Furthermore, Younan and colleagues's[61] study of youth in Los Angeles found that exposure to greenspace within 1000 m was associated with reduced aggressive behaviors. Considering these findings in aggregate, team sports played outdoors may be ideal for youth with ADHD.

Physical exercise tends to be deemphasized relative to medication and psychosocial treatments in ADHD treatment planning. This is not surprising given evidence of only mild to moderate effect when this treatment is studied in isolation. There are also the inherent challenges associated with encouraging, and families successfully implementing, lifestyle changes. However, when thoughtfully designed, programs to enhance physical activity in children with ADHD and their families are both feasible and acceptable.[62] In addition to specific benefits for children with ADHD, physical activity's broader benefits on brain health should also be considered. Physical activity is positively associated with global fractional anisotropy, decreased P300 latency and increased P300 amplitude by EEG, decreased cortisol, increased serotonin, and increased brain-derived neurotrophic factor (BDNF) and insulin-like growth factor 1 (IGF-1) in young people.[63–65] It also seems to have a protective effect on children and adolescents in times of extreme stress. During the Fukushima Daiichi disaster, children in the evacuation zone who had lower rates of physical activity had higher total difficulties scores on the Strengths and Difficulties Questionnaire.[66] Emerging research from the coronavirus disease-2019 pandemic suggests a similar effect.[67] In summary, the combination of low side effects, brain health benefits, and positive effects on well-being support its role as a safe, sensible, and cost-effective complementary treatment.

Sleep Hygiene

ADHD is independently associated with a variety of sleep problems including prolonged sleep latency, sleep phase delay, increased periodic limb movements, problems staying asleep and reduced total sleep duration.[68] Sleep problems are also a common adverse effect of both methylphenidate and amphetamine-based psychostimulants.[69,70] Sleep deprivation negatively impacts attention, working memory, reward/incentive processing, emotion discrimination/expression, and learning. Neurobiological correlates of sleep deprivation include altered functioning of the DLPFC, DMN, mesolimbic system, and hippocampus.[71]

Distinguishing between characteristics of ADHD, contributions from comorbid conditions, exacerbating environmental factors, and adverse effects from treatment is challenging.[72] Treatment can also be a challenge. There are currently no FDA-approved medications for sleep problems in youth. Furthermore, pharmacologic treatment of insomnia in ADHD runs the risk of additional adverse effects while potentially masking medication-related adverse effects that could be better addressed through dose/timing optimization. Behavioral interventions for insomnia in youth can be safe and effective.[73,74] Yet access to specialized therapeutic interventions such as cognitive-behavioral therapy for insomnia (CBT-I) is limited in many communities. Sleep hygiene is a set of behavioral, environmental, and cognitive modifications to improve sleep, including emphasis on a bedtime routine, electronic media restriction, caffeine restriction, exposure to morning light, scheduling physical activity during the day, and optimization of the sleep environment.[75] Nilkes and colleagues[76] conducted a systematic review of the effectiveness of sleep hygiene in children with ADHD that included 16 articles, only 4 of which are RCTs. All but one showed a small effect. This consistent pattern of benefit combined with safety and negligible cost lowers the threshold for recommendation.

Traditional Chinese Medicine

TCM refers to an ancient system of medical practice that combines herbal treatments, acupuncture, tui na, tai chi chuan, and diet.[77] It is practiced widely in Asia, but remains poorly understood in western medical practice. Ni and colleagues[77] published a useful review of this practice in the treatment of ADHD in 2014. According to the authors, TCM views ADHD as arising from imbalance of yin-yang and the dysfunction of Zang-fu (viscera); the heart, liver, sleep, and kidney are the systems most implicated. TCM is a holistic system that is highly individualized, which creates challenges for empirical study. Ni and colleagues[77] cites several Chinese-language randomized trials comparing treatment with various herbal preparations against methylphenidate, concluding similar effect and better tolerability.

Within the English-language literature, acupuncture and acupressure have been the most studied. Underscoring the inherent challenges related to standardization and blinding in TCM, the authors of a Cochrane Review of acupuncture for ADHD in 2011 identified 14 potential studies for inclusion but ended up excluding all and declaring an inadequate evidence base.[78] A meta-analysis by Lee MS published the same year found only 3 trials meeting their inclusion criteria but came to a similar conclusion after considering risk for bias.[79] Chen and colleagues's[80] meta-analysis included 10 studies and concluded benefit and tolerability superior to that of methylphenidate, but tempered these findings by highlighting the included studies' high risk for bias and variable quality.

Emerging Treatments

Two emerging first-of-their-kind treatments deserve mention here. Both have the potential for expanding the landscape of non-medication treatment options for ADHD. The first, EndeavorRx, is a game-based digital therapeutic designed to improve attention in inattentive and combined type ADHD. In June of 2020, the FDA permitted marketing of EndeavorRx as an adjunctive treatment for ADHD.[81] The approval came through the agency's medical device De Novo pathway, which has a lower threshold for efficacy than would be demanded of pharmaceutical, biologic or other treatments. Approval was based on a 1-month randomized, double-blind, parallel-group controlled trial composed of 348 children aged 8 to 12 years with ADHD.[82] The active treatment was a game-like activity based around Go-No-Go-style challenges with the capability of real-time adaptation based on performance. A digital spelling task with progressive difficulty was the control condition. The main outcome measure was change on the Test of Variables of Attention - Attention Performance Index Test of Variables of Attention (TOVA)-Attention Performance Index (API), a computerized continuous performance test designed to measure attention and inhibitory control. Secondary outcome measures included changes on TOVA non-composite scores, Cambridge Neuropsychological Test Automated Battery, as well as the more common clinical scales attention-deficit/hyperactivity disorder rating scale IV (ADHD-RS-IV), Clinical Global Impressions-Improvement (CGI-I), and the Behavior Rating Inventory of Executive Function (BRIEF). Results included a small but significant change in the TOVA-API. However, changes on all secondary outcome measures were non-significant. These findings of course raise questions about generalizability of benefit beyond the laboratory setting. Despite limitations, the size and power of this study represents a real step forward for the study of digital therapeutics. Additional studies will be necessary to replicate findings, clarify clinical benefit, and determine longitudinal effects.

A second emerging treatment of note, trigeminal nerve stimulation, is a non-invasive neuromodulation intervention. The FDA approved the Monarch external Trigeminal Nerve Stimulation (eTMS) system in April of 2019.[83] The treatment involves a small stimulator worn during sleep that emits a low-level current via an electrode placed on the forehead over branch V_1 of the trigeminal nerve. The treatment had been approved in Canada and Europe for adults with treatment-resistant depression and epilepsy but had not been considered for children with ADHD until recently. Building on a successful open-label feasibility study, McGough and colleagues completed a double-blind, sham-controlled pilot study with 62 children aged 8 to 12 randomized to 4 weeks of nightly treatment.[84,85] The sham condition followed the same schedule and instructions as the active condition but without emitting current. The primary

Table 1
Summary of high-level evidence

Treatment	Strength of Recommendation Based on Benefit and Safety	Level of Certainty Based on Benefit and Quality of Evidence	Evidence Base in Youth	Evidence-based or Meets SECS Criteria	Personal Recommendations of the Reviewer
I. Dietary Intervention					
a. Restriction/Elimination (Kavale & Forness et al, 1983[8], 23 studies, N = 875) (Nigg et al, 2012[14], N = 2220) (Sonuga-Barke et al, 2013[22], 8 studies, N = 407)	B	Moderate	3 meta-analyses	SECS	Small to moderate effect for restricting artificial color, eliminating food additives in setting of known sensitivity. Adjunctive rather than primary treatment.
b. Artificial Food Color Exclusion (Sonuga-Barke et al, 2013[22], 7 studies, N = 294)	B	Moderate	1 meta-analysis	EB	Small to moderate effect. Low threshold for recommending, as foods with artificial food colors also tend to have very low nutrient density.
II. Nutritional Optimization					
a. Omega-3 PUFAs (Bloch & Qawasmi et al, 2011[20], 10 studies, N = 699) (Sonuga-Barke et al, 2013[20], 11 studies, N = 723) (Hawkey & Nigg et al, 2014[23], 16 studies, N = 1408) (Catala-Lopez et al, 2017[41], 3 studies, N = 124) (Cooper et al, 2016[24], 10 studies) (Chang et al, 2018[25], 8 studies, N = 664)	B	Moderate	6 meta-analyses	EB	Small to moderate effect, minimal side effects. Deploy as adjunctive rather than primary treatment. Guiding families toward foods rich in this nutrient may be preferable to supplementation.

b. Iron (Cortese et al, 2012[40], 20 studies) (Catala-Lopez et al, 2017[41], 1 study, N = 18)	C	Low	1 systematic review. 1 RCT included in larger network analysis of multiple interventions	EB only if iron-insufficient	Limited evidence other than in setting of deficiency. Can have collateral benefits on sleep.
c. Zinc (Ghanizadeh et al,[86] 2013, 3 studies, N = 496) (Catala-Lopez et al, 2017[41], 1 study)	C	Low	1 meta-analysis, 1 RCT included in	Neither	Few well-designed trials. Limited evidence other than in deficiency.
d. Broad-spectrum Micronutrients (Rucklidge et al, 2018[30], N = 93, age 6-12) (Johnstone et al, 2021[29], N = 126, age 6-12)	B	Moderate	2 RCTs	Nutritional Optimization	Significantly better than placebo on CGI-I, not parent symptom rating. Requires 3–4 capsules TID.
III. Neurofeedback					
(Sonuga-Barke et al, 2013[22], 7 studies, N = 273) (Hodgson et al, 2014[39], 5 studies) (Micoulaud-Franchi et al, 2014[38], 5 studies, N = 263) (Catala-Lopez et al, 2017[41], 4 studies, N = 110) (Cortese et al, 2016[40], 13 studies, N = 540) (Bussalb et al, 2019[37], 33 studies, N = 846) (Van Doren et al, 2019 36, 10 studies, N = 506)	C	Moderate	7 meta-analyses	Neither	Strong rationale, but studies are heterogeneous and evidence mixed. Best blinded show no significant advantage over control.

(continued on next page)

Table 1
(continued)

Treatment	Strength of Recommendation Based on Benefit and Safety	Level of Certainty Based on Benefit and Quality of Evidence	Evidence Base in Youth	Evidence-based or Meets SECS Criteria	Personal Recommendations of the Reviewer
IV. Mind-body Activities					
a. Yoga (Krisanaprakornkit et al, 2010[46], 2 studies, N = 36) (Chimiklis et al, 2018[45], 5 studies)	C	Low	2 meta-analyses	SECS	Few well-designed studies, with mixed evidence. But side effects minimal for average youth; may have additional benefits for health and well-being.
b. Meditation (Krisanaprakornkit et al, 2010[46], 2 studies, N = 47) (Chimiklis et al, 2018[45], 8 studies) (Zhang et al, 2018[48], 14 studies, N = 609) (Cairncross et al, 2020[44], 10 studies, N = 195)	C	Low	4 meta-analyses	SECS	Strong rationale, but few well-designed studies. Minimal side effects, and may have additional benefits for health, well-being.
V. Physical Exercise (Cerrillo-Urbina et al, 2015[54], 8 studies, N = 249) (Zang et al, 2019[56], 14 studies, N = 574) (Seiffer et al, 2022[57], 11 studies, N = 448)	B	Moderate	3 meta-analyses	EB	Small but significant benefits for ADHD, and clear benefits for general brain/body health.

VI. Sleep Hygiene					
(Nikles et al, 2020[76], 16 studies, N = 1469)	B	Low	1 systematic review	SECS	Consistent but small effects. Low-cost, minimal risk, and potential benefits beyond ADHD lower the threshold for recommending.
VII. Traditional Chinese Medicine					
a. Acupuncture (Li et al, 2011[78], 0 studies met inclusion criteria) (Lee et al, 2011[79], 3 studies, N = 308) (Chen et al, 2021[80], 10 studies, N = 876)	C	Low	3 meta-analyses	Neither	Studies are of variable quality, with high bias risk. Quality of implementation and fidelity to TCM practice highly practitioner-dependent.

Strength of Recommendations based on benefit and safety:

A=Recommend Strongly. There is a high certainty that the net benefit is substantial **and safe.**

B=Recommend. There is a high certainty that the net benefit is moderate or there is moderate certainty that the net benefit is moderate to substantial **and safe.**

C=Neutral (offer or provide this service for selected patients depending on individual circumstances, based on professional judgment and patient preferences). There is at least moderate certainty that the net benefit is small.

D=Discourage. There is moderate or high certainty that the service has no net benefit or that the harms outweigh the benefits

I = Insufficient (if the service is offered, patients should understand the uncertainty about the balance of benefits and harms) Current evidence is insufficient to assess the balance of benefits and harms of the service. Evidence is lacking, of poor quality, or conflicting, and the balance of benefits cannot be determined.)

Level of certainty regarding quality:

HIGH Level of Evidence with robust positive data meta-analyses or meta-reviews involving 2 or more RCTs of excellent, robust quality. The available evidence usually includes consistent results from well-designed, well-conducted RCTs in representative child, adolescent or young adult (18-24 years old) populations, assessing the effects on mental health outcomes. **MODERATE** Level of Evidence with robust positive data involving 2 or more RCTs of excellent, robust quality. The available evidence usually includes consistent results from well-designed, well-conducted RCTs in representative child, adolescent or young adult (18-24 years old) populations, assessing the effects on mental health outcomes.

LOW Level of evidence with less than 2 RCTs with good or average quality. The available evidence is insufficient to assess the effects on mental health outcomes.

SECS Criteria:

A guide to clinical decisions is that Interventions that are Safe, Easy, Cheap, **and** Sensible (SECS) require less evidence to justify individual trials than those that are Risky, Unrealistic, Difficult, **or** Expensive (RUDE). Because some of the treatments do not have much solid, compelling evidence but would be reasonable to try with a lower bar of evidence, this criterion is also taken into account. Being risky, unrealistic, difficult **OR** expensive (RUDE) disqualifies from SECS. The bolded conjunctions are essential in applying this guide.

efficacy outcome was a mean change on ADHD-RS. Secondary measures included qualitative EEG (qEEG) CGI-I, BRIEF, Conners Global Index, Children's Sleep Habits Questionnaire (CSHQ), Affective Reactivity Index (ARI), Multidimentional Anxiety Scale for Children (MASC), Children's Depression Rating Scale (CDRS-R), the computer-based Spatial Working Memory Test and Attention Network Task. Results included a moderate decrease in ADHD-RS (Cohen's $d = 0.5$), an effect similar to that of non-stimulant medication. The active treatment also showed increased broadband power on qEEG compared with sham. There was no attrition due to adverse effects, but weight and pulse were higher in the active group than in sham. The data are encouraging, but larger controlled studies will be needed.

A summary of these studies can be found in (**Table 1**) using the United States Preventative Services Task Force ratings for the strength of the recommendation and level of certainty for each study. (See **Table 1**).

SUMMARY

The complex nature and holistic perspectives that characterize and bring value to many CIM interventions for ADHD also present inherent challenges for controlled scientific study. Heterogeneity of method, inadequate blinding, and risk of bias are common. So despite the existence of multiple studies reported in the literature for some of the approaches described above, their limitations can make it difficult to come to definitive conclusions about efficacy. Exceptions include omega-3 supplementation, restriction of artificial food additives and physical activity, the evidence for which have progressed to the point that these CIM interventions can be considered evidence-based.

So where does that leave the thoughtful medical professional when evaluating CIM interventions which are not yet considered evidence-based? When the existing evidence base is not sufficient to clarify the benefits for a proposed treatment, the SECS versus RUDE criteria can be a useful framework to determine if an intervention is reasonable to recommend. SECS stands for 'safe, easy, cheap *and* sensible', whereas RUDE denotes those treatments which are "risky, unrealistic, difficult *or* expensive." A treatment that is safe, sensible and affordable might reasonably lower the threshold for recommendation even if the evidence base is limited. However, if any single element of the RUDE criteria is met, a treatment should not be considered advisable without convincing efficacy evidence.

Utilizing the evidence-based classification for efficacy above along with the SECS versus RUDE criteria for those interventions that cannot yet be considered evidence-based, several modalities are worth highlighting. Increasing consumption of foods rich in omega-3 PUFAs and decreasing consumption of foods containing artificial food coloring are reasonable dietary interventions. Of mind–body activities, meditation and yoga can similarly be recommended. Patients and their families should also be encouraged to practice sleep hygiene and seek out opportunities for regular physical activity. For those patients with co-morbid emotional dysregulation, broad-spectrum micronutrients could also be considered. Although none of these should be considered replacements for first-line psychopharmacologic and psychosocial strategies to manage inattention and hyperactivity, all offer a reasonable expectation of adjunctive benefit with minimal associated risk while conferring additional health benefits.

DISCLOSURE

Dr D.A. Russell is currently a co-investigator on studies funded by National Institute of Health/National Institute of Mental Health and the University of Washington's Garvey

Institute for Brain Health Solutions. Dr L.E. Arnold has received research funding from Supernus Pharmaceuticals, Roche/Genentech Pharmaceuticals, Otsuka Pharmaceuticals, Axial, and YoungLiving Essential Oils and National Institute of Health (USA, R01 MH 100144), has consulted with Pfizer Pharmaceuticals and CHADD, and been on advisory boards for Otsuka and Roche/Genentech.

REFERENCES

1. Danielson ML, Bitsko RH, Ghandour RM, et al. Prevalence of parent-reported ADHD Diagnosis and associated treatment Among U.S. Children and adolescents, 2016. J Clin Child Adolesc Psychol 2018;47(2):199–212.
2. Sayal K, Prasad V, Daley D, et al. ADHD in children and young people: prevalence, care pathways, and service provision. Lancet Psychiatry 2018;5(2):175–86.
3. Wolraich ML, Hagan JF Jr, Allan C, et al. Clinical practice Guideline for the Diagnosis, evaluation, and treatment of attention-deficit/hyperactivity disorder in children and adolescents. Pediatrics 2019;144(4).
4. Brinkman WB, Simon JO, Epstein JN. Reasons Why children and adolescents with attention-deficit/hyperactivity disorder Stop and Restart Taking medicine. Acad Pediatr 2018;18(3):273–80.
5. Coletti DJ, Pappadopulos E, Katsiotas NJ, et al. Parent perspectives on the decision to initiate medication treatment of attention-deficit/hyperactivity disorder. J Child Adolesc Psychopharmacol 2012;22(3):226–37.
6. DuPaul GJ, Evans SW, Mautone JA, et al. Future Directions for psychosocial interventions for children and adolescents with ADHD. J Clin Child Adolesc Psychol 2020;49(1):134–45.
7. Feingold BF. Why Your child is hyperactive. New York, NY: Random House; 1974.
8. Kavale KA, Forness SR. Hyperactivity and diet treatment: a meta-analysis of the Feingold hypothesis. J Learn Disabil 1983;16(6):324–30.
9. Bateman B, Warner JO, Hutchinson E, et al. The effects of a double blind, placebo controlled, artificial food colourings and benzoate preservative challenge on hyperactivity in a general population sample of preschool children. Arch Dis Child 2004;89(6):506–11.
10. McCann D, Barrett A, Cooper A, et al. Food additives and hyperactive behaviour in 3-year-old and 8/9-year-old children in the community: a randomised, double-blinded, placebo-controlled trial. Lancet 2007;370(9598):1560–7.
11. Food Standards agency. Food additives. 2019. Available at: https://www.food.gov.uk/safety-hygiene/food-additives#food-colours-and-hyperactivity. Accessed May 16, 2022.
12. Stevenson J, Sonuga-Barke E, McCann D, et al. The role of histamine degradation gene polymorphisms in moderating the effects of food additives on children's ADHD symptoms. Am J Psychiatry 2010;167(9):1108–15.
13. Pelsser LM, Frankena K, Toorman J, et al. Effects of a restricted elimination diet on the behaviour of children with attention-deficit hyperactivity disorder (INCA study): a randomised controlled trial. Lancet 2011;377(9764):494–503.
14. Nigg JT, Lewis K, Edinger T, et al. Meta-analysis of attention-deficit/hyperactivity disorder or attention-deficit/hyperactivity disorder symptoms, restriction diet, and synthetic food color additives. J Am Acad Child Adolesc Psychiatry 2012;51(1):86–97 e88.
15. Chalon S. Omega-3 fatty acids and monoamine neurotransmission. Prostaglandins Leukot Essent Fatty Acids 2006;75(4–5):259–69.

16. Vancassel S, Leman S, Hanonick L, et al. n-3 polyunsaturated fatty acid supplementation reverses stress-induced modifications on brain monoamine levels in mice. J Lipid Res 2008;49(2):340–8.
17. Colter AL, Cutler C, Meckling KA. Fatty acid status and behavioural symptoms of attention deficit hyperactivity disorder in adolescents: a case-control study. Nutr J 2008;7:8.
18. Howard AL, Robinson M, Smith GJ, et al. ADHD is associated with a "Western" dietary pattern in adolescents. J Atten Disord 2011;15(5):403–11.
19. LaChance L, McKenzie K, Taylor VH, et al. Omega-6 to omega-3 fatty acid Ratio in patients with ADHD: a meta-analysis. J Can Acad Child Adolesc Psychiatry 2016;25(2):87–96.
20. Bloch MH, Qawasmi A. Omega-3 fatty acid supplementation for the treatment of children with attention-deficit/hyperactivity disorder symptomatology: systematic review and meta-analysis. J Am Acad Child Adolesc Psychiatry 2011;50(10): 991–1000.
21. Gillies D, Sinn J, Lad SS, et al. Polyunsaturated fatty acids (PUFA) for attention deficit hyperactivity disorder (ADHD) in children and adolescents. Cochrane Database Syst Rev 2012;(7):CD007986.
22. Sonuga-Barke EJ, Brandeis D, Cortese S, et al. Nonpharmacological interventions for ADHD: systematic review and meta-analyses of randomized controlled trials of dietary and psychological treatments. Am J Psychiatry 2013;170(3): 275–89.
23. Hawkey E, Nigg JT. Omega-3 fatty acid and ADHD: blood level analysis and meta-analytic extension of supplementation trials. Clin Psychol Rev 2014;34(6): 496–505.
24. Cooper RE, Tye C, Kuntsi J, et al. The effect of omega-3 polyunsaturated fatty acid supplementation on emotional dysregulation, oppositional behaviour and conduct problems in ADHD: a systematic review and meta-analysis. J Affect Disord 2016;190:474–82.
25. Chang JP, Su KP, Mondelli V, et al. Omega-3 polyunsaturated fatty acids in youths with attention deficit hyperactivity disorder: a systematic review and meta-analysis of clinical trials and biological studies. Neuropsychopharmacology 2018;43(3):534–45.
26. Abdullah M, Jowett B, Whittaker PJ, et al. The effectiveness of omega-3 supplementation in reducing ADHD associated symptoms in children as measured by the Conners' rating scales: a systematic review of randomized controlled trials. J Psychiatr Res 2019;110:64–73.
27. Visioli F, Rise P, Barassi MC, et al. Dietary intake of fish vs. formulations leads to higher plasma concentrations of n-3 fatty acids. Lipids 2003;38(4):415–8.
28. U.S. Department of Agriculture. FoodData Central. 2016. Available at: https://fdc.nal.usda.gov/index.html. Accessed May 19, 2022.
29. Johnstone JM, Hatsu I, Tost G, et al. Micronutrients for attention-deficit/hyperactivity disorder in youths: a placebo-controlled randomized clinical trial. J Am Acad Child Adolesc Psychiatry 2021;61(5):647–61.
30. Rucklidge JJ, Eggleston MJF, Johnstone JM, et al. Vitamin-mineral treatment improves aggression and emotional regulation in children with ADHD: a fully blinded, randomized, placebo-controlled trial. J Child Psychol Psychiatry 2018; 59(3):232–46.
31. Checa-Ros A, Jerez-Calero A, Molina-Carballo A, et al. Current evidence on the role of the gut microbiome in ADHD Pathophysiology and therapeutic implications. Nutrients 2021;13(1).

32. Rianda D, Agustina R, Setiawan EA, et al. Effect of probiotic supplementation on cognitive function in children and adolescents: a systematic review of randomised trials. Benef Microbes 2019;10(8):873–82.
33. Mattfeld AT, Gabrieli JD, Biederman J, et al. Brain differences between persistent and remitted attention deficit hyperactivity disorder. Brain 2014;137(Pt 9):2423–8.
34. Whitfield-Gabrieli S, Wendelken C, Nieto-Castanon A, et al. Association of Intrinsic brain Architecture with changes in attentional and Mood symptoms during Development. JAMA Psychiatry 2020;77(4):378–86.
35. Rubia K, Criaud M, Wulff M, et al. Functional connectivity changes associated with fMRI neurofeedback of right inferior frontal cortex in adolescents with ADHD. Neuroimage 2019;188:43–58.
36. Van Doren J, Arns M, Heinrich H, et al. Sustained effects of neurofeedback in ADHD: a systematic review and meta-analysis. Eur Child Adolesc Psychiatry 2019;28(3):293–305.
37. Bussalb A, Congedo M, Barthelemy Q, et al. Clinical and Experimental factors Influencing the efficacy of neurofeedback in ADHD: a meta-analysis. Front Psychiatry 2019;10:35.
38. Micoulaud-Franchi JA, Geoffroy PA, Fond G, et al. EEG neurofeedback treatments in children with ADHD: an updated meta-analysis of randomized controlled trials. Front Hum Neurosci 2014;8:906.
39. Hodgson K, Hutchinson AD, Denson L. Nonpharmacological treatments for ADHD: a meta-analytic review. J Atten Disord 2014;18(4):275–82.
40. Cortese S, Ferrin M, Brandeis D, et al. Neurofeedback for attention-deficit/hyperactivity disorder: meta-analysis of clinical and neuropsychological outcomes from randomized controlled trials. J Am Acad Child Adolesc Psychiatry 2016;55(6):444–55.
41. Catala-Lopez F, Hutton B, Nunez-Beltran A, et al. The pharmacological and non-pharmacological treatment of attention deficit hyperactivity disorder in children and adolescents: a systematic review with network meta-analyses of randomised trials. PLoS One 2017;12(7):e0180355.
42. Neurofeedback Collaborative Group. Double-blind placebo-controlled randomized clinical trial of neurofeedback for attention-deficit/hyperactivity disorder with 13-month follow-up. J Am Acad Child Adolesc Psychiatry 2021;60(7):841–55.
43. Tang YY, Holzel BK, Posner MI. The neuroscience of mindfulness meditation. Nat Rev Neurosci 2015;16(4):213–25.
44. Cairncross M, Miller CJ. The effectiveness of mindfulness-based therapies for ADHD: a meta-analytic review. J Atten Disord 2020;24(5):627–43.
45. Chimiklis A, Dahl V, Spears A, et al. Yoga, mindfulness, and meditation interventions for youth with ADHD: systematic review and meta-analysis. J Child Fam Stud 2018;27.
46. Krisanaprakornkit T, Ngamjarus C, Witoonchart C, et al. Meditation therapies for attention-deficit/hyperactivity disorder (ADHD). Cochrane Database Syst Rev 2010;(6):CD006507.
47. Xue J, Zhang Y, Huang Y. A meta-analytic investigation of the impact of mindfulness-based interventions on ADHD symptoms. Medicine (Baltimore) 2019;98(23):e15957.
48. Zhang J, Diaz-Roman A, Cortese S. Meditation-based therapies for attention-deficit/hyperactivity disorder in children, adolescents and adults: a systematic review and meta-analysis. Evid Based Ment Health 2018;21(3):87–94.

49. Evans S, Ling M, Hill B, et al. Systematic review of meditation-based interventions for children with ADHD. Eur Child Adolesc Psychiatry 2018;27(1):9–27.

50. Caldwell DM, Davies SR, Hetrick SE, et al. School-based interventions to prevent anxiety and depression in children and young people: a systematic review and network meta-analysis. Lancet Psychiatry 2019;6(12):1011–20.

51. Pandey A, Hale D, Das S, et al. Effectiveness of Universal self-regulation-based interventions in children and adolescents: a systematic review and meta-analysis. JAMA Pediatr 2018;172(6):566–75.

52. Tomporowski PD, Davis CL, Miller PH, et al. Exercise and children's Intelligence, cognition, and academic achievement. Educ Psychol Rev 2008;20(2):111–31.

53. Wigal SB, Emmerson N, Gehricke JG, et al. Exercise: applications to childhood ADHD. J Atten Disord 2013;17(4):279–90.

54. Cerrillo-Urbina AJ, Garcia-Hermoso A, Sanchez-Lopez M, et al. The effects of physical exercise in children with attention deficit hyperactivity disorder: a systematic review and meta-analysis of randomized control trials. Child Care Health Dev 2015;41(6):779–88.

55. Watson A, Timperio A, Brown H, et al. Effect of classroom-based physical activity interventions on academic and physical activity outcomes: a systematic review and meta-analysis. Int J Behav Nutr Phys Act 2017;14(1):114.

56. Zang Y. Impact of physical exercise on children with attention deficit hyperactivity disorders: evidence through a meta-analysis. Medicine (Baltimore) 2019;98(46): e17980.

57. Seiffer B, Hautzinger M, Ulrich R, et al. The efficacy of physical activity for children with attention deficit hyperactivity disorder: a meta-analysis of randomized controlled trials. J Atten Disord 2022;26(5):656–73.

58. Chekroud SR, Gueorguieva R, Zheutlin AB, et al. Association between physical exercise and mental health in 1.2 million individuals in the USA between 2011 and 2015: a cross-sectional study. Lancet Psychiatry 2018;5(9):739–46.

59. Hosker DK, Elkins RM, Potter MP. Promoting mental health and Wellness in youth through physical activity, nutrition, and sleep. Child Adolesc Psychiatr Clin N Am 2019;28(2):171–93.

60. Thygesen M, Engemann K, Holst GJ, et al. The association between Residential green space in childhood and Development of attention deficit hyperactivity disorder: a population-based cohort study. Environ Health Perspect 2020;128(12): 127011.

61. Younan D, Tuvblad C, Li L, et al. Environmental Determinants of aggression in adolescents: role of Urban Neighborhood greenspace. J Am Acad Child Adolesc Psychiatry 2016;55(7):591–601.

62. Ola C, Gonzalez E, Tran N, et al. Evaluating the feasibility and Acceptability of the lifestyle Enhancement for ADHD program. J Pediatr Psychol 2021;46(6):662–72.

63. Azevedo KPM, de Oliveira VH, Medeiros G, et al. The effects of exercise on BDNF levels in adolescents: a systematic review with meta-analysis. Int J Environ Res Public Health 2020;17(17).

64. Heinze K, Cumming J, Dosanjh A, et al. Neurobiological evidence of longer-term physical activity interventions on mental health outcomes and cognition in young people: a systematic review of randomised controlled trials. Neurosci Biobehav Rev 2021;120:431–41.

65. Rodriguez-Ayllon M, Derks IPM, van den Dries MA, et al. Associations of physical activity and screen time with white matter microstructure in children from the general population. Neuroimage 2020;205:116258.

66. Itagaki S, Harigane M, Maeda M, et al. Exercise Habits are important for the mental health of children in Fukushima after the Fukushima Daiichi disaster. Asia Pac J Public Health 2017;29(2_suppl):171S–81S.

67. Qin Z, Shi L, Xue Y, et al. Prevalence and risk factors associated with self-reported psychological distress Among children and adolescents during the COVID-19 pandemic in China. JAMA Netw Open 2021;4(1):e2035487.

68. Bondopadhyay U, Diaz-Orueta U, Coogan AN. A systematic review of sleep and circadian rhythms in children with attention deficit hyperactivity disorder. J Atten Disord 2022;26(2):149–224.

69. Punja S, Shamseer L, Hartling L, et al. Amphetamines for attention deficit hyperactivity disorder (ADHD) in children and adolescents. Cochrane Database Syst Rev 2016;2:CD009996.

70. Storebo OJ, Ramstad E, Krogh HB, et al. Methylphenidate for children and adolescents with attention deficit hyperactivity disorder (ADHD). Cochrane Database Syst Rev 2015;(11):CD009885.

71. Krause AJ, Simon EB, Mander BA, et al. The sleep-deprived human brain. Nat Rev Neurosci 2017;18(7):404–18.

72. Corkum P, Moldofsky H, Hogg-Johnson S, et al. Sleep problems in children with attention-deficit/hyperactivity disorder: impact of subtype, comorbidity, and stimulant medication. J Am Acad Child Adolesc Psychiatry 1999;38(10):1285–93.

73. Lunsford-Avery JR, Bidopia T, Jackson L, et al. Behavioral treatment of insomnia and sleep Disturbances in school-aged children and adolescents. Child Adolesc Psychiatr Clin N Am 2021;30(1):101–16.

74. Morgenthaler TI, Owens J, Alessi C, et al. Practice parameters for behavioral treatment of bedtime problems and night wakings in infants and young children. Sleep 2006;29(10):1277–81.

75. American Academy of sleep medicine. Healthy sleep Habits. 2020. Available at: https://sleepeducation.org/healthy-sleep/healthy-sleep-habits/. Accessed May 15, 2022.

76. Nikles J, Mitchell GK, de Miranda Araujo R, et al. A systematic review of the effectiveness of sleep hygiene in children with ADHD. Psychol Health Med 2020;25(4):497–518.

77. Ni X, Zhang-James Y, Han X, et al. Traditional Chinese medicine in the treatment of ADHD: a review. Child Adolesc Psychiatr Clin N Am 2014;23(4):853–81.

78. Li S, Yu B, Zhou D, et al. Acupuncture for attention deficit hyperactivity disorder (ADHD) in children and adolescents. Cochrane Database Syst Rev 2011;(4):CD007839.

79. Lee MS, Choi TY, Kim JI, et al. Acupuncture for treating attention deficit hyperactivity disorder: a systematic review and meta-analysis. Chin J Integr Med 2011;17(4):257–60.

80. Chen YC, Wu LK, Lee MS, et al. The efficacy of acupuncture treatment for attention deficit hyperactivity disorder: a systematic review and meta-analysis. Complement Med Res 2021;28(4):357–67.

81. U.S. Food and Drug Adminstration. FDA permits marketing of first game-based digital therapeutic to improve attention function in children with ADHD. 2020. Available at: https://www.fda.gov/news-events/press-announcements/fda-permits-marketing-first-game-based-digital-therapeutic-improve-attention-function-children-adhd. Accessed March 19, 2022.

82. Kollins SH, DeLoss DJ, Canadas E, et al. A novel digital intervention for actively reducing severity of paediatric ADHD (STARS-ADHD): a randomised controlled trial. Lancet Digit Health 2020;2(4):e168–78.

83. U.S. Food and Drug Administration. FDA permits marketing of first medical device for treatment of ADHD. 2019. Available at: https://www.fda.gov/news-events/press-announcements/fda-permits-marketing-first-medical-device-treatment-adhd. Accessed March 20, 2022.

84. McGough JJ, Loo SK, Sturm A, et al. An eight-week, open-trial, pilot feasibility study of trigeminal nerve stimulation in youth with attention-deficit/hyperactivity disorder. Brain Stimul 2015;8(2):299–304.

85. McGough JJ, Sturm A, Cowen J, et al. Double-blind, sham-controlled, pilot study of trigeminal nerve stimulation for attention-deficit/hyperactivity disorder. J Am Acad Child Adolesc Psychiatry 2019;58(4):403–411 e403.

86. Ghanizadeh A, Berk M. Zinc for treating of children and adolescents with attention-deficit hyperactivity disorder: a systematic review of randomized controlled clinical trials. Eur J Clin Nutr 2013;67(1):122–4.

Complementary and Integrative Medicine for Anxiety in Children, Adolescents, and Young Adults

Deborah R. Simkin, MD, DFAACAP[a,1], Shayna Swick, MD[b,1], Krishna S. Taneja, MD, MBA[c], Noshene Ranjbar, MD[a,*]

KEYWORDS

- Integrative psychiatry • Complementary and alternative medicine • Anxiety
- Nutraceuticals • Mind–body medicine

KEY POINTS

- An integrative approach to treatment of child and adolescent anxiety disorders requires a person-centered biopsychosocial-spiritual framework, considering potential mechanisms involved including gut–brain connection, nutritional and physical activity components, as well as social determinants of health, genetic, epigenetic, and environmental factors.
- Several treatment approaches such as mindfulness, biofeedback, omega-3 supplementation, and N-acetylcysteine, among others are thought to be effective at least partly through an anti-inflammatory mechanism.
- Based on the current review, the following approaches have some evidence and can be considered in the care of the appropriate patient: multiple micronutrient supplementation in anxious youth with inadequate diets; chamomile and lavender oil for generalized anxiety in young adults, saffron for separation anxiety in young adults, galphimia for social phobia in young adults, N-acetylcysteine for obsessive compulsive disorder, L-theanine for sleep satisfaction, omega-3 fatty acids to counteract proinflammatory effects of anxiety, acupuncture for overactive gag reflex during dental procedures; and biofeedback for tension or migraine headache (which can be associated with anxiety).
- Treatment recommendations are best made on an individual basis, considering each patient and family's needs and preferences, while explaining the current state of the evidence, and accessibility.

[a] Department of Psychiatry, Emory University School of Medicine, 8955 Highway 98 West, Suite 204, Miramar Beach, FL 32550, USA; [b] University of Arizona College of Medicine, 2800 E Ajo Way, Behavioral Health Pavilion, 3rd Floor, Tucson, AZ 85713, USA; [c] Southern Illinois University School of Medicine, 319 E Madison Street, Springfield, IL 62701, USA
[1] Shared first authorship.
* Corresponding author.
E-mail address: noshene@psychiatry.arizona.edu

Child Adolesc Psychiatric Clin N Am 32 (2023) 193–216
https://doi.org/10.1016/j.chc.2022.08.006
1056-4993/23/© 2022 Elsevier Inc. All rights reserved.

INTRODUCTION

A recent review of evidence-based strategies to treat youth anxiety concluded that cognitive behavioral therapy and selective serotonin reuptake inhibitors (SSRIs) have the strongest evidence base for treating anxiety in youth.[1] An integrative approach to anxiety in children takes a multifaceted approach that considers all aspects of a child's health and well-being. Childhood stress increases the risk of developing anxiety.[2,3] Early life stress may translate into anxiety via epigenetic mechanisms, the adoption of maladaptive coping tendencies (poor eating, sedentary life, substance use), and dysregulation of central autonomic nervous system function.[4] Each of these mechanisms may increase inflammatory markers.[5–7]

Recent research elucidates the importance of inflammation in the pathophysiology of childhood anxiety, and inflammation and social behavior are powerful coregulators of one another.[8,9] Examples of strategies with anti-inflammatory effects include mindfulness; biofeedback (through enhancement of self-regulation); acupuncture; dietary factors, including nutrient supplements; omega-3 fatty acids (by producing anti-inflammatory eicosanoids); chamomile; and N-acetylcysteine.[10–17] Several of the strategies examined have the additional advantage of improving the regulation of the central autonomic nervous system (mindfulness, biofeedback, acupuncture), and some enhance coping strategies (mindfulness, biofeedback, yoga, and improving diet). In this article, the efficacy of these Complementary and Integrative Medicine interventions will be explored. Of note, trauma-related mechanisms and approaches on post-traumatic stress disoder (PTSD) and CIM are not covered in this article, as these are covered in a separate article in these series.

PATHOPHYSIOLOGY

The pathophysiology of the various anxiety disorders is complex and multifaceted. Our understanding continues to evolve as new research emerges. An integrative approach is primarily aimed at understanding and treating anxiety disorders with a biopsychosocial-spiritual framework in mind. Recent updates in the field lend credence to this conceptualization of mental illness, particularly as they emerge in and are influenced by the developing child and their environment. Current areas of interest within the realm of anxiety disorders are environmental stressors, inflammation, epigenetics, and the interplay among these three. A review of the most recent evidence is detailed below.

Social-Environmental Determinants of Health

A meta-analysis and systematic review of 111 studies including 264,967 children analyzed the relationship between children whose parents had migrated without them and the risk and prevalence of health outcomes.[18] The results revealed a wide range of impacts on left-behind children's health but in the interest of this review, we will look specifically at the risk of anxiety development. This meta-analysis revealed that these children had a significantly higher risk of anxiety, with a relative risk of 1.85, translating to an overall 85% increased risk of anxiety. Interestingly, the risk of anxiety was not significantly different between children who had one parent migrate and those who had both parents migrate. Of note, most of the studies included in this meta-analysis analyzed populations in China. More research to evaluate other populations and cultures need to be done. However, this meta-analysis provides strong support for the notion that societal and environmental stressors in childhood and adolescence are significantly associated with the development of anxiety disorders.

Inflammation

Exposure to high levels of inflammation has been proposed as a potential contributor to the pathophysiology and development of anxiety disorders. Recent research has attempted to uncover what specific inflammatory processes may be at play in various anxiety disorders.

The best-studied anxiety disorder associated with inflammation is obsessive compulsive disorder (OCD). A recent meta-analysis of 12 studies examined the association between OCD and plasma serum levels of proinflammatory cytokines.[19] The authors found an association between OCD and lower levels of Interleukin-1 (IL-1) and beta. There was no significant difference in IL-6 or tumor necrosis factor (TNF)-α in the overall group; however, when broken down by age and medication usage, the data revealed lower levels of IL-6 in children on psychotropic medications. Elevated TNF-α was associated with anxiety disorders with comorbid depression. As there were many confounding variables within the various studies included in this meta-analysis, no firm conclusions may be drawn. However, there seems to be some degree of inflammatory dysregulation involved in the pathophysiology of OCD. More research is needed to reveal what specific pathways are most critical and how these contribute to the behaviors seen in OCD.

Inflammation in regard to pediatric autoimmune neuropsychiatric disorders associated with strep (PANDAS) has provided additional insight into the inflammation in OCD. Gliosis is a brain response to injury or infection in the brain that involves both proliferation and morphologic changes of glia. The range of functions for activated microglia and astroglia may include producing cytokines, complement proteins, reactive oxygen species (ROS), and proteinases, as well as removing debris and synaptic remodeling. Gliosis is often viewed as an inflammatory response but it has a range of severity and may be used by the brain to respond to the more modest intensity of injury such as neurodegeneration.[20]

Translocator protein imaging (TSPO) in neuropsychiatric illness is a method to detect mainly activated microglia and, to a lesser extent, astroglia. TSPO is overexpressed on outer mitochondrial membranes during inflammatory changes, such as the activation of microglia and astroglia.[21] TSPO is mainly found on outer mitochondrial membranes, and it is overexpressed during inflammatory changes. This method identified more excellent TSPO binding in the corticostriatal-thalamo-cortical circuit in OCD (not just in PANDAS), providing a direct brain measure of an essential component of inflammation.

In an attempt to find biochemical markers of TSPO in OCD, researchers have found that ratios of TNFα/C-Reactive Protein (CRP), prostaglandin E (PGE)$_2$/CRP, which replicated across diagnoses, or PGF$_2$/CRP, which accounted for a very high proportion of variance in dorsal caudate TSPO V_T in OCD, may be applied in clinical trials to advance participant stratification to detect those with greater gliosis to match to new therapeutics targeting neuroinflammation for OCD.[22]

The link between oxidative stress and the severity of OCD was seen in a study by Chakraborty and colleagues, 2009.[23] Thiobarbituric acid reacting substances (TBARSs) are products formed because of free radical-induced lipid peroxidation in the human body. The study investigated the correlation between TBARS and the clinical severity of OCD as indicated by the Yale-Brown Obsessive Compulsive Scale (YBOCS). Serum TBARS was estimated in 39 newly diagnosed drug-free OCD patients and 33 disease-free control subjects. Mean values for serum TBARS were found to be significantly higher ($P < .001$) in cases than in controls. Among cases, a strong positive correlation (rs = 0.757, $P < .01$) between the lipid peroxidation marker TBARS and the disease severity indicator YBOCS was found. A significant positive correlation was also found between TBARS and the obsessive and compulsive subscales of YBOCS.

Role of Cortisol

A systemic review and meta-analysis that included 6 studies and 275 patients evaluated the relationship between cortisol levels (associated with inflammation) and response to psychotherapy.[24] Of note, those with PTSD and OCD were excluded from this meta-analysis. Also excluded were patients requiring pharmacotherapy and psychiatric management. Included were separation anxiety disorder, specific phobia, social anxiety disorder, panic disorder and agoraphobia, generalized anxiety disorder (GAD), and adjustment disorder with anxiety. The authors found that basal cortisol levels were not related to psychological treatment response in patients with the included anxiety disorders. This meta-analysis included one study in children aged 8 to 16 years, which also found no difference in cortisol and the response to treatment with psychotherapy. In those with specific phobias, the level of cortisol level spike when exposed to a stressor was not predictive of response to treatment. Patients included in this study had relatively mild forms of anxiety, which did not necessitate psychiatric treatment. Therefore, caution must be used when generalizing these findings to patients often seen in psychiatric clinics. Further studies to reveal if cortisol has a role in the development of and response to both psychological and pharmacologic treatments in more acute and severely ill populations would be a worthy endeavor.

Epigenome

Several studies have investigated the effect of environmental stressors and their influences on genome expression. Epigenetics has recently gained much interest in psychiatry as possibly being a key contributor to the development and biological underpinnings of various psychiatric illnesses. Childhood, particularly adolescence, seems to be a developmental window in which individuals are susceptible to epigenetic changes that can increase the risk of developing anxiety disorders.[25] For an interesting and thorough review of the current state of epigenetics, please see Cavalli's study in Nature.[26]

A recent meta-analysis evaluated genetic associations with OCD.[27] The study revealed that no single nucleotide polymorphisms were associated with OCD at a genome-wide significant level. However, the authors found significantly increased methylation quantitative trait loci (mQTL) and frontal lobe expression QTL (eQTL) in those with OCD. A QTL is a region of DNA associated with the relationship between the genotype and expressed phenotype. More specifically, QTLs are noncoding sections of genes that affect RNA transcription. Methylation of QTLs influence gene expression by way of the binding of methyl groups close to promoter regions, whereas eQTLs are the amount of messenger RNA transcript for a gene that is thought to be related to noncoding sections of the genome that exert an effect on the promoter region. QTLs, therefore, seem to play a key role in the risk associated with the development of certain complex traits and diseases.[28] Thus, OCD seems to be a result of gene and environmental interactions mediated by epigenetic factors and genetic sequences in the noncoding regions of genes.

COMPLEMENTARY AND INTEGRATIVE APPROACHES TO ANXIETY
Mindfulness for Generalized Anxiety Disorder

A meta-analysis analyzing studies investigating mindfulness interventions in youth was promising. The meta-analysis demonstrated that mindfulness interventions have the possibility of improving psychopathology in childhood.[29] This meta-analysis used Kabat-Zinn's definition of mindfulness, stating "paying attention in a particular way, on purpose, in the present moment, and non-judgmentally." The concept of mindfulness has gained traction over the years. Two of the most known are mindfulness-based stress reduction (MBSR) and mindfulness-based cognitive therapy (MBCT). The studies used in this meta-analysis were peer-reviewed, investigated interventions with mindfulness as the primary intervention component and had a sample population with an age range of 6 to 21 years. Of note, studies that included participants 18 years and older had age ranges with a minimum at or younger than 17 years of age. Interventions that focused on a specific concentration (such as transcendental meditation) and those with mindfulness as one component of a multicomponent intervention were excluded. In total, 20 articles were included in the meta-analysis with the following intervention breakdown: 3 MBSR, 3 MBCT, 5 using one component of MBSR, and 9 using a different mindfulness intervention. Of note, only 4 studies used a clinical sample, with the rest coming from nonclinical settings, such as school programs. Overall, the meta-analysis revealed that, on average, the mindfulness intervention resulted in greater overall improvement than active control conditions ($P < .0001$). Of particular interest was the finding that the most significant improvement was seen in the clinical population, effect size nearly 3-fold more than nonclinical samples, meaning those with diagnosed mental health disorders. Even more reassuring was the more significant effect on psychopathology symptoms when compared with the nonclinical population. It is reasonable to extrapolate from this information that mindfulness has a greater positive impact on those with diagnosed mental illness and may be a reasonable adjunctive therapy for children with GAD.

The mindfulness-based meta-analysis did not demonstrate iatrogenic harm and provided a small-to-moderate primary omnibus effect ($P < .0001$). Therefore, it is reasonable to incorporate mindfulness-based practices into the management of GAD in the pediatric population. Mindfulness-based practices can decrease the frequency and intensity of ruminating thoughts, which are thought to contribute to GAD. Successfully practicing mindfulness requires a level of commitment to learn and incorporate these skills. Therefore, the most likely group to benefit from mindfulness-based practices is motivated adolescents.

Yoga for Anxiety

A meta-analysis of yoga in children and young adults with anxiety was done by James-Palmer and colleagues, 2020.[30] Twenty-seven studies involving youth with varying health statuses were reviewed (aged 3–21 years, n = 1262). Intervention characteristics varied considerably across studies revealing multiple factors that may affect intervention efficacy; however, 70% of the studies overall showed improvements. For studies assessing anxiety and depression, 58% showed reductions in both symptoms, whereas 25% showed reductions in anxiety only. Additionally, 70% of studies assessing anxiety alone showed improvement. Studies may have included the additional elements of breathing, meditation, and relaxation but if studies included only breathing and/or meditation practices, they were not included in this review. Overall, 70% of the studies showed some improvement in anxiety and/or depression symptoms. For studies assessing anxiety and depression, 58% showed improvement in both symptoms, whereas 25% showed improvements in anxiety only. For studies only assessing anxiety, 70% showed improvements, and 40% of studies only assessing depression showed improvements. Overall, the methodological quality of evidence was weak, which can be attributed to a lack of randomization, blinding, and limited analysis. Although the variety of intervention characteristics made it challenging to recommend specific intervention parameters, it showed that yoga, defined here by the practice of postures, generally leads to some reductions in anxiety and depression regardless of type, other yoga elements practiced, delivery method, and setting. Future research will aid in the development of optimal dosage and intervention parameters.

Multiple Micronutrient Supplementation

Multiple factors may play a role in nutrient deficiency, including the prevalence of highly processed diets with low vegetable, fruit, and whole-grain intake, topsoil erosion, and a decline of nutrient levels in the soil, and food insecurity or limited access to healthy foods and variety.[31] Micronutrient malnutrition, or deficiencies in one or more crucial vitamins or minerals, may negatively affect both physical and mental health and potentially leading to chronic illness. To compound the issue, chronic psychological and environmental stress may negatively influence micronutrient concentrations in the body, leading to micronutrient depletion.[32] A randomized clinical trial (RCT) evaluated the effect of multiple micronutrient supplementation (MMS) on anxiety in children living in rural China.[33] The MMS contained 5 mg of ferrous sulfate and 20 other vitamins and minerals. The concept was based on prior study findings where anemia was positively correlated with anxiety. The study had 2730 fourth grade students attending elementary school in various areas of the northwest region of China. Participants in the intervention group took one MMS per day for a total of 36 weeks, minus a couple of weeks during winter break when the school could not supply the MMS supplement. The 2 primary outcomes evaluated were hemoglobin levels and anxiety measured by mental health test (MHT) scores. Results showed that the mean change in hemoglobin levels between the beginning and end of the study were significantly higher in the intervention group compared with the control group $(P < .01)$. MHT scores were lower, indicating less anxiety in the treatment group compared with the control group, with a mean score difference of 1.6 points $(P < .05)$. Of note, when subcategories of anxiety were evaluated, the only significant score reduction was in personal and body anxiety. Overall, MMS use in children had a small-to-medium effect size on anxiety and hemoglobin levels. Due to this study being conducted under financial constraints, the effects of the other micronutrients were not evaluated. Therefore, the role of the other 20 vitamins and minerals remains unknown. At this point, it is difficult to extrapolate this data to a more general pediatric population; however, given the increase in hemoglobin, it is reasonable to give supplementation to children who are deficient.

Melatonin

Before blood draw–anticipatory anxiety

This double-blind RCT looked at the effect of oral melatonin, compared with placebo, to reduce blood draw anxiety in children.[34] The study had a total of 60 participants, ages ranging from 1 to 14 years, who were either given 0.5 mg/kg (maximum total of 5 mg) of melatonin or a placebo of 5% glucose solution 30 minutes before a blood draw. To properly assess the effect of melatonin on anxiety, children were assessed by a parent and blinded resident before the blood draw using the children's anxiety and pain scales (CAPS). The CAPS evaluates pain using faces on a 0 to 5 scale. Postprocedural pain and anxiety were evaluated 5 minutes after the procedure using the face, legs, activity, cry, and the consolability scale for children under 3 years of age, the faces pain scale for children aged 3 to 8 years, and a numeric rating scale for those more than 8 years of age. Notably, there was a significant difference between anxiety and pain scores in the melatonin and placebo groups, where those given melatonin had significantly lower scores than placebo ($P < .0005$) indicating a reduction in anxiety and pain. Of note, children younger than 3 years of age had the greatest reduction in pain ($P < .0002$); however, this may be due to the need to have adults score the child based on observation. Overall, this is a small study with significant results indicating a possible treatment of preblood draw anxiety. However, it should also be noted that other studies using melatonin have found contradictory results. For this reason, relaxation and distraction techniques may be equally useful for blood draw anxiety.

Before Procedure

Anxiety during dental procedures can reduce the effectiveness of procedures and negatively affect dental health. Therefore, there is interest in therapies targeting this specific form of anxiety.[35] Midazolam is a commonly used sedative for dental procedures; however, due to its potential for side effects, including paradoxic reactions of anxiety and agitation as well as delayed recovery and bradycardia, an alternative treatment is of interest. An RCT compared the role of melatonin to midazolam as an anxiolytic in combination with nitrous oxide/oxygen sedation before and during dental procedures in children aged 3 to 8 years. There were 4 comparator groups, 2 of different melatonin doses (3 mg and 0.5 mg/kg), a 0.75 mg midazolam group, and then a control group of 3 mL of normal saline given orally. Based on prior studies evaluating the time of onset for melatonin and midazolam, melatonin was given 60 minutes before the procedure, and midazolam, or placebo, was given 15 minutes before the procedure. Anxiety was assessed using the Frankl Behavioral Scale. Due to the physical effects of sedation, vitals were monitored and documented as well. Results indicated that melatonin was no better than the control at reducing anxiety. In contrast, midazolam was found to have more of an effect on anxiety and overall patient satisfaction. It is important to note that those given midazolam had a significantly lower heart rate during the procedure, indicating these participants were more sedated, likely reducing overall anxiety and improving patient satisfaction. Vitals in the melatonin groups were no different than those of the control. Based on this study, midazolam is a better option for dental procedure anxiety, even if it has a more extensive side effect profile than melatonin. It may be worthwhile to use distraction and relaxation techniques in these patients if midazolam use is unwanted. At this point, melatonin is not recommended for dental procedure anxiety in children.

Acupuncture for Hyperactive Gag Reflex (Dental Procedures)

Gagging during dental procedures can compromise overall procedure quality and dental health. Therefore, evaluating possible interventions for children who suffer from gagging is essential. Interestingly, gagging can be psychological or somatic, or both in origin. Therefore, it is worthwhile to investigate therapies targeting the psychological component.[36] Acupuncture, specifically at the pericardium 6 location (anterior midline portion of the wrist), is beneficial for reducing nausea. Given this study was evaluating pediatric patients who may not tolerate needle acupuncture, the researchers used a laser form of acupuncture that has similar benefits without the invasive nature of a needle. This study had a total of 40 subjects, ranging in age from 4 to 14 years, who required an impression of the maxillary arch and were deemed to have a hyperactive gag reflex based on Dickinson's criteria. Anxiety from gag reflex was evaluated after the impression procedure using the faces version of the Modified Child Dental Anxiety Scale. Other markers that were assessed included heart rate and oxygen saturation. The subjects were assigned to 1 of 2 groups: group A had the laser acupuncture before the second impression, and group B had the laser acupuncture before the first impression; therefore, each group had one impression with acupuncture and one without. Results showed a significant reduction in heart rate and improvement in oxygen saturation during the second impression for group A and the first impression for group B, indicating that laser acupuncture reduced heart rate and improved oxygen saturation. These vitals indicate participants were more comfortable or less anxious, with the impression when the laser acupuncture preceded it. Of equal importance, the gag reflex was absent in one patient during the non-acupuncture impression of group A. In contrast, the gag reflex was absent in 17 out of 20 patients during the acupuncture impression. Similar results were shown in group B, with gag reflex being absent in all 20 patients during the acupuncture impression, and it was only absent in 4 subjects during the nonacupuncture impression. Not only did the acupuncture reduce gag reflex but it also significantly reduced anxiety scores ($P < .001$). Overall, there are no side effects with laser acupuncture, and it was well tolerated in this study. Therefore, this is a reasonable option for children with gag reflex anxiety undergoing dental procedures. More studies need to be conducted given the small sample size of this study; however, if laser acupuncture is available and the patient is interested, it is reasonable to pursue this treatment route.

N-acetylcysteine for Obsessive Compulsive Disorder

Glutamine and glutamate are 2 amino acids in our bodies. Glutathione is a powerful antioxidant that is made from glutamine and 2 other amino acids cysteine and glycine. Glutathione is then used to neutralize ROS and thus reduce oxidized stress (**Fig. 1**). N-acetylcysteine (NAC), as a powerful antioxidant, is used as a nutritional supplement for different disorders. NAC is a precursor of L-cysteine, which donates cysteine and combines with glutamine and glycine to form more glutathione when more glutathione is needed to combat oxidative stress. Psychiatric disorders allegedly related to oxidative stress include schizophrenia, bipolar disorder, as well as psychiatric syndromes characterized by impulsive/compulsive symptoms (eg, trichotillomania, pathologic nail-biting, gambling, substance misuse) and OCD severity.[37]

NAC may modulate pathophysiological processes that are involved in multiple psychiatric and neurologic disorders, including oxidative stress, neurogenesis and apoptosis, mitochondrial dysfunction, neuroinflammation, and dysregulation of

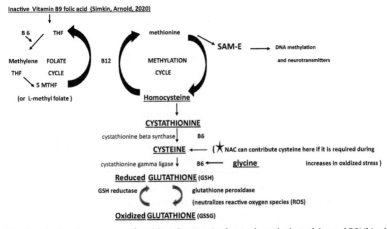

Fig. 1. The best measure of oxidized stress is the reduced glutathione (GSH)/oxidized glutathione (GSSG) ratio. A low ratio indicates increased oxidized stress.

glutamate and dopamine neurotransmitter systems.[38,39] Early magnetic resonance spectroscopy studies suggested that children with OCD have elevated glutamate/glutamine levels in the striatum, and reduced glutamate/glutamine in the anterior cingulate cortex.[40,41] Therefore, using CIM interventions that modulate glutamate, such as NAC, has been found to be helpful.

In a 12-week randomized, double-blind, placebo-controlled, 2-center, parallel-assignment clinical trial (N = 82, aged 18–45 years), participants in the intervention group received an initial dosage of 600 mg/d of NAC, which doubled weekly to a maximum dose of 2400 mg/d depending on the Clinical Global Impression Improvement (CGI-I) scale scores and the patients' tolerance.[42] Participants were those with a primary OCD diagnosis who failed clinical response to at least 12 weeks of high-dose treatment with a SSRI or clomipramine without any history of bipolar disorder. NAC-assigned patients showed significantly improved mean Y-BOCS score ($P = .003$) and CGI Severity of Illness scale score ($P = .01$) but not on the CGI-I scale score at study endpoint. Of the patients in the NAC group, 52.6% were full responders at the end of the study, which was significantly higher than 15% of the patients in the placebo group ($P = .013$). This trial suggests that NAC may be a safe and effective option to augment standard treatment in patients with refractory OCD.

In a double-blind, placebo-controlled trial (DBPCT) of NAC on children and young adults (aged 10–21 years, n = 29) with refractory OCD to at least one SSRI, one group received citalopram (20–40 mg/d) and NAC (titrated up to 2400 mg/d), and the other group received citalopram (20–40 mg/d) plus placebo.[43] One patient in the NAC group received fluoxetine during this trial (20 mg/d). Two other patients in NAC received fluvoxamine (50 mg/d) or sertraline (100 mg/d). The dose of NAC during the first week of the trial was 600 mg/d, which increased to 1200 mg/d in 2 divided doses in the second week. The patients were administered 1800 mg/d during weeks 4 and 5. The daily dose for NAC from week 6 to the end of this trial was 2400 mg/d (week 12). The YBOCS score decreased from 21.0 (8.2) to 11.3 (5.7) in the NAC group during this trial. The change of score in the placebo group was from 22.5 (8.4) to 19.7 (9.7). The Cohen's d effect size was 0.83. The mean score of change for resistance/control to compulsion in the NAC and placebo groups was 2.3(1.8) and 0.9(2.3), respectively ($t = 2.5$, df = 32, $P < .04$). The score decreased from 4.7(1.7) to 3.6(2.6) in the placebo group, whereas it decreased from 4.7(1.9) to 2.3(1.6) in the NAC group. There were no between-group differences in resistance to obsessions. The changes in different domains of quality of life scores showed that the emotional functioning and social functioning scores, except for physical function, decreased in both groups during this trial. This trial suggests that NAC adds to the effect of citalopram in improving resistance/control to compulsions in OCD children and adolescents.

Although the dosages, pharmacologic strategies (monotherapy vs augmentation), and long-term risks are not fully evident, NAC seems to be a promising, relatively low-risk intervention for OCD.

L-Theanine for Generalized Anxiety Disorder

L-theanine is a nonproteinogenic amino acid derived from tea leaves (Camellia sinensis).[44] It is an analog of glutamate. Studies have found L-theanine to pass freely through the blood–brain barrier, reduce presynaptic glutamate release increase inhibitory neurotransmitter γ-aminobutyric acid (GABA), and enhance glycine and serotonin and dopamine release.[45–47] L-theanine's mood regulating properties and balance of neurotransmission are hypothesized to directly result from elevated glycine. Additionally, L-theanine administration reduces cortisol levels and increases brain derived neurotrophic factor (BDNF) levels, resulting in improved neurogenesis and neuroplasticity, positive mood regulation, motivation, cognition, and memory. Increased anxiety gives rise to escalating cortisol levels, which adjusts the brain wave patterns to reflect a state of stress by increased coupling between delta and beta waves.[48] Increased cortisol levels strengthen this coupling.[49] However, alpha wave activity is inversely correlated with cortisol levels.[50] Alpha wave patterns arise in the wakeful relaxation state—a state of composure, alertness, and improved concentration without the edge of anxiety.[51] Mindfulness, meditation, and yoga are not the only practices that induce alpha wave activity.[52–54] L-theanine also induces a resting state of alpha wave activity without causing drowsiness due to unchanged theta waves[55] (**Fig. 2**).

In a DBPCT participants received adjunctive L-theanine (450–900 mg) or a matching placebo for 8 weeks.[56] Participants (aged 18–75 years, N = 19 in the control group and 18 years in the placebo group) included those with a Diagnostic and Statistical Manual of Mental Disorders 5 (DSM-5) primary diagnosis of a GAD, a Hamilton Anxiety Rating Scale ([HAMA] score of 16 or greater) and those taking an antidepressant medication at a stable dose for a minimum of 4 weeks. Results revealed that adjunctive L-theanine did not outperform placebo for anxiety reduction on the HAMA ($P = .73$) nor insomnia severity on the Insomnia Severity Index (ISI; $P = .35$). However, L-theanine treated participants reported greater self-reported sleep satisfaction than placebo (ISI item 4; $P = .015$).

Kava for Generalized Anxiety Disorder

There have been many studies showing that Kava can help with mild anxiety. It contains alpha-pyrones (kavalactones), which increases GABA transmission, noradrenaline and dopamine reuptake inhibition. However, the best study to date with significant effects looked at genetic subtypes of the GABA gene and the norepinephrine transporter gene.[57] Two subtypes of the GABA gene (GABA transporter genes rs2601126 and rs2697153) were identified in patients who had a significant effect of kava on GAD. A double-blind, randomized, controlled trial (DBRCT) (N = 58, aged 18–65 years) using aqueous extract of kava (120/240 mg of kavalactones per day depending on response) versus placebo. GABA and noradrenaline transporter polymorphisms were also analyzed as potential pharmacogenetic markers of response. Reduction in anxiety was measured using the HAMA as the primary outcome. Results revealed a significant reduction in anxiety for the kava group compared with the placebo group with a moderate effect size ($P = .046$, Cohen $d = 0.62$). Among participants with moderate-to-severe *Diagnostic and Statistical Manual of Mental Disorders*–diagnosed GAD, this effect was larger ($P = .02$; $d = 0.82$). At conclusion of the controlled phase, 26% of the kava group were classified as remitted (HAMA

NEUROMODULATORY EFFECTS OF L-THEANINE

1. Inhibits the Glutamate receptors (NMDA, AMPG & mGluR) from astrocytes which stimulates the release of :

GABA   and   Glycine (from pre-synaptic neurons)

2. ↑Glycine and ↑ GABAwhich triggers the release of :

SEROTONIN and DOPAMINE

3. In addition it decreases CORTISOL and ↑ Brain-Derived Neurotrophic Factor (BDNF)

4. ↑ ALPHA WAVES to produce a relaxed state

Fig. 2. Neuromodulatory effects of L-theanine.

≤ 7) compared with 6% of the placebo group (P = .04). Within the kava group, GABA transporter polymorphisms rs2601126 (P = .021) and rs2697153 (P = .046) were associated with HAMA reduction. Kava was well tolerated, and aside from more headaches reported in the kava group (P = .05), no other significant differences between groups occurred for any other adverse effects, nor for liver function tests.

Several cases of liver toxicity have been reported. It seems that liver toxicity became a problem when the extraction solvent was changed from ethanol to the acetone preparation of Kava.[58] Factors for possible hepatotoxic effects include hepatic insufficiency to metabolize kavalactones, preparations low in glutathione, use of aerial parts or root peelings (higher in alkaloids) in preparations, or the use of acetonic or ethanolic kava extracts.[59] An analysis was done of 6 kavalactones (kavain, dihydrokavain, methysticin, dihydromethysticin, yangonin, and desmethoxyyangonin) and 2 flavokavains (flavokavains A and B) and their contents in 28 different kava products in the form of capsules, tinctures, traditional aqueous suspensions, and dried powders. The results demonstrated a great variation in terms of the total and relative abundance of the analyzed kavalactones and flavokavains among the analyzed kava preparations. In the final recommendation, more rigorous and comprehensive quality control of kava products is required with respect to the content of individual kavalactones and flavokavains. Therefore, safety concerns limit the use of Kava for anxiety at this time.[60] It should be noted that the form of kava used in the Sarris study was neither nonacetonic nor ethanolic extract. It was an aqueous extract, which is considered safer.

Chamomile (Matricaria recutita or Chamomilla recutita) for GAD

Chamomile has many flavonoid components that may produce anxiolytic activity by affecting GABA and GABA pathways.[61] It also has antioxidant, antimicrobial, antidepressant, and anti-inflammatory effects.[62]

In a DBPCT study of oral chamomile for GAD (DSM IV Axis), participants were considered to have a good response if they had a 50% or greater improvement on the HAMA.[63] There were 57 participants (chamomile n = 28 and placebo n = 29, aged 18 years or older). Chamomile or placebo therapy was initiated at one capsule daily for the first week and increased to 2 capsules daily during the second week of therapy. Patients with a 50% or less reduction in total HAMA score (vs baseline) were increased to 3 capsules daily during week 3, and then to 4 capsules daily during week 4 of therapy. Patients who continued to have a 50% or greater reduction in baseline HAMA score were increased to 5 capsules daily during study weeks 5 through 8 of therapy. Dose reductions could occur at any time based on drug tolerability. Outcome measurements were obtained at baseline and after 2, 4, 6, and 8 weeks of treatment. There was a somewhat greater proportion of HAMA responders to chamomile (57.13%) versus placebo (37.93%; P = .146). Finally, the overall percentage change was numerically greater for chamomile (−52.97%) versus placebo (−34.92%) on the HAMA (P = .085), for chamomile (−42.48%) versus placebo (−20.79%) on the Beck Anxiety Inventory (P = .142), and for chamomile (27.58%) versus placebo (17.64%) on the Psychological General Well Being (P = .344). However, it was speculated that a more robust result could have occurred at a higher dose for a longer period. There is no recommended dose for chamomile.

The first long-term RCT using a higher dose was done by Mao and colleagues, 2016.[64] In an RCT, of chamomile in patients with a DSM-IV diagnosis of GAD (18 years or older, n-93, placebo, n = 47 or chamomile continuation, n = 46), participants were treated with 1500 mg (3 capsules daily) of open-label chamomile extract for up to 12 weeks. Individuals who had successfully attained a clinical response to treatment (defined as a reduction in GAD-7 score from baseline of at least 50% and a score of 3 or less on the CGI–Severity [CGI-S] scale) during 12 weeks were then randomized to either continuation chamomile or placebo for an additional 26 weeks. Relative to participants randomized to placebo, those who continued on chamomile experienced a lesser increase in GAD-7 symptoms ($P = .0032$) and had overall better psychological well-being ($P = .013$), specifically in anxiety impacts on well-being ($P = .0094$). Anxiety symptoms measured by the HAMA and Beck Anxiety Inventory (BAI) showed the same trends but were not significant. During the 26-week follow-up period after randomization, 7 (15.2%) in the chamomile group compared with 12 (25.5%) in the placebo group relapsed ($P = .15$). The mean time to relapse was 11.4 ± 8.4 weeks in the chamomile group versus 6.3 ± 3.9 weeks for placebo. These studies demonstrate that chamomile may be helpful as an adjunct for the treatment of GAD in young adults. However, chamomile can trigger an allergic reaction because it belongs to the ragweed family.

Lavender Oil for Generalized Anxiety Disorder

A DBRCT multicenter trial comparing silexan, a new oral lavender oil capsule preparation, versus a benzodiazepine (lorazepam) was conducted by Woelk and colleagues, 2010 for 6 weeks, with a 2 week taper from week 7 to 8.[65] The study included patients aged 18 to 65 years (n = 77, silexan: = 40 patients, lorazepam: = 37). Patients received either 1 × 1 capsule filled with 80 mg silexan *and* 1 × 1 capsule filled with lorazepam placebo representing the silexan group, or 1 × 1 capsule of 0.5 mg lorazepam *and* 1 × 1 capsule filled with silexan placebo, representing the lorazepam group. The mean of the HAMA-total score decreased clearly and to a similar extent in both groups (by 11.3 ± 6.7 points [45%] in the silexan group and by 11.6 ± 6.6 points (46%) in the lorazepam group, from 25 ± 4 points at baseline in both groups). During the active treatment period, the 2 HAMA subscores "somatic anxiety" (HAMA subscore I) and "psychic anxiety" (HAMA subscore II) also decreased clearly and to a similar extent in both groups. The changes in other subscores measured during the study, such as the Self–rating Anxiety Scale, Penn State Worry Questionnaire, Short Form (SF) 36 Health survey Questionnaire and CGIs of severity of disorder (CGI item 1, CGI item 2, CGI item 3), and the results of the sleep diary demonstrated comparable positive effects of the 2 compounds.

Results suggest that this new compound of lavender oil may be as effective for GAD as lorazepam for adults. In children and adolescents, use of lavender oil should be approached with caution given the lipophilic estrogenic components of lavender accumulation in adipose tissue, which can act as an endocrine disruptor. Clinicians must be aware that gynecomastia has been reported with the use of topical lavender oil in prepubertal boys and girls.[66,67]

Currently, given lack of studies in children, and these safety concerns, the use of oral lavendar is not recommended.

Saffron for Separation Anxiety and Social Phobia

Saffron is a spice derived from the *Crocus sativus* flower. It has several pharmacologic actions including anti-inflammatory, antioxidant, and neuroprotective properties.[68] It also acts as an anxiolytic effect probably through their interaction with the benzodiazepine binding site at the $GABA_A$ receptor.[69] In a DBPCT, 68 participants (aged 12–16 years) received saffron (produced in a tablet called affron with 3.5% Lepticrosalides) twice a day for 8 weeks.[70] On the Revised Child Anxiety and Depression Scale (RCADS) for youth, significant univariate time × group interactions were found for the following subscale scores: separation anxiety (F2.68,196 = 5.03, $P = .003$), social phobia (F2.92,213 = 3.27, $P = .023$), depression (F2.68,206 = 3.70, $P = .016$), and near significance for generalized anxiety ($F2.79,204 = 2.48, P = .067$). An independent samples T-test confirmed significance between group differences at varying time points for generalized anxiety, and obsessions/compulsions. RCADS parent scores were also significantly different in the saffron (40%) and placebo (26%) conditions ($T73 = 2.27; P = .026$). However, a Pearson's Chi-Square analysis revealed no differences in percentage of treatment responders in the saffron and placebo conditions (29% vs 24%) ($\chi2(1) = 0.205, P = .424$, 95% CI [.787, .802], OR = 1.27). Cohen's d effect sizes ranged from small effect size of 0.25 on the obsessions/compulsions subscale to a moderate effect size of more than 0.57 on the panic subscale score. Thus, saffron extract showed improvement in youth with mild-moderate anxiety and depressive symptoms. These beneficial effects were inconsistently corroborated by parents but positively reported from the adolescent's perspective.

Galphimia

The plant species *Galphimia glauca* is a native species of Mexico. The effects produced by *G glauca* are selective for the dopaminergic neurons that, besides not interacting with the GABAergic system, are capable of blocking the effects produced by glutamate on the *N*-methyl-D-aspartate (NMDA) ionotropic receptors.[71] A DBPCT trial was done comparing galphimia to sertraline for social phobia. The trial was carried out, using 50 mg of sertraline as a control. Patients of both sexes (aged 18–35 years) with moderate or severe social anxiety were included. The experimental group was treated daily (orally), for 10 weeks, with an extract from *G glauca* containing 0.374 mg/dose of Galphimine-B (G-B, active compound). All patients were evaluated every 2 weeks. Another assessment was done 1 month after the end of the administration period. A total of 34 patients were included, 17 in each group. In patients who received the *G glauca* standardized extract, a significant reduction in anxiety was observed, with a value (in the Brief Social Phobia Scale) of 41.1 ± 10.3 points at the start and 11.2 ± 5.6 points at the end of treatment, whereas patients treated with sertraline had a value of 37.7 ± 7.3 points at the beginning and 11.1 ± 5.2 points at the end. No significant difference was observed between the treated groups. In a similar way, the health scale showed a gradual and continuous improvement in each of the 5 evaluations. In conclusion, the 10-week oral administration of *G glauca* standardized extract showed efficacy and safety in patients with social anxiety disorder, without showing a significant difference from patients treated with sertraline.[72]

Omega-3 Supplementation for Anxiety in Autism Spectrum Disorder

Autism spectrum disorder (ASD) is a neurodevelopmental disorder with a variety of symptoms ranging from deficits in social interaction to repetitive and restrictive patterns of behavior. Anxiety is a common comorbidity of ASD and can greatly negatively influence quality of life.[73] Given the findings of omega-3 supplementation reducing inflammation and the positive correlation between inflammation and anxiety, it is reasonable to consider the role of omega-3 fatty acids in the management of anxiety in ASD.[74] Prior studies have found a reduced concentration of omega-3 fatty acids in children with ASD. A meta-analysis evaluating 5 RCTs (n = 183) sought clarification on the role of omega-3 fatty acids in the management of children with ASD; of note, these studies evaluated a variety of symptoms of ASD and not anxiety exclusively.[75] These RCTs had a participant age range of 2 to 7 years who were diagnosed with ASD using a variety of validated scales including autism diagnostic interview-revised, autism diagnostic observation schedule, childhood autism rating scale (score greater than or equal to 30), fourth edition of DSM, and social communication questionnaire (score >12). The dose of omega-3 fatty acids ranged from 0.2 g docosahexaenoic acid (DHA)/d only to 1.5 g eicosapentaenoic acid (EPA) and DHA/d, given in the form of fish oil or algal oil. Placebos used in the RCTs included medium chain triglycerides, safflower, corn, soybean, olive, and coconut plus fish oil. The length of intervention ranged from 6 weeks (2 studies), 12 weeks (1 study), and 6 months (2 studies).

The effects of intervention were assessed via a variety of scale scores that were assessed by teachers, parents, as well as clinicians. Two RCTs (n = 69) used the aberrant behavior checklist scoring system and found that although there were no significant differences between experimental and control interventions when teachers and clinicians provided the scores, there was a significant difference in lethargy when parents completed the scoring (pooled MD 1.98, 95% CI 0.32, 3.63). This suggests that omega-3 fatty acids may improve lethargy in children with ASD; however, it was only noticeable in 1 of the 3 settings, therefore more studies will need to be conducted. The Behavior Assessment System for Children (BASC) scores found significant worsening in externalizing behavior (pooled mean difference (MD): −6.22; 95% CI: −10.9, −1.59) but not internalizing. This was the only significant finding when using the BASC scores. Both the clinical global impression-improvement scores and the social responsiveness scale scores did not have any significant differences between the interventional and placebo groups.

Overall, the findings from this meta-analysis show minimal to no effect of omega-3 fatty acid supplementation on the symptoms of ASD. That being said, the adverse events were similar in both the experimental and control groups, indicating that omega-3 fatty acids are low risk for causing harm in this population. It is difficult to assess the accuracy of this meta-analysis due to the small sample size; therefore, more studies and data points are needed to truly evaluate the role of omega-3 fatty acids in this population. That being said, the anti-inflammatory effects of omega-3 fatty acids and the evidence that anxiety may be related to a proinflammatory state, it may still be reasonable to provide omega-3 supplementation to children with ASD, particularly if they have symptoms of anxiety.[75] Although there are conflicting results about omega-3s, some studies have found improved scores in hyperactivity, lethargy, and stereotypies in children with ASD. Most clinical trials have used dosages of 1.3 to 1.5 g, with duration of 16 to 24 weeks. Although not clearly delineated for ASD, most studies of omega-3s for mental health conditions have demonstrated a 2:1 ratio of EPA:DHA as optimal. Of note, some clinical findings that have been correlated with omega-3 fatty acid deficiency include dry and scaly skin, dry eyes, and eczema.[76]

Biofeedback for Anxiety with Comorbid Headaches

Biofeedback is one of the most useful adjuncts for reducing physiological hyperarousal in GAD; it can also be beneficial for exposure sensitization in panic disorder and PTSD. It can also complement cognitive/behavioral therapies to help reduce fearful anticipation triggers. Headaches are a common comorbidity with anxiety disorders, therefore discussed here.

Tension Headaches

A meta-analysis evaluated 53 studies looking at the role of various types of biofeedback on tension headaches.[77] Of note, only 9 of these studies evaluated a pediatric population who ranged from 11 to 19 years of age and had an average headache duration of 3.5 years. The primary outcome was headache pain and was evaluated through structured headache diaries. Across all studies, there was a medium-large effect size (d = 0.73; 95% CI = 0.61, 0.84) in biofeedback groups when compared with placebo that proved stable over an average follow-up phase of 15 months. Overall, the average

Table 1
Complementary/integrative treatments for child/adolescent anxiety

Treatment Population	Recommendation Strength	Certainty (US Prevention Task Force (PTF)	Evidence Base in Youth	Evidence-Based or SECS Criteria met	Reviewer Recommendations
Anxiety Disorder or Anxiety as a Symptom					
I. GAD					
a. Mindfulness (Zoogman, 2015, N=1914, age <18 y)[29]	B	Moderate	Meta-analysis (13 RCTs)	EB	Recommend
b. TMS	I		None		Await further trials
c. Lavender oil (Woelk et al., 2010, N= 77, aged 18–65 y)[65]	I for children, C for young adults	Low for children; moderate for young adults	DBRCT		Consider for young adults with GAD; await trials for children
d. Chamomile (Amsterdam et al., 2009, N=57, age >18 y; Mao et al., 2016, N=93, age >18 y)[63,64]	I for children, C for young adults	Low for children; moderate for young adults	DBRCT		Consider for young adults with GAD; await trials for children
e. Kava (Sarris J et al., 2013, N=58 aged 18–65 y)[57]	I	low for children; moderate for young adults	DBRCT		Await further safety trials
II. Unspecified Anxiety					
a. MMS children with inadequate diets (Zhang, 2013, N=2740, aged 10–12 y)[33]	C	Low	RCT	SECS	Inquire into diet, consider supplementation with OTC multivitamin if diet inadequate
b. Yoga (James- Palmer, 2020, N=1262, aged 3–21 y)[30]	B	Moderate	Systematic review (6 RCTs)	SECS	Consider, given low risk of harm and many documented benefits of exercise
OCD					

(continued on next page)

Table 1
(continued)

Treatment Population	Recommendation Strength	Certainty (US Prevention Task Force (PTF)	Evidence Base in Youth	Evidence-Based or SECS Criteria met	Reviewer Recommendations
a. NAC (Ghanizadeh, 2017, N=29 age 10–21)[43]	C	Low	DBPCT	SECS	Consider as augmentation to SSRI, given low risk of harm and some evidence of improvement in resistance/control to compulsions
IV. Separation Anxiety and Social Phobia					
a. Saffron (Lopresti, 2018, N=68, aged 12–16 y)[70]	C	Low	DBPCT	SECS	Consider for augmentation in children
b. Galphimia (Romero-Cerecero, 2018, N=34, aged 18–65 y)[72]	C	Low	RCT	Does not pass SECS-formulation has to be studied more	Weak evidence in RCT More research needed before recommending in young adults. No studies in children Not recommended
V. Preprocedural/procedural anxiety					
a. Melatonin before blood draw (Marseglia, 2015, N=60, aged 1–14 y)34	I	Low	RCTs		Would not recommend; distraction/relaxation likely more effective
b. Melatonin for preprocedural anxiety (Isik, 2008, N=60, children)[35]					
c. Acupuncture for hyperactive gag reflex during dental procedures (Goel, 2017, N=40, aged 4–14 y)[36]	C, but not risky	Low	Clinical trial, crossover design		Promising. Await further studies; may consider for patients with hyperactive gag reflex for dental procedures when available

Issues and Populations Related to/Overlapping With Anxiety

VI. Headache (which may be associated with anxiety)

a. Biofeedback-tension headache (Nestoriuc, 2008, N=1532, adults and children)[74]	C	Moderate	Meta-analysis (6 youth studies)	SECS	Although level C, Recommend for tension headache
b. Biofeedback- migraine headache (Hermann, 1995, aged 5–18 y, N=68)[75]	C	Low	Meta-analysis	SECS	Recommend for migraine headache

Strength of Recommendations based on benefit and safety:

A=**Recommend strongly.** There is a high certainty that the net benefit is substantial and safe.

B=**Recommend.** There is a high certainty that the net benefit is moderate or there is moderate certainty that the net benefit is moderate to substantial and safe. There is at least moderate certainty that the net benefit is small.

C=**Neutral** (offer or provide this service for selected patients depending on individual circumstances, based on professional judgment and patient preferences).

D=**Discourage.** There is moderate or high certainty that the service has no net benefit or that the harms outweigh the benefits. Recommend strongly

I = **Insufficient** (if the service is offered, patients should understand the uncertainty about the balance of benefits and harms). Current evidence is insufficient to assess the balance of benefits and harms of the service. Evidence is lacking, of poor quality, or conflicting, and the balance of benefits cannot be determined.)

Level of certainty regarding quality:

HIGH level of evidence with robust positive data meta-analyses or meta-reviews involving 2 or more RCTs of excellent, robust quality. The available evidence usually includes consistent results from well-designed, well-conducted RCTs in representative child, adolescent, or young adult (aged 18–24 y) populations, assessing the effects on mental health outcomes.

MODERATE level of evidence with robust positive data involving 2 or more RCTs of excellent, robust quality. The available evidence usually includes consistent results from well-designed, well-conducted RCTs in representative child, adolescent, or young adult (aged 18–24 y) populations, assessing the effects on mental health outcomes.

LOW level of evidence with less than 2 RCTs with good or average quality. The available evidence is insufficient to assess the effects on mental health outcomes.

SECS Criteria:

* Headache is included here because of comorbidity with anxiety disorders.

A guide to clinical decisions is that interventions that are Safe, Easy, Cheap, and Sensible (SECS) require less evidence to justify individual trials than those that are Risky, Unrealistic, Difficult, or Expensive (RUDE). Because some of the treatments do not have much solid, compelling evidence but would be reasonable to try with a lower bar of evidence, this criterion is also taken into account. Being risky, unrealistic, difficult OR expensive (RUDE) disqualifies from SECS. The bolded conjunctions are essential in applying this guide.

effect for headache index was significantly higher in the biofeedback group when compared with the medication use group. The most effective version of biofeedback was the electromyography-feedback (EMG-FB) plus relaxation techniques. EMG-FB was also effective; however, to a lesser extent compared with when it was combined with relaxation techniques. Excitingly, biofeedback was more effective in the pediatric population in comparison to adults. Across all 53 studies, an average of 11 sessions were conducted which is reasonable and translatable to clinical care. The low dropout rate suggested EMG-FB was well tolerated and accepted by patients. Secondary outcomes highlighted the improvement in psychological health that occurs with headache reduction, including improvement in self-efficacy, reduced anxiety and depression, as well as a reduction in muscle tension. This meta-analysis suggests the beneficial role of EMG-FB in the management of tension headaches; however, more studies need to be conducted to evaluate the role of EMG-FB in conjunction and/or in replacement of pharmacotherapy, specifically in the pediatric population. Given the low risk and highly tolerable nature of EMG-FB, combined with the beneficial effect on reducing tension headaches, it is reasonable to use this therapy in the management of tension headaches in the pediatric population.

Migraine Headaches

A meta-analysis evaluating the role of biofeedback on children with migraines found that thermal biofeedback and progressive muscle relaxation (PMR) were the most effective overall biofeedback forms.[78,79] Other variations investigated included PMR with EMG, cognitive therapy, autogenic training, autogenic training combined with PMR, hypnosis, psychological placebo, waitlist control, and multicomponent, which combined at least 3 treatment varieties. When comparing psychological interventions, all had significantly more headache reduction than placebo or waitlist control; however, there was no significant difference between these interventions when compared with pharmacologic interventions. Of note, this meta-analysis was published in 1995; therefore, all data should be interpreted with caution. That being said, there was evidence in some studies indicating that thermal biofeedback was more effective than serotonergic drugs, the most popular migraine medications used today. Overall, biofeedback is a low-risk intervention and has been found to provide benefit to children with migraines; therefore, it may be considered as an adjunctive, or potentially alternative, therapy for the management of migraines in the pediatric population. This therapy will likely be most effective in the motivated population as biofeedback does require multiple sessions.

SUMMARY

The CIM interventions that have enough evidence to pass the Safe, Easy, Cheap, and Sensible (SECS) criterion to recommend for anxiety are mindfulness techniques and yoga. Those that have some evidence for selected patients include MMS in anxious youth with inadequate diets; kava, chamomile, galphimia, and lavender oil for generalized anxiety, saffron for separation anxiety and depressive symptoms, NAC for OCD, L-theanine for sleep satisfaction, omega-3 fatty acids to counteract proinflammatory effects of anxiety, acupuncture for overactive gag reflex during dental procedures; and biofeedback for tension or migraine headache (which can be associated with anxiety). Those needing further studies before making a recommendation include transcranial magnetic stimulation (TMS); and L-theanine for generalized anxiety. At this time, the use of melatonin for preprocedural anxiety is not recommended. Overall, there are limited studies on CIM interventions for anxiety, even more so in children.

It is recommended to make treatment recommendations on an individual basis, considering each patient and family's needs and preferences, while explaining the current state of the evidence, and considering what treatments are accessible. Looking at lifestyle entities that may perpetuate inflammation and continue to worsen anxiety and mood disorders or put individuals at risk for developing these disorders is extremely important (**Table 1**) for recommendations.

DISCLOSURE

Authors have no disclosures, no commercial or financial conflicts of interest, and no funding sources.

REFERENCES

1. Walter HJ, Bukstein OG, Abright AR, et al. Clinical practice Guideline for the assessment and treatment of children and adolescents with anxiety disorders. J Am Acad Child Adolesc Psychiatry 2020;59(10):1107–24. https://doi.org/10.1016/j.jaac.2020.05.005.
2. Lee HY, Kim I, Nam S, et al. Adverse childhood experiences and the associations with depression and anxiety in adolescents. Child Youth Serv Rev 2020;(104850):111. https://doi.org/10.1016/j.childyouth.2020.104850.
3. Elmore AL, Crouch E. The association of adverse childhood experiences with anxiety and depression for children and youth, 8 to 17 Years of age. Acad Pediatr 2020;20(5):600–8. https://doi.org/10.1016/j.acap.2020.02.012.
4. Boullier M, Blair M. Adverse childhood experiences. Paediatrics Child Health 2018;28(3):132–7. https://doi.org/10.1016/j.paed.2017.12.008.
5. Danese A, Lewis J. Psychoneuroimmunology of Early-life stress: the Hidden Wounds of childhood trauma? Neuropsychopharmacology 2017;42(1):99–114. https://doi.org/10.1038/npp.2016.198.
6. Takizawa R, Danese A, Maughan B, et al. Bullying victimization in childhood predicts inflammation and obesity at mid-life: a five-decade birth cohort study. Psychological. Medicine 2015;45(13):2705–15. https://doi.org/10.1017/S0033291715000653.
7. Wolf JM, Miller GE, Chen E. Parent psychological states predict changes in inflammatory markers in children with asthma and healthy children. Brain Behav Immun 2009;22(4):433–41. https://doi.org/10.1016/j.bbi.2007.10.016.
8. Capuron L, Miller AH. Immune system to brain signaling: neuropsychopharmacological implications. Pharmacology & therapeutics 2011;130(2):226–38. https://doi.org/10.1016/j.pharmthera.2011.01.014.
9. Eisenberger NI, Moieni M, Inagaki TK, et al. In Sickness and in health: the Co-regulation of inflammation and social behavior. Neuropsychopharmacology 2017;42(1):242–53. https://doi.org/10.1038/npp.2016.141.
10. Rosenkranz MA, Davidson RJ, Maccoon DG, et al. A comparison of mindfulness-based stress reduction and an active control in modulation of neurogenic inflammation. Brain Behav Immun 2013;27(1):174–84. https://doi.org/10.1016/j.bbi.2012.10.013.
11. Morgan N, Irwin MR, Chung M, et al. The effects of mind-body therapies on the immune system: meta-analysis. PLOS One 2014;9(7):1–14. https://doi.org/10.1371/journal.pone.0100903.
12. Lehrer P, Eddie D. Dynamic processes in regulation and some implications for biofeedback and Biobehavioral interventions. Appl Psychophysiology Biofeedback 2013;38(2):143–55.

13. Liang F, Koya D. Acupuncture: is it effective for treatment of insulin resistance? Diabetes Obes Metab 2010;12(7):555–69. https://doi.org/10.1111/j.1463-1326. 2009.01192.x.

14. Blampied M, Bell C, Gilbert C, et al. Broad spectrum micronutrient formulas for the treatment of symptoms of depression, stress, and/or anxiety: a systematic review. Expert Rev Neurotherapeutics 2020;20(4):351–71. https://doi.org/10.1080/ 14737175.2020.1740595.

15. Furman D, Campisi J, Verdin E, et al. Chronic inflammation in the etiology of disease across the lifespan. Nat Med 2019;25(12):1822–32. https://doi.org/10.1038/ s41591-019-0675-0.

16. Basu A, Devaraj S, Jialal I. Dietary factors that Promote or Retard inflammation. Arteriosclerosis, Thromb Vasc Biol 2006;26(5):995–1001. https://doi.org/10. 1161/01.ATV.0000214295.86079.d1.

17. Tenório MCdS, Graciliano NG, Moura FA, et al. N-acetylcysteine (NAC): impacts on human health. Antioxidants 2021;10(6):967. https://doi.org/10.3390/ antiox10060967.

18. Fellmeth G, Rose-Clarke K, Zhao C, et al. Health impacts of parental migration on left-behind children and adolescents: a systematic review and meta-analysis. Lancet 2018;392(10164):2567–82.

19. Gray SM, Bloch MH. Systematic review of proinflammatory cytokines in obsessive-compulsive disorder. Curr Psychiatry Rep 2012;14(3):220–8. https:// doi.org/10.1007/s11920-012-0272-0.

20. Pekny M, Pekna M. Reactive gliosis in the pathogenesis of CNS diseases. Biochim Biophys Acta (Bba) - Mol Basis Dis 2016;1862(3):483–91.

21. Meyer J. Inflammation, obsessive-compulsive disorder, and related disorders. Curr Top Behav Neurosci 2021;49:31–53. https://doi.org/10.1007/7854_ 2020_210.

22. Atwells S, Setiawan E, Wilson AA, et al. Replicating predictive serum correlates of greater translocator protein distribution volume in brain. Neuropsychopharmacology 2020;45(6):925–31. https://doi.org/10.1038/s41386-019-0561-y.

23. Chakraborty S, Singh OP, Dasgupta A, et al. Correlation between lipid peroxidation-induced TBARS level and disease severity in obsessive-compulsive disorder. Prog Neuropsychopharmacol Biol Psychiatry 2009;33(2): 363–6. https://doi.org/10.1016/j.pnpbp.2009.01.001.

24. Fischer S, Cleare AJ. Cortisol as a predictor of psychological therapy response in anxiety disorders-Systematic review and meta-analysis. J Anxiety Disord 2017; 47:60–8. https://doi.org/10.1016/j.janxdis.2017.02.007.

25. Nieto SJ, Patriquin MA, Nielsen DA, et al. Don't worry; be informed about the epigenetics of anxiety. Pharmacol Biochem Behav 2016;146-147:60–72. https://doi. org/10.1016/j.pbb.2016.05.006.

26. Cavalli G, Heard E. Advances in epigenetics link genetics to the environment and disease. Nature 2019;571(7766):489–99.

27. Stewart S, Yu D, Scharf J. Genome-wide association study of obsessive-compulsive disorder. Mol Psychiatry 2013;18(7):788–98. https://doi.org/10. 1038/mp.2012.85.

28. Umans BD, Battle A, Gilad Y. Where are the disease-associated eQTLs? Trends Genet 2021;37(2):109–24. https://doi.org/10.1016/j.tig.2020.08.009.

29. Zoogman S, Goldberg SB, Hoyt WT, et al. Mindfulness interventions with youth: a meta-analysis. Mindfulness 2015;6(2):290–302.

30. James-Palmer A, Anderson EZ, Zucker L, et al. Yoga as an intervention for the reduction of symptoms of anxiety and depression in children and adolescents:

a systematic review. Front Pediatr 2020;8:78. https://doi.org/10.3389/fped.2020.00078.

31. U.S. Department of health and human Services and U.S. Department of Agriculture. 2015 – 2020 dietary Guidelines for Americans. 8th edition. 2015. Available at: https://health.gov/our-work/food-nutrition/previous-dietary-guidelines/2015.

32. Lopresti AL. The effects of psychological and environmental stress on micronutrient concentrations in the body: a review of the evidence. Adv Nutr 2020; 11(1):103–12.

33. Zhang L, Kleiman-Weiner M, Luo R, et al. Multiple micronutrient supplementation reduces anemia and anxiety in rural China's elementary school children. J Nutr 2013;143(5):640–7. https://doi.org/10.3945/jn.112.171959.

34. Marseglia L, Manti S, D'Angelo G, et al. Potential use of melatonin in procedural anxiety and pain in children undergoing blood withdrawal. J Biol Regul Homeost Agents 2015;29(2):509–14.

35. Isik B, Baygin O, Bodur H. Premedication with melatonin vs midazolam in anxious children. Paediatr Anaesth 2008;18(7):635–41. https://doi.org/10.1111/j.1460-9592.2008.02608.x.

36. Goel H, Mathur S, Sandhu M, et al. Effect of low-level LASER therapy on P6 Acupoint to control gag reflex in children: a clinical trial. J Acupunct Meridian Stud 2017;10(5):317–23. https://doi.org/10.1016/j.jams.2017.07.002.

37. Sansone RA, Sansone LA. Getting a Knack for NAC: N-Acetyl-Cysteine. Innov Clin Neurosci 2011;8(1):10–4. PMID: 21311702; PMCID: PMC3036554.

38. Dean O, Giorlando F, Berk M. N-acetylcysteine in psychiatry: current therapeutic evidence and potential mechanisms of action. J Psychiatry Neurosci 2011;36(2):78–86.

39. Samuni Y, Goldstein S, Dean OM, et al. The chemistry and biological activities of N-acetylcysteine. Biochim Biophys Acta 2013;1830(8):4117–29. https://doi.org/10.1016/j.bbagen.2013.04.016.

40. Rosenberg DR, MacMillan SN, Moore GJ. Brain anatomy and chemistry may predict treatment response in paediatric obsessive–compulsive disorder. Int J Neuropsychopharmacol 2001;4(2):179–90. https://doi.org/10.1017/S1461145701002401.

41. Rosenberg DR, Mirza Y, Russell A, et al. Reduced anterior cingulate glutamatergic concentrations in childhood OCD and major depression versus healthy controls. J Am Acad Child Adolesc Psychiatry 2004;43(9):1146–53. https://doi.org/10.1097/01.chi.0000132812.44664.2d.

42. Afshar H, Roohafza H, Mohammad-Beigi H, et al. N-acetylcysteine add-on treatment in refractory obsessive-compulsive disorder: a randomized, double-blind, placebo-controlled trial. J Clin Psychopharmacol 2012;32(6):780–97. https://doi.org/10.1097/JCP.0b013e318272677d.

43. Ghanizadeh A, Mohammadi MR, Bahraini S, et al. Efficacy of N-acetylcysteine augmentation on obsessive compulsive disorder: a Multicenter randomized double blind placebo controlled clinical trial. Iran J Psychiatry 2017;12(2):134–41. PMID: 28659986.

44. Syu KY, Lin CL, Huang HC, et al. Determination of theanine, GABA, and other amino acids in green, oolong, black, and Pu-erh teas with dabsylation and high-performance liquid chromatography. J Agric Food Chem 2008;56(17):7637–43. https://doi.org/10.1021/jf801795m.

45. Kimura R, Murata T. Influence of alkylamides of glutamic acid and related compounds on the central nervous system. I. Central depressant effect of theanine. Chem Pharm Bull (Tokyo) 1971;19(6):1257–61. https://doi.org/10.1248/cpb.19.1257.

46. Kakuda T, Hinoi E, Abe A, et al. Theanine, an ingredient of green tea, inhibits [3H] glutamine transport in neurons and astroglia in rat brain. J Neurosci Res 2008; 86(8):1846–56. https://doi.org/10.1002/jnr.21637.

47. Nathan PJ, Lu K, Gray M, et al. The neuropharmacology of L-theanine(N-ethyl-L-glutamine): a possible neuroprotective and cognitive enhancing agent. J Herb Pharmacother 2006;6(2):21–30. PMID: 17182482.

48. White DJ, de Klerk S, Woods W, et al. Anti-stress, Behavioural and Magnetoencephalography effects of an L-theanine-based nutrient Drink: a randomised, double-blind, placebo-controlled, Crossover trial. Nutrients 2016;8(1):53. https://doi.org/10.3390/nu8010053.

49. Schutter DJ, van Honk J. Salivary cortisol levels and the coupling of midfrontal delta-beta oscillations. Int J Psychophysiol 2005;55(1):127–9. https://doi.org/10.1016/j.ijpsycho.2004.07.003.

50. Kamei T, Toriumi Y, Kimura H, et al. Decrease in serum cortisol during yoga exercise is correlated with alpha wave activation. Percept Mot Skills 2000;90(3 Pt 1): 1027–32. https://doi.org/10.2466/pms.2000.90.3.1027.

51. Churchland PA. Touching A Nerve. New York: W.W. Norton & Company; 2013.

52. Jung M, Lee M. The effect of a mindfulness-based Education program on brain waves and the autonomic nervous system in University students. Healthcare (Basel) 2021;9(11):1606. https://doi.org/10.3390/healthcare9111606.

53. Stapleton P, Dispenza J, McGill S, et al. Large effects of brief meditation intervention on EEG spectra in meditation novices. IBRO Rep 2020;27(9):290–301. https://doi.org/10.1016/j.ibror.2020.10.006.

54. Kamei T, Toriumi Y, Kimura H, et al. Decrease in serum cortisol during yoga exercise is correlated with alpha wave activation. Percept Mot Skills 2000;90: 1027–32. https://doi.org/10.2466/pms.2000.90.3.1027.

55. Williams J, Kellett J, Roach PD, et al. L-theanine as a functional food additive: its role in disease Prevention and health promotion. Beverages 2016;2(2):13.

56. Sarris J, Byrne GJ, Cribb L, et al. L-theanine in the adjunctive treatment of generalized anxiety disorder: a double-blind, randomized, placebo-controlled trial. J Psychiatr Res 2019;110:31–7. https://doi.org/10.1016/j.jpsychires.2018.12.014.

57. Sarris J, Con Stough, Bousman CA, et al. Kava in the treatment of generalized anxiety disorder. J Clin Psychopharmacol 2013;33(5):643–8. https://doi.org/10.1097/JCP.0b013e318291be67.

58. Thomsen M, Schmidt M. Health policy versus kava (Piper methysticum): anxiolytic efficacy may be instrumental in restoring the reputation of a major South Pacific crop. J Ethnopharmacol 2021;268:113582. https://doi.org/10.1016/j.jep.2020.113582.

59. Ulbricht C, Basch E, Boon H, et al. Safety review of kava (Piper methysticum) by the natural standard research Collaboration. Expert Opin Drug Saf 2005;4(4): 779–94. https://doi.org/10.1517/14740338.4.4.779.

60. Mamallapalli J, Raju KSR, Corral P, et al. Characterization of different forms of kava (Piper methysticum) products by UPLC-MS/MS [published online ahead of print, 2021 Nov 28]. Planta Med 2021. https://doi.org/10.1055/a-1708-1994.

61. Savage K, Firth J, Stough C, et al. GABA-modulating phytomedicines for anxiety: a systematic review of preclinical and clinical evidence. Phytother Res 2018; 32(1):3–18. https://doi.org/10.1002/ptr.5940.

62. Miraj S, Alesaeidi S. A systematic review study of therapeutic effects of Matricaria recuitta chamomile (chamomile). Electron Physician 2016;8(9):3024–31. https://doi.org/10.19082/3024.

63. Amsterdam JD, Li Y, Soeller I, et al. A randomized, double-blind, placebo-controlled trial of oral Matricaria recutita (chamomile) extract therapy for generalized anxiety disorder. J Clin Psychopharmacol 2009;29(4):378–82. https://doi.org/10.1097/JCP.0b013e3181ac935c.

64. Mao JJ, Xie SX, Keefe JR, et al. Long-term chamomile (Matricaria chamomilla L.) treatment for generalized anxiety disorder: a randomized clinical trial. Phytomedicine 2016;23(14):1735–42. https://doi.org/10.1016/j.phymed.2016.10.012.

65. Woelk H, Schläfke S. A multi-center, double-blind, randomised study of the Lavender oil preparation Silexan in comparison to Lorazepam for generalized anxiety disorder. Phytomedicine 2010;17(2):94–9. https://doi.org/10.1016/j.phymed.2009.10.006.

66. Henley DV, Lipson N, Korach KS, et al. Prepubertal gynecomastia linked to lavender and tea tree oils. N Engl J Med 2007;356(5):479–85. https://doi.org/10.1056/NEJMoa064725.

67. Ramsey JT, Li Y, Arao Y, et al. Lavender products associated with Premature Thelarche and prepubertal gynecomastia: Case Reports and endocrine-Disrupting Chemical activities. J Clin Endocrinol Metab 2019;104(11):5393–405. https://doi.org/10.1210/jc.2018-01880.

68. Lopresti AL, Drummond PD. Saffron (Crocus sativus) for depression: a systematic review of clinical studies and examination of underlying antidepressant mechanisms of action. Hum Psychopharmacol 2014;29(6):517–27. https://doi.org/10.1002/hup.2434.

69. El Midaoui A, Ghzaiel I, Vervandier-Fasseur D, et al. Saffron (Crocus sativus L.): a source of nutrients for health and for the treatment of neuropsychiatric and age-related diseases. Nutrients 2022;14(3):597. https://doi.org/10.3390/nu14030597.

70. Lopresti AL, Drummond PD, Inarejos-García AM, et al. Affron®, a standardized extract from saffron (Crocus sativus L.) for the treatment of youth anxiety and depressive symptoms: a randomized, double-blind, placebo-controlled study. J Affect Disord 2018;232:349–57. https://doi.org/10.1016/j.jad.2018.02.070.

71. Tortoriello J, Ortega A, Herrera-Ruíz M, et al. Galphimine-B modifes electrical activity of ventral tegmental area neurons in rats. Planta Med 1998;64(4):309–13.

72. Romero-Cerecero O, Islas-Garduño AL, Zamilpa A, et al. Therapeutic effectiveness of Galphimia glauca in young People with social anxiety disorder: a Pilot study. Evid Based Complement Alternat Med 2018;2018:1716939.

73. Zaboski BA, Storch EA. Comorbid autism spectrum disorder and anxiety disorders: a brief review. Future Neurol 2018;13(1):31–7. https://doi.org/10.2217/fnl-2017-0030.

74. Kiecolt-Glaser JK, Gouin JP, Weng NP, et al. Childhood adversity heightens the impact of later-life caregiving stress on telomere length and inflammation. Psychosomatic Med 2011;73(1):16–22.

75. Horvath A, Łukasik J, Szajewska H. ω-3 fatty acid supplementation does not affect autism spectrum disorder in children: a systematic review and meta-analysis. J Nutr 2017;147(3):367–76. https://doi.org/10.3945/jn.116.242354.

76. Chang JP, Su KP. Nutritional Neuroscience as Mainstream of psychiatry: the evidence- based treatment Guidelines for using omega-3 fatty acids as a new treatment for psychiatric disorders in children and adolescents. Clin Psychopharmacol Neurosci 2020;18(4):469–83. https://doi.org/10.9758/cpn.2020.18.4.469.

77. Nestoriuc Y, Rief W, Martin A. Meta-analysis of biofeedback for tension-type headache: efficacy, specificity, and treatment moderators. J Consult Clin Psychol 2008;76(3):379–96. https://doi.org/10.1037/0022-006X.76.3.379.

78. Hermann C, Kim M, Blanchard EB. Behavioral and prophylactic pharmacological intervention studies of pediatric migraine: an exploratory meta-analysis. Pain 1995;60(3):239–55. https://doi.org/10.1016/0304-3959(94)00210-6.
79. Simkin D, Arnold LE. The roles of inflammation, oxidative stress, and the gut-brain Axis in treatment-refractory depression in youth. OBM Integr Complement Med 2020;5(4):040. ISSN 2573-4393). http://www.lidsen.com/journals/icm/icm-05-04-040.

Substance Use Disorders and Role of Complementary and Integrative Medicine/Functional Medicine

Shikha Verma, MD, FAPA[a,b,*]

KEYWORDS

- Substance use disorders • Addiction • Drug use • Adolescents
- Complementary medicine • Integrative medicine

KEY POINTS

- Drug use-related concerns continue to increase among adolescents.
- Traditional treatment options are still limited in this population.
- Complementary and integrative medicine is expanding but few studies have been done. Many of these options are safe, easy, and readily available.

INTRODUCTION

Substance use disorders (SUDs) are a public health crisis in the country, particularly opioid use. Alcohol, marijuana, and nicotine are adolescents' most commonly used substances. Almost two-thirds of students have tried alcohol by 12th grade, and half of 9th to 12th graders have tried marijuana.[1] In addition, the Center for Disease Control and Prevention (CDC) reported a 28% increase in drug overdose-related deaths in youths aged between 15 to 24 years in 2015 to 2016.[2,3]

In October 2020, CDC reported that 15% of high school students used illicit or injection drugs, and 14% of the students misused prescription opioids (CDC[4,5]). Such substance use (SU) can be directly related to high-risk behaviors, from sharing needles or risky sexual behaviors. Youth are at risk for contracting blood-transmissible diseases such as human immunodeficiency virus (HIV), hepatitis B, hepatitis C, increased violence, triggering or exacerbating mental illness, and drug-related overdose (CDC[4,5]).

There are limited evidence-based treatment options among youth, and most evidence comes from research on adults. Overall, treatment of SUDs has shifted in all

[a] Evolve-PC Residential Treatment Centers, CA; [b] Department of Psychiatry and Behavioral Health, Rosalind Franklin University of Medicine and Science, IL
* Evolve Treatment Centers, El Segundo, CA.
E-mail address: sverma@evolvetreatment.com

Child Adolesc Psychiatric Clin N Am 32 (2023) 217–241
https://doi.org/10.1016/j.chc.2022.08.007
1056-4993/23/© 2022 Elsevier Inc. All rights reserved.

childpsych.theclinics.com

age groups. Because SUDs are a chronic condition, besides managing the withdrawal symptoms after acute abstinence, reducing cravings and relapse prevention (RP) are gaining attention among the researchers.

Very few medications are approved in adolescents for acute withdrawal or maintenance phase of SU. Perhaps that is why there is increasing interest in complementary and integrative medicine (CIM) treatment approaches for adolescent SUDs. Moreover, the evidence for these CIM approaches is growing in this population. Still, most of the evidence comes from studies on adults.

Diagnostic Dilemmas in Adolescents

A large subset of adolescents engages in the experimental use of substances. Many switch or replace one substance with another based on availability and access to it rather than using their substance of choice. These adolescents might show a pattern of short-lasting multiple SU or even taking a large quantity (binge-use) of a substance but only for a handful of times; however, the use of a particular substance might not be sufficient to give a definitive diagnosis for an SUD. These at-risk SU behaviors can continue for a while before being recognized, translating to severe SU or resulting in accidental overdose and death.

Neurophysiology of Substance Use Disorders

Repeated use of illicit substances affect the mesolimbic-dopamine system constituting the nucleus accumbens and ventral tegmental area, also called the brain's reward pathway. This pleasure-reinforcing pathway is reinforced through increased glutamate and dopamine levels.[6] Hence, medications that downregulate glutamate and dopamine levels are suggested to decrease cravings, promote abstinence, and reduce risks for relapse.

There are 2 critical factors to remember in terms of SUD in adolescents. First is the neurobiology of the adolescent brain that puts them at increased risk of using. Second is the epigenetic events that increase the risk of using illicit substances.

The nucleus accumbens matures when hormones come on board during adolescence. However, the prefrontal cortex (PFC), which provides top–down inhibition, does not mature until about 24 years of age. Therefore, the heightened responsiveness to rewards and immaturity in behavioral control areas may bias adolescents to seek immediate rather than long-term gains, perhaps explaining their increase in risky decision-making and impulsive behaviors. Imaging studies indicate an increased activation of the nucleus accumbens when making risky choices,[7] which is exaggerated in adolescents. Typically, when someone has a pleasurable experience, such as eating ice cream, the amygdala recognizes this as a motivational event, which triggers the PFC to determine salience. The PFC then influences the nucleus accumbens, which mediates behavior.[8,9] When the adolescent begins to depend on addictive drugs for self-soothing, the salience of the drug will become more significant than the salience associated with the pleasure in the PFC, for instance, eating an ice cream. Unlike adults, the overactivation of the nucleus accumbens in adolescents will drive the desire to immediately seek this reward with very little ability to inhibit this desire. This occurs in the acute phase of addiction. As use continues, the hypothalamus–pituitary -axis (HPA) becomes overactivated, and this causes increased sensitivity to stress, thus increasing the desire to use substances to relieve the stress. This process also occurs during withdrawal, increasing the drive to use. This increased sensitivity to stress is more prominent in adolescents with a history of trauma. Early trauma causes epigenetic changes that also increase the sensitivity to stress in the HPA, thus putting these individuals at more risk for developing an SUD. Thus, taken together, adolescence is a period where the desire to use drugs and the risk of developing an SUD is enhanced.[10,11]

Many available treatments influence these pathways by reducing withdrawal symptoms or ameliorating substance cravings. The table at the end of this article compares traditional treatment approaches with CIM options regarding the evidence base, safety, ease of administration, cost, and sensibility.

Traditional Treatment Approaches

There is a need for furthering addiction-related treatment in general. Addiction medicine has seen advances in treatment approaches for several drugs, particularly alcohol, nicotine, and opioid use among adults. However, evidence in adolescent addiction medicine is limited, and only a few medications are approved or have indications for use.

Medications

Buprenorphine and buprenorphine/naloxone are the only United States Food and Drug Administration (FDA)-approved medication-assisted treatment of opioid use disorders in adolescents aged older than 16 years.[3] Buprenorphine is a partial agonist at opioid mu receptors, is a delta receptor agonist, and is a weak kappa receptor antagonist. Its effects on mu receptors can produce some euphoria and respiratory depression at low-to-moderate doses. The combination of buprenorphine and naloxone reduces the risks of diversion of buprenorphine because naloxone is an opioid receptor antagonist with the strongest affinity for mu receptors. Marsch[12] studied 36 adolescents from 13 to 18 years of age in a double-blind, parallel groups randomized controlled trial. Patients were assigned randomly to medication-assisted treatment with buprenorphine or centrally active alpha-2-adrenergic blocker clonidine. It was evident that only 36% of adolescents receiving clonidine stayed in treatment compared with 72% of adolescents who received buprenorphine.

Naltrexone: Naltrexone is a mu-opioid receptor antagonist. In a randomized, double-blind, placebo-controlled, crossover study by Miranda,[13] 22 adolescents (aged 15–19 years) were observed comparing Naltrexone 50 mg with placebo. Naltrexone demonstrated a reduction in drinking alcohol, heavy alcohol consumption, reduced cravings, and altered subjective responses to alcohol.

Bupropion: Leischow[14] studied the effects of bupropion 150 and 300 mg with placebo in 312 adolescents (aged 14–17 years) smoking more than 6 cigarettes daily who were willing to quit and had tried quitting at least twice in the past. The study concluded effectiveness of bupropion in adolescent smoking cessation was closely related to medication adherence.

Noncomplementary and integrative medicine psychotherapy interventions (family-based and cognitive behavioral therapy)

Goldstein[15] studied the effects of family-focused treatment in 10 adolescents with bipolar disorder and comorbid SU. These adolescents were followed for 21 sessions during 12 months. There was an improvement in global functioning and a reduction in manic symptoms, depressive symptoms, and cannabis use but the reduction in cannabis use was not significant. This was a small study with total of 10 participants aged between 13 years 0 months and 18 years 11 months.

Danielson and colleagues[16] conducted a randomized control trial (RCT) on adolescents with cooccurring SU concerns and posttraumatic stress disorder (PTSD) symptoms. They studied risk reduction by using exposures through family therapy on 124 adolescents (aged 13–18 years), who were followed for 18 months. The treatment group showed greater improvement in SU concerns and PTSD symptoms (hyper-arousal and avoidance) than treatment as usual (TAU) group.

Multidimensional family therapy and brief strategic family therapy can be efficacious treatments. In addition, family behavioral therapy, functional family therapy, and multi-systemic treatment are also promising.

Esposito-Smythers and colleagues[17] completed a randomized controlled trial on 40 adolescents (mean age 15 years, with cooccurring alcohol or other drug [AOD] use and suicidality) and their families. This group was selected from inpatient psychiatric hospitalization, and they were assigned to either integrated outpatient cognitive behavioral intervention (I-CBT) for AOD use and suicidality or enhanced treatment as usual (E-TAU) group. They were followed at up to 18 months after enrollment. I-CBT group showed to reduce heavy drinking day and cannabis use when compared with E-TAU but this reduction was not observed in fewer drinking days. Individuals in I-CBT group also had less global impairment, psychiatric hospitalization, emergency room visits, suicide attempts, and arrests.

In 2014, Godley and colleagues[18] published a randomized controlled trial completed on 337 adolescents (aged 12–18 years) who met criteria for AOD use and were admitted to residential treatment centers. Individuals were divided into 4 intervention groups: contingency management (CM), assertive continuing care (ACC), combined (CM + ACC), and usual continuing care (UCC). These individuals were followed for 12 months after discharge. CM group and ACC group independently showed greater reduction in heavy alcohol use, any alcohol use, AOD use, and higher remission rates as compared with UCC group. However, combined (CM + ACC) groups did not show significant difference in outcome when compared with UCC group.

Cognitive-behavioral therapy can help in improving adolescents coping skills, reducing SU urges, and enhancing the improved ability for interpersonal connection and problem-solving, leading to a reduction in risk-taking behaviors. Fadus[19] concluded that family therapy, cognitive behavioral therapy, and multicomponent approaches have the most supporting evidence for efficacious treatment modalities in SUDs among adolescents.

Brief Intervention, 12-Step Programs, and Motivational Interviewing

Goti and colleagues[20] studied effects of brief interventions in adolescents (aged 12–17 years) admitted to psychiatric department. This RCT included 237 participants (n = 237) and brief interventions were compared with the control group (or TAU). Patients included in brief interventions reported increased knowledge about psychoactive substances and increased awareness of risks related to SU. TAU group also had increased knowledge but the difference between brief intervention group and TAU group was statistically significant, favoring brief intervention group.

Winters[21] conducted an RCT on 284 adolescents aged from 13 to 17 years. They assigned them to adolescent only (aged 13–17 years) brief intervention group, adolescent and parent brief intervention group, and control conditions. Both adolescent-only and adolescent and parent brief intervention groups showed reductions in SU behaviors, particularly cannabis outcome measures.

In 2016, Kelly and colleagues[22] incorporated an integrated 12-step facilitation (TSF) program which included TSF along with motivational interviewing (MI) and cognitive behavioral therapy elements in 36 adolescents (mean age 17 years) in an outpatient setting. Outcomes showed excellent feasibility and acceptability of these interventions. In addition, programs were attended consistently, and results indicated greater abstinence from SU in this age group.

In another RCT, Colby[23] compared MI with brief advice in 162 adolescents aged between 14 to 18 years. There was reduction in cigarettes smoked per day at 1 month but it did not change to smoking abstinence. MI was also able to address misperceptions around adult and peer smoking. However, overall MI seemed to be more helpful as an adjunct approach to other intense interventions and not a standalone treatment.

Complementary and Integrative Medicine Approaches

N-acetylcysteine

N-acetylcysteine (NAC) is an over-the-counter antioxidant medication that can upregulate the glutamate transporter (GLT)-1. It is proposed that the upregulation of GLT-1 removes excess glutamate from the nucleus accumbens, which can aid in reversing neural dysfunction of SUDs. Roberts-Wolfe, in 2015,[24] completed a review of 108 studies on GLT-1 as a target for SUDs. Most of the studies on NAC are in adults, and these reviews suggest NAC can effectively treat several SUDs, including cocaine, alcohol, cannabis, and stimulants (cocaine and methamphetamine).

Rhodes and colleagues, 2017,[25] reviewed 7 studies in which NAC seems well-tolerated and has mild side effects of nausea, vomiting, sedation, and diarrhea. However, due to suboptimal reporting and documentation, Rhodes recommended the need for continued research.

Cannabis Use Disorders

Gray and colleagues, 2012,[26] did an 8-week double-blind RCT on 116 youths aged between 15 to 21 years with cannabis use disorder (CUD). In this placebo-controlled trial, groups received 1200 mg of NAC or a placebo twice daily, CM, and brief weekly cessation counseling for 10 minutes. NAC-receiving participants had twice the odds for negative urine cannabinoid results as compared with participants receiving placebo, concluding with positive primary cannabis cessation as an outcome. A secondary analysis of this study demonstrated that low impulsivity, NAC treatment, medication adherence, and baseline negative cannabinoid testing were associated with increased rates of abstinence in adolescents seeking treatment of CUD. However, highly impulsive (HI) individuals adherent to NAC had increased odds of having negative urine cannabinoid test results compared with HI individuals nonadherent to NAC over treatment (OR = 8.08 95% CI = 1.43–45.70, χ^2 = 5.6, P = .018, n = 18). In contrast, for low-impulsive individuals, adherence to NAC did not have the same effect on abstinence rates (χ^2 = 0.2, P = .892). Therefore, adhering to recommended NAC treatment in HI individuals may increase negative urine tests for cannabinoids.[23]

Stimulant Use Disorders

LaRowe and colleagues, 2013,[27] studied 111 participants (mean age 43.2 years) with cocaine use disorders. They compared 2 doses of NAC, 1200 and 2400 mg, with a placebo for 8 weeks. When participants were not abstinent at the beginning of the treatment, there was no noticeable reported reduction in cravings or cocaine use. However, individuals abstinent at the beginning of treatment were more likely to remain abstinent for longer periods and had lower cravings.

Similarly, Mousavi and colleagues, 2015,[28] reported the benefits of 1200 mg of NAC in reducing methamphetamine cravings compared with placebo in 32 participants (no age given) with methamphetamine use disorder during 4 weeks. However, on crossover, these benefits were not observed.

Tobacco Use Disorders

Prado and colleagues, 2015,[29] completed a 12-week double-blind study on 34 participants (aged 18–65 years) with tobacco use disorders. All participants took a deep breath, held their breath for 20 seconds, and exhaled completely through a mouthpiece. A cutoff point for exhaled carbon monoxide (CO_{EXH}) levels of 6 ppm or greater was used as a criterion for smoking cessation. The group receiving NAC 1500 mg twice daily reported fewer cigarette use and lower carbon monoxide levels than the placebo group. There was a significant correlation between the Δ CO_{EXH} and Δ daily cigarette usage ($r = 0.705$, $P < .001$, $n = 31$). In NAC-treated subjects, there was a significantly greater quit rate (as defined by $CO_{EXH} < 6$ ppm), that is, 8/17 ($P = .008$), whereas in placebo-treated patients no such effect was found, that is, 3/14 ($P = .250$). As a secondary outcome, there was a significant effect of NAC reducing the Hamilton Depression Rating Scale (HDRS) score as compared with placebo. This effect was not correlated to the CO_{EXH} levels or the number of daily cigarettes. Therefore, NAC's effects on the HDRS may be due to its direct effect on mood disorders.

Alcohol Use Disorders

Sqeuglia and colleagues, 2016,[30] studied 116 youth from 15 to 21 years of age with alcohol and cannabis use for 8 weeks. One group received NAC 1200 mg twice daily, and the other received a placebo. Youth in the NAC group showed decreased number of drinks per week and a reduction in cannabis use. The placebo group showed no changes in the amount of alcohol use. Less *marijuana use* (measured via urine *cannabinoid* levels) was associated with less alcohol use in the NAC-treated group but not in the placebo-treated group ($P = .016$).

Herbal medicines

Several Chinese, Indian, and American herbal treatment options are explored in managing SUDs, specifically opioid use disorders. Most of the studies are done on animals and few on adults. They are mentioned because they may prove promising to use in research.

Opioid alkaloids (codeine, morphine, noscapine, papaverine, and thebaine) from poppy (*Papaver somniferum*) can activate endogenous opioid systems. This endogenous opioid system activation can affect many systems in the body resulting in euphoria, pain relief, and addiction. Medications that interfere with mu opioid receptors activation can help reduce drug-seeking behaviors. Doosti and colleagues, 2013,[31] completed an extensive review of several other herbal medications and their available evidence to treat SUDs.

In a double-blind clinical trial, Hao and colleagues, 2000,[32] studied 42 heroin-dependent individuals. Each group had 21 participants. One group received buprenorphine, and the other received WeineCom. Both groups tolerated treatment but the WeineCom group showed a more significant reduction in cravings and withdrawal signs. This study did not have a placebo group.

Lu and colleagues, 1997,[33] compared a hundred heroin-dependent individuals who received Qingjunyin for 10 days with 2 groups of 50 patients, each receiving clonidine, and methadone. Methadone results were superior to Qingjunyin but clonidine and Quinjunyin showed a comparable decrease in abstinence symptoms after the first 3 days.

Composite Dong Yuan Gao (CDYG), another Chinese herbal medication, was studied by Wu and colleagues, 1995,[34] for morphine withdrawal symptoms in mice. The results were compared with sustained morphine and the control group. CDYG was noticed to have a more significant increase in weights and reduced jumping in mice after naloxone administration, and these benefits were dose-dependent.

Wang and colleagues, 2007[35] used asafetida, a typical Chinese and Indian herb, in a clinical study on heroin-dependent individuals. They compared asafetida with the groups of positive control (receiving phenoxyimidazoline hydrochloride) and negative control (receiving saline). Asafetida was shown to decrease abstinence-related withdrawal symptoms and weight loss.

Kulkarni and colleagues, 1992[36] studied mental, a combination of 8 Indian herbs. Mental also showed a reduction in tolerance to analgesic effects of morphine in mice.

Similarly, Tiwari and colleagues, 2001,[37] studied a brownish exudate from decomposing plants and animals, shilajit, a rejuvenator and antiaging compound, found in Ayurvedic medicine. Shilajit also resulted in decreasing tolerance to morphine's analgesic effects in mice. Bansal and colleagues, 2016,[38] also described the antianxiety properties of shilajit. Their study also noted shilajit to ameliorate alcohol withdrawal and reduce dependence in the mice population by altering cortico-hippocampal dopamine.

Withania somnifera (WS), known as "Rasayana," "Ashwagandha," or "Indian Ginseng" in Ayurveda, was studied in mice for alcohol dependence and withdrawal symptoms by Marathe and colleagues, 2021.[39] The WS group was compared with naltrexone and control (normal saline), and results from the WS group were comparable to naltrexone in increasing gamma aminobutyric acid (GABA) and decreasing dopamine levels in the brain. This study suggests that WS can protect animals from alcohol relapse and influence brain neurotransmitters to reduce alcohol dependence. Bansal and colleagues, 2016,[38] also observed decreased alcohol dependence and withdrawal symptoms (including withdrawal-associate anxiety) in mice when given WS by increasing GABA and serotonin levels.

Yang and colleagues, 1983,[40] studied Yukgunja-tang (YGT/NPI-025), which has 8 other drugs, in 300 people for 10 years and concluded that it could decrease withdrawal symptoms and cravings as compared with individuals who did not receive any treatment.

In the American Society of Addiction Medicine guidelines, 2013, Lee[41] discussed using *Corydalis yanhusuo*. It is one of the 5 herbal plants in NPI-025, and its chemical fractionation produces L-tetrahydropalmatine that has an affinity for D1 and D5 dopamine receptors.

Lu and colleagues, 2009,[42] reported *Radix puerariae* as having high efficacy in treating alcoholism by acting through Daidzin. Daidzein inhibits mitochondrial aldehyde dehydrogenase 2 and leads to disulfiram-like alcohol reactions.

Albaugh, 1974,[43] mentioned that Peyote is known to have some evidence in treating alcohol use disorders (AUDs) among Native Americans. The use of Peyote is one of the ancient Native-American practices. Secondary to its addictive potential, it would not be recommended as a treatment of substance dependence.

Some studies did not confirm the advantages of these herbal treatment options. For example, Caputi, 2018,[44] reported that WS and *Salvia miltiorrhiza* have no proven efficacy but were noticed to reduce morphine-related tolerance in animals by gene expression changes.

Hence, despite these recent efforts, current clinical trials for these herbal medications have limitations. Their pharmacokinetic and pharmacodynamics are not entirely elucidated. Furthermore, these herbs might not be well tolerated or can result in toxicity. Hence, trials of these herbal medications are further limited in children and adolescents.

Meditation and mindfulness

Mindfulness meditation is one of the most-studied approaches and centers on developing present-focused and nonjudgmental awareness about oneself. Mindfulness meditation facilitates awareness of one's body, sensations, and changes experienced within. Garland and colleagues, 2018,[45] discussed how mindfulness-based interventions could impact self-regulation and reward processing due to their effect on cognition, emotions, sensations, perception, and psychosocial processes. These changes can reduce substance misuse and cravings for several substances, including alcohol, nicotine, opioids, heroin, and cocaine.

Focused attention and constant monitoring are 2 components of practicing mindfulness without perseverating on thoughts related to the past or future. Besides mindfulness-based stress reduction and mindfulness-based cognitive therapy, 2 other approaches are tailored explicitly toward the treatment of SUDs. The approaches include mindfulness-based relapse prevention (MBRP) and mindfulness-oriented recovery enhancement (MORE). MBRP is a manualized treatment that integrates formal mindfulness practice (eg, meditation and mindful breathing exercises), MI, and RP cognitive therapy.[46] MORE is a manualized treatment that integrates aspects of formal mindfulness training, CBT, and positive psychology principles into a cohesive therapeutic approach.[45] Mindfulness-based approaches enhance cognitive control and are inversely proportional to cravings and subsequent use.[46–49] In addition, as one becomes more aware of their own body, these techniques promote long-term lifestyle changes during the acute phase and withdrawals and can prevent relapses. Further advancements in the field are likely to be more geared toward standardizing the delivery approaches, optimizing the treatment, studying dose and response relationships, and reproducibility of the results to confirm the effectiveness of these approaches.

Many recent studies are suggesting exploring the use of these safe, cheap, and sensible techniques.

In an RCT by Chaplin and colleagues, 2021,[50] 96 mothers of 11 to 17-year-olds were randomly assigned to a mindfulness intervention for parents (the parenting mindfully [PM] intervention) or a brief parent education [PE] control group. A preintervention, postintervention, 6-month follow-up, and 1-year follow-up were done. The PM intervention prevented increases in adolescent SU over time, relative to the PE control group. The PM intervention also prevented increases in mother-reported externalizing symptoms over time relative to the PE control group. PM had an indirect effect on adolescent-reported externalizing symptoms, suggesting mother mindfulness as a potential intervention mechanism. Notably, although mothers reported high satisfaction with PM, intervention attendance was low (31% of mothers attended zero sessions). Secondary analyses with mothers who attended more than 50% of the interventions ($n = 48$) found significant PM effects on externalizing symptoms but not SU. Overall, findings support mindfulness training for parents as a promising intervention and future studies should work to promote accessibility for stressed parents.

In a study by Russell,[51] 27 high school students were given mindfulness interventions in small groups to help improve emotional regulation. The study had a comparison group without SUD (n = 29). Postintervention influences on depression in students who were in recovery and on 2 separate measures of impulsivity ($t22 = 2.358$. $P < .05$; $t20 = 2.358$, $P < .05$; $t17 = 3.979$, $P < .01$) respectively was significant. Because impulsivity may be a factor in recovery in adolescents, mindfulness interventions may be a helpful adjunct. The study was promising but the authors recommended the dose of the technique and the effect of small groups requires more investigation.

Alizadehgoradel and colleagues, 2019,[52] completed a randomized controlled trial on 40 adolescents and young adults (aged 18–21 years) with methamphetamine use disorder. Twenty each were assigned to the experimental and control group. Mindfulness-Based Substance Use Treatment (MBSUT) was provided in 12 sessions. Individuals were assessed before, immediately after, and 1-month posttreatment. The MBSUT group was noted to improve executive functioning as compared with the control.

An RCT completed by Bowen and colleagues[53] evaluated the long-term efficacy of MBRP in reducing relapse compared with cognitive-behavioral RP and TAU, which included a 12-step programming and psychoeducation program during a 12-month follow-up period. A total of 286 eligible individuals who successfully completed initial treatment of SUDs were randomized to 8 weekly group sessions of MBRP, RP, or TAU aftercare and monitored for 12 months. Participants were aged 18 to 70 years; 71.5% were men, and 42.1% were of ethnic/racial minority. Variables were assessed at baseline and at 3-month, 6-month, and 12-month follow-up points. Measures used included self-report of relapse and urinalysis drug and alcohol screenings. Compared with TAU, participants assigned to MBRP and RP reported a significantly lower risk of relapse to SU and heavy drinking and, among those who used substances, significantly fewer days of SU and heavy drinking at the 6-month follow-up. Cognitive-behavioral RP showed an advantage over MBRP in time to first drug use. At the 12-month follow-up, MBRP participants reported significantly fewer days of SU and significantly decreased heavy drinking compared with RP and TAU.[53]

A systemic review and meta-analysis of randomized controlled trials of mindfulness treatments for substance misuse were done by Li and colleagues, 2017.[54] Forty-two pertinent studies were identified (aged 14 years and older, N = 4,123 of which 905 were adolescents and college students). Meta-analytic results revealed significant small-to-large effects of mindfulness treatments in reducing the frequency and severity of substance misuse, the intensity of craving for psychoactive substances, and the severity of stress. Virtually all studies found that mindfulness treatments were associated with superior substance misuse treatment outcomes at posttreatment and follow-up assessments compared with comparison conditions. Specifically, mindfulness treatment was superior to control conditions (eg, TAU, RP treatment, CBT, and active support group) in reducing the frequency and amount of alcohol and drug use, number of alcohol and drug-related problems, and level of craving for SU, and in increasing abstinence rates. Five RCTs compared mindfulness treatment combined with TAU to TAU alone in samples of adults and adolescents with alcohol and drug misuse problems. MBRP participation moderated the mediation effects of craving on SU outcome; compared with TAU recipients, MBRP recipients were less likely to experience craving in response to depressive symptoms at 2-month follow-up, and the attenuated reactivity to depressive symptoms and reduced craving led to significantly fewer days of SU at 4-month follow-up among MBRP recipients. One study compared a brief mindfulness treatment that consisted of an "urge surfing" exercise and mindfulness meditation to an inactive control condition in university students with binge drinking problems. Students who received mindfulness training had a significantly greater decrease in the number of binge drinking episodes during the 4-week follow-up compared with students who received no intervention. Contrary to the positive findings, 3 RCTs evaluating mindfulness treatments in alcohol-misusing adults did not observe significant effects of mindfulness treatments vis-a-vis decreasing alcohol consumption compared with CBT, electromyography (EMG) Biofeedback, and running exercises.

Transcendental meditation was used in addiction treatment as early as the 1970s. Transcendental meditation achieves a state of restful alertness by using mantras that assist in calming the mind and thoughts. It can be practiced once or twice daily for 20 to 30 minutes where an individual reaches a state of self-awareness while thoughts are quieter. Transcendental meditation allows a sense of increased satisfaction and being content with self. Inner gratification can decrease the need for seeking other external means, including recreational substances, without directly targeting behavioral changes, beliefs, or attitudes. A qualitative review by Hawkins, 2003,[55] and a quantitative review by Myers and colleagues, 1974,[56] reported promising outcomes in reducing SU by using transcendental meditation techniques. Haaga and colleagues, 2011,[57] reported providing transcendental meditation instructions led to a decrease in alcohol use in male university students but no such decrease was noticed in females students. Both groups demonstrated lowering of blood pressure. However, accounting for only self-report was one of the limitations of this study because results were not corroborated by any biochemical markers monitoring, self-monitoring, or detailed interviewing.

Vipassana meditation is a spirituality-based concept that includes mindfulness approaches. It aids in self-transformation by self-observation by focusing on the deep connection between mind and body. Vipassana is observed to be promising in reducing alcohol and SU-related symptoms in incarcerated individuals in India.[58,59] Inmates practicing vipassana meditation also demonstrated an increase in positive behaviors, lower rates to reoffend, and a decrease in other mental health symptoms.[58] In the general population, vipassana is shown to decrease impulsiveness and improve distress tolerance in the event of a stressor.[60] Vipassana allows one to cognitively understand the root cause of the physical and mental state, including cravings from substances and being able to perceive and experience the events as impermanent.

The benefits of these interventions on physical and emotional health are noticeable. Different levels of these mindfulness and meditation-based activities can also help in tailoring the needs of an individual, depending on their ability to get involved. The outcomes of many of these mindfulness and meditation-based interventions in SUD can vary on several factors, some of them being methods of delivering the instructions, amount of time spent by an individual, and symptom monitoring. Hence, further research is needed to ensure the results can be reproduced.

YOGA

Yoga is a mind–body practice that originated in India. Yoga can improve physical and emotional health and decrease perceived stress and anxiety. There are 8 components of yoga, abstinence/yama, discipline (observances)/niyama, withdrawal of senses/pratyahara, postures/asanas, breathing exercises/pranayama, concentration/dharana, meditation/dhyana, and absorption/samadhi.

Yoga has been used as adjunctive therapy for SUDs and psychiatric disorders. There have been mixed results about the benefits of yoga in youth with SUDs.

Nicotine use disorders

Kochupillai and colleagues, 2005,[61] studied 82 adult cancer participants who were introduced to Sudarshan kriya and pranayama. Ninety-five percent of individuals reported quitting tobacco and reducing cravings. Shahab and colleagues, 2013,[62] conducted an RCT on 96 participants who smoked cigarettes. Yoga breathing exercises were introduced to one group, and the other arm included a video control group. Yoga breathing exercises led to a significant reduction in nicotine cravings but these benefits were not observed at 24 hours. Sidhu and colleagues, 2016,[63] completed a quasi-experimental design that included motivational enhancement, yoga/meditation, and a control group, assessing 624 Indian students aged between 16 and 18 years for tobacco use. Motivational enhancement had a preventative effect but yoga/meditation was most likable by the group. In an RCT, Butzer and colleagues, 2017 randomly assigned 117 seventh graders to yoga or a physical education class. The yoga group had 32 sessions of yoga. Six-month and 1-year assessments demonstrated that the yoga group was less likely to engage in cigarette smoking and that women had more emotional control.[64] However, a quasi-experimental design by McDaniel[65] assessed the impact of yoga as a moderator on substance abuse treatment effectiveness and concluded that it did not result in improving the severity of treatment effectiveness.

Alcohol use disorders

The Sudarshan kriya yoga demonstrated a decrease in the Beck Depression Inventory, plasma cortisol, and adrenocorticotrophic levels in 60 adult patients with AUD in an RCT conducted by Vedamurthachar and colleagues in 2006.[66] Reddy and colleagues, 2014,[67] introduced Kripalu-based Hatha yoga to 38 adult female participants with PTSD with alcohol use. Patients in the yoga sessions scored significantly less on the AUD Identification Test and the Drug Use Disorder Identification Test (DUDIT), whereas scores increased for individuals in the control group.

Exercise

Schuzany and colleagues, 2014,[68] also conducted a meta-analysis of 29 studies with 1111 participants (mean age 42.1 years). They looked into the strength of association of exercise on brain-derived neurotrophic factor (BDNF) levels and its effect on mood and cognition. They observed BDNF levels in 3 different models of delivering exercise, a single session of exercise, a session of exercise followed by a program of regular exercise, and resting levels of BDNF after following a program of exercise. A single session of exercise led to a moderate effect size in increasing BDNF levels.

A meta-analysis completed by Wang and colleagues in 2014[69] suggested that 22 RCTs (aged 18 years or older) done between 1990 and 2013 showed a reduction in anxiety, depression decrease or subsiding of withdrawal symptoms in individuals using alcohol, cocaine, heroin, nicotine, or polysubstance. Exercise increased the abstinence rate (OR = 1.69 [95% CI: 1.44, 1.99], z = 6.33, P = 0.001), ease withdrawal symptoms (SMD = 21.24 [95% CI: 22.46, 20.02], z = 22, P= 0.05), and reduce anxiety (SMD = 20.31 [95% CI: 20.45, 20.16], z = 24.12, P = 0.001) and depression (SMD = 20.47 [95% CI: 20.80, 20.14], z = 22.76, P = 0.01). It is proposed that exercise can stimulate the production of BDNF that promotes neurogenesis, sustaining neural connections, and new neurons. Some other studies did not show robust changes.

More and colleagues[70], 2017, completed a review suggesting that exercise could be helpful in adolescents with SUDs or even at-risk or delinquent youth.

The benefits of exercise in SUD among adolescents still need to be determined fully. The challenges in existing studies remain around maintaining consistencies while delivering treatment, individuals involved in the study, and if type and intensity of exercise would produce different results or outcomes.

Acupuncture

As Wittenauer describes, acupuncture follows traditional Chinese medicine principles focusing on correcting the flow of energy or "qi." It involves inserting needles in certain meridians of the body, which are considered to be obstructed.[71] There are some studies suggesting acupuncture decreases dopamine release in nucleus accumbens and brings their levels to be normal in mesolimbic regions of morphine and alcohol-sensitized rats.[72,73] Some studies also indicate acupuncture leads to postsynaptic activation in the striatum and nucleus accumbens, which aid in alcohol and nicotine use disorder treatment.[72] These are small studies, and there is a need for continued research and further exploration.

Table 1
Summarizing treatments by an adapted version of the U.S. Preventative Services Task Force (USPSTF) principles

Treatment	Level of certainty by USPTF definitions	Strength of recommendation based on Benefit and Safety	Evidence of Base in Youth	Personal Recommendations of the Reviewer
COMPLEMENTARY AND INTEGRATIVE APPROACHES				
I. Mind–Body Activities				
a. Mindfulness-based interventions				
1. Mothers of substance abusing adolescents (aged 11–17 y) (Chaplin et al, 2021[50], N 5 48)	Low	C	1. RCT	Possible adjunct treatment 1. >50% of the interventions (n = 48) found significant parent mindfulness effects on externalizing symptoms but not substance use in adolescents. But attendance was low (31%) More studies needed. Recommend as adjunct. Passes SECS
2. High school students in recovery vs control without SUD (Russell et al, 2021[51], N = 27)	Low	C	2. RCT	2. Scores on depression (t22 = 2.358. $P < .05$; t20 = 2.358) and separate measures of impulsivity, ($P < .05$; t17 = 3.979, $P < .01$) were significant. Recommend as adjunct. Passes SECS
3. Mindfulness-based substance use treatment of methamphetamine, (ages 18–21 y), 12 sessions of mindfulness, N = 20 in study and control group (Alizadehgoradel et al, 2019[52])	Low	C	3. RCT	3. Improved executive function Recommend as adjunct in young adults. Passes SECS
4. Aftercare 12 sessions Mindfulness-Based Relapse	Low	C	4. RCT	4. MBRP and RP reported a significantly lower risk of

Prevention (RP) vs Cognitive Behavior Relapse Prevention (CBRP) vs Treatment as Usual (TAU), (Bowen et al, 2014[46] n = 286, ages 18–70 y)				relapse to substance use and heavy drinking 12 mo = MBRP and RP reported a significantly lower risk of relapse to substance use and heavy drinking Recommend as adjunct in young adults. Passes SECS
5. Study of preventing substance misuse (14 y and older and among those adolescents and college students = 905) (Li et al, 2017[54], N = 4123)	Moderate	5. Meta-analysis and systemic review (41 studies)	B	5. Five RCTs compared mindfulness treatment combined with TAU to TAU alone in samples of adults and adolescents with alcohol and drug misuse problems. MBRP participation moderated the mediation effects of craving on substance use outcome; compared with TAU recipients, MBRP recipients were less likely to experience craving in response to depressive symptoms at 2-mo follow-up, and the attenuated reactivity to depressive symptoms and reduced craving led to significantly fewer days of substance use at 4-mo follow-up among MBRP recipients Recommended as an adjunct treatment of adolescents and young adults Passes SECS

(continued on next page)

Table 1
(continued)

Treatment	Level of certainty by USPTF definitions	Strength of recommendation based on Benefit and Safety	Evidence of Base in Youth	Personal Recommendations of the Reviewer
b. Yoga				
1. Yoga group vs physical education group in preventing cigarette use, (N = 117, N = 94, seventh graders) Butzer et al, 2017[64]	1. Low	1. C minimal risk	1. RCT	1. After 32 sessions, 1 y later yoga group had less engagement with cigarettes and women had more emotional control. Recommend as adjunct. Passes SECS
2. Motivational enhancement, yoga/meditation for prevention of tobacco use (N-614, ages 16–18 y) Sidhu et al, 2016[63]	2. Low	2. C	2. RCT	2. Motivational enhancement > Yoga in prevention. Recommend as adjunct. Passes SECS
3. Rhythmic breathing exercise reducing stress, smoking, and improving immune functions. (N = 82, adult patients with cancer) Kochupillai et al, 2005[61]	3. Low	3. C	3. RCT	3. Improvement in tobacco habits in 21% participants at 6 mo along with increase in natural killer cells by 24 wk. Needs more study in adolescents Passes SECS
4. Acute effects of yogic breathing on reducing smoking cravings and withdrawal. (N = 96, adults) Shahab et al, 2013[62]	4. Low	4. C	4. RCT	4. All carving measures reduced in yogic breathing group as compared with video control group in immediate follow-up but effects were not sustained at 24-h follow-up. Needs more study in adolescents. Passes SECS
5. Sudarshan kriya yoga's effects in alcohol use disorders. (N = 60, adults) Vedamurthachar et al, 2006[66]	5. Low	5. C	5. RCT	5. Decrease in cortisol level, ACTH levels, and Beck Depression inventory in individuals with alcohol use disorders. Recommend as adjunct for comorbid depression. Needs more evidence in adolescents. Passes SECS

6. Kripalu-based hath yoga in PTSD and alcohol use. (N = 38, adult women) Reddy et al, 2014[67]	6. Low	6. C	6. RCT	6. Yoga sessions group scored significantly less on the Alcohol Use Disorder Identification Test and the Drug Use Disorder Identification Test, as compared with the control group. Yoga passes SECS. Recommended as an adjunct treatment Needs further evidence in adolescents
c. Exercise (22 RCTs, age >18 y) Wang et al, 2014[69]	1. Moderate	1. B	1. Meta-analysis	1. Decreased ease of withdrawal, increased abstinence rates, and decreased anxiety and depression in young adults and adults Recommended for young adults Passes SECS
2. (Reviewed 127 articles) More et al, 2017[70]	2. Low	2. C	2. Review	2. No RCTs review of best approaches Exercise needs further evidence in adolescents Recommend as an adjunctive treatment Passes SECS
II. Acupuncture (10 articles) Wittenauer et al, 2015[71]	Low	C (small benefit)	Review	Overall safe but results are inconclusive so far. Hence, cost, ease of use, and sensibility of this treatment needs further investigation Does not pass SECS

(continued on next page)

Table 1
(continued)

Treatment	Level of certainty by USPTF definitions	Strength of recommendation based on Benefit and Safety	Evidence of Base in Youth	Personal Recommendations of the Reviewer
III. Animal-assisted therapy				
(N = 31, age 12–17 y) Trujillo et al, 2020[73]	Low	C	Prepost comparison group design	Limited studies. Can be easy; however, safety, cost, and sensibility are questionable. Does not pass SECS
IV. Technology-based interventions/digital interventions				
(N = 714, age 12–18 y) Walton et al, 2014[74]	Low	C	RCT	Could help adjunctively to other treatments Does not pass SECS-expensive
V. Herbal Remedies				
a. Comparing WeineCom with Buprenorphine in heroin dependence (N = 42, adults) Hao et al, 2000[32]	Low	I	Double-blind clinical trial	WeineCom group showed greater reduction in cravings and withdrawal than Buprenorphine. No RCTs in adolescents. Safety yet to be determined. Does not pass SECS
b. Qingjunyin compared with clonidine and methadone in heroin-dependent individuals. (N = 200, adults.) Lu et al, 1997[33]	Low	I	Clinical trial	Methadone results were superior to Qingjunyin but clonidine and Quinjunyin showed a comparable decrease in abstinence symptoms after the first 3 d Minimal to no studies in adolescents. Safety yet to be determined Does not pass SECS

VI. N-acetylcysteine

a. Cannabis Use Disorder (N-116, ages 15–21 y) Gray et al, 2012[26]	Low	C	RCT	1. Nonsignificant effect posttreatment but a follow-up study did show a significant effect for abstinence in low impulsive and NAC adhering individuals with a negative drug test before treatment. Those with high impulsivity had a high abstinence rate if adherent to NAC. Recommend-Passes SECS
b. Stimulant Use Disorder (1. Cocaine N = 111, mean age 43.2 y) LaRowe et al, 2013[27]	b. 1. Low	b. 1. C	b. 1. RCT	b. 1. No significant decrease in cocaine use. Needs more studies. Not recommended. Passes SECS b.
(2. Methamphetamine cravings, N = 32, no age given) Mousavi et al, 2015[28]	b. 2. Low	b. 2. C	b. 2. DBPC crossover trial	b. 2. No significant change in cravings. Needs more studies. Not recommended. Passes SECS
c. Tobacco Use Disorder-NAC and group behavioral therapy (N = 34, ages 18–65 y) Prado et al, 2015[29]	Low	C	DBPCT	3. Significant decrease in daily cigarette use and number who quit. Recommend. Passes SECS
d. Alcohol Use Disorder (N = 116, age 15–21 y) Sqeuglia et al, 2016[30]	Low	D	RCT	4. Less marijuana use (measured via urine cannabinoid levels) was associated with less alcohol use in the NAC-treated group but not in the placebo-treated group ($P = .016$). Recommend Passes SECS

(continued on next page)

Table 1
(continued)

Treatment	Level of certainty by USPTF definitions	Strength of recommendation based on Benefit and Safety	Evidence of Base in Youth	Personal Recommendations of the Reviewer
VII. *TRADITIONAL TREATMENT*				
a. *Psychotherapy Interventions*				
1. Brief Intervention (N = 237, age 12–17 y) Goti et al, 2010 (N = 284, Age 13–17 y) Winters et al, 2014[20]	Low	C	RCT	Passes SECS
2. 12-steps program (N = 74, mean age 17 y) Kelly et al, 2012[22]	Low	C	RCT	Possibly efficacious but palatability problems for some adolescents Passes SECS
3. Motivational Interviewing (N = 162, age 14–18 y) Colby et al, 2012[23]	Low	C	RCT	Probably efficacious Passes SECS
a. Goldstein et al, 2014[15] b. Danielson et al, 2020[16]	4. a. Low 4. b. Low	4. a. c 4. b. c	4. a. non RCT pilot study 4. b. c RCT	Well established, efficacious Passes SECS
5. Cognitive Behavioral Therapy (N = 40, mean age =15) Esposito-Smythers et al, 2011[17]	Low	C	RCT	Well-established efficacious standalone treatment Passes SECS
6. Multicomponent interventions. (N = 337, age 12–18 y) Godley et al, 2014[18]	Low	C	RCT	Well-established, efficacious Passes SECS
b. *Non CIM Psychotropic Medication*				
1. Buprenorphine or Buprenorphine/Naloxone vs clonidine for retention rates (N = 36, age 13–18 y) Marsch et al, 2005[12]	Low	C	DBPCT	Retention rates better than clonidine. It can be safe and sensible option but might not be cheap or easy

2. Naltrexone to reduce alcohol use (N = 22, age 15–22 y) Miranda et al, 2013[13]	Low	C	RCT	Reduced alcohol use and cravings. Be cautious in individuals with Kidney problems Passes SECS. Off-label use in adolescents
3. Bupropion for cessation of cigarette smoking (N = 312, age 14–17 y) Leischow et al, 2015[14]	Low	C	RCT	Decreased smoking correlated to compliance with medication Passes SECS if insurance pays for medication. It can be safe, easy, and sensible option but might not be cheap. Off label use in adolescents

Strength of recommendations based on benefit and safety

A = Recommend strongly. There is a high certainty that the net benefit is substantial and safe. B = Recommend. There is a high certainty that the net benefit is moderate or there is moderate certainty that the net benefit is moderate to substantial and safe. C = Neutral (offer or provide this service for selected patients depending on individual circumstances, based on professional judgment and patient preferences). There is at least moderate certainty that the net benefit is small. D = Discourage. There is moderate or high certainty that the service has no net benefit or that the harms outweigh the benefits. I = Insufficient (if the service is offered, patients should understand the uncertainty about the balance of benefits and harms). Current evidence is insufficient to assess the balance of benefits and harms of the service. Evidence is lacking, of poor quality, or conflicting, and the balance of benefits cannot be determined.

Level of certainty regarding quality

HIGH level of evidence with robust positive data meta-analyses or meta-reviews involving 2 or more RCTs of excellent, robust quality. The available evidence usually includes consistent results from well-designed, well-conducted RCTs in representative child, adolescent, or young adult (aged 18–24 years) populations, assessing the effects on mental health outcomes.

MODERATE level of evidence with robust positive data involving 2 or more RCTs of excellent, robust quality. The available evidence usually includes consistent results from well-designed, well-conducted RCTs in representative child, adolescent, or young adult (aged 18–24 years) populations, assessing the effects on mental health outcomes.

LOW level of evidence with less than 2 RCTs with good or average quality. The available evidence is insufficient to assess the effects on mental health outcomes.

Safe, Easy, Cheap, and Sensible Criteria:

A guide to clinical decisions is that interventions that are safe, easy, cheap, and sensible (SECS) require less evidence to justify individual trials than those that are risky, unrealistic, difficult, or expensive (RUDE). Because some of the treatments do not have much solid, compelling evidence but would be reasonable to try with a lower bar of evidence, this criterion is also considered. Being RUDE disqualifies from SECS. The bolded conjunctions are essential in applying this guide.

Technology-Based/Digital Interventions

With growing use and reliance on technology, digital interventions to deliver SU-related treatment are gaining momentum. There is increasing evidence that digital recovery support services can have utility in preventing SU, complementing/supporting existing treatments, and possibly improving recovery-related outcomes.

Walton and colleagues, 2014,[74] completed a randomized controlled trial on 714 adolescents (aged 12–18 years). They compared the efficacy of brief intervention by therapist-based intervention, computer-based intervention, and a control group in a cannabis universal prevention program in a primary care setting. The computer-based intervention and therapist-based intervention seemed to prevent and reduce cannabis use and other risky behaviors but results decreased over time.

Doumas and colleagues, 2015,[75] conducted web-based personalized feedback among 159 adolescents (aged 13–16 years) from 2 high schools to determine their alcohol use, beliefs, attitudes, and perception of parent attitude and parent–teen communication. The study indicated that web-based feedback could be implemented safely, was inexpensive, and maintained high fidelity.

Most of these studies have been observational or qualitative, and there is a need for further establishing and confirming the efficacy of these treatment delivery methods, particularly in youths.

Animal-assisted Interventions

Animal-assisted Interventions: Trujillo and colleagues, 2020,[76] conducted a quasi-experimental design to study treatment engagement and outcomes in 31 adolescents 12 to 17 years old with SUDs and psychiatric comorbidities. Fourteen were provided with animal-assisted therapy (AAT), and 17 constituted a control with no AAT. The AAT group showed improved treatment engagement and overall well-being.

A summary of these studies can be found in **Table 1** using the United States Preventative Services Task Force ratings for the strength of the recommendation and level of certainty for each study. (See **Table 1**).

SUMMARY

Substance use disorders present challenges that are unique to adolescence. Evidence in this population is significantly behind compared with the adult groups, and treatment options, particularly pharmacologic options, are further scarce due to limited evidence. NAC is gaining evidence in reducing cravings and promoting abstinence, particularly in low impulsive youth with CUD and alcohol use disorders (AOL). In highly impulsive youth, adherence to NAC may increase abstinence to CUD and AUD. Family therapy and cognitive behavioral therapy are known efficacious approaches. Some other techniques such as mindfulness, meditation, yoga, exercise, acupuncture, digital interventions, and animal-assisted therapy options can also have relevance in adjunctively treating adolescents with SU. Adolescents develop their nucleus accumbens before the frontal lobes have the ability to inhibit it. Therefore, overactivation of the nucleus accumbens in adolescents will drive the desire to immediately seek a reward with very little ability to inhibit this desire, especially in regards to SUD. Given the impact of self-regulation and reward processing with mindfulness interventions, more studies using this technique should be incorporated into treatment of adolescents with SUD. The maximal effect required in dose and time needs to be evaluated for each substance (**Table 1**).

CLINICS CARE POINTS

- Prefrontal cortex matures later than nucleus accumbens hence there is a lag in top-down inhibition.

- There is a growing evidence for N-acetylcysteine for cannabis, stimulants, tobacco, and alcohol use disorders.

- Most of the other studies on herbal interventions are on animals and few on adults. Evidence in adolescent population is lacking.

- Mindfulness techniques have most evidence in substance use disorders in adolescents but yoga, exercise, and acupuncture like interventions are being explored as well.

DISCLOSURE

The author has nothing to disclose.

REFERENCES

1. Johnson LD, O'Malley PM, Bachman JG, et al. Monitoring the Future national survey results on drug use, 1975-2013: volume 1, Secondary school students. Ann Arbor, MI: Institute for Social Research, University of Michigan; 2014. p. 32–6.
2. Hedegaard H, Warner M, Miniño AM. Drug overdose deaths in the United States, 1999–2016. NCHS Data Brief, no 294. Hyattsville, MD: National Center for Health Statistics; 2017.
3. Verma S. Opioid use disorder in adolescents: an overview. Curr Psychiatry 2020; 19(2):12–4, 16-21.
4. Center for Disease Control and Prevention (CDC). Youth risk behavior surveillance United States, 2019. MMWR Suppl 2020;69(1):1–83.
5. Center for Disease Control and Prevention (CDC). Division of adolescent and school health, national center for HIV/AIDS, viral hepatitis, STD, and TB prevention. Youth risk behavior survey data summary & trends report, 2009–2019 pdf icon[PDF – 31 MB]. Atlanta, GA: U.S. Department of Health and Human Services, Centers for Disease Control and Prevention, Office of Infectious Diseases; 2020. NCHHSTP.
6. McFarland K, Lapish CC, Kalivas PW. Prefrontal glutamate release into the core of the nucleus accumbens mediates cocaine-induced reinstatement of drug-seeking behavior. J Neurosci 2003;23(8):3531–7.
7. Matthews SC, Simmons AN, Lane SD, et al. Selective activation of the nucleus accumbens during risk-taking decision making. Neuroreport 2004;15(13):2123–7.
8. Koob G. The neurobiology of addiction: a neuroadaptational view relevant for diagnosis. Addiction 2006;101(Suppl 1):23–30.
9. Kalivas PW, Volkow ND. The neural basis of addiction: a pathology of motivation and choice. Am J Psychiatry 2005;162:1403–13.
10. Casey BJ, Cannonier T, Conley MI, et al. ABCD imaging acquisition workgroup. The adolescent brain cognitive development (ABCD) study: imaging acquisition across 21 sites. Dev Cogn Neurosci 2018;32:43–54.
11. Simkin D. Neurobiology of addiction from a developmental perspective" chapter 102. In: Richard K Ries MD, Shannon C, Miller FASAM, et al, editors. Principles of addiction medicine. 4th Edition. MPH, FACP, FASAM; 2018. p. 1391–409.

12. Marsch LA, Bickel WK, Badger GJ, et al. Comparison of pharmacological treatments for opioid-dependent adolescents: a randomized controlled trial. Arch Gen Psychiatry 2005;62(10):1157–64.

13. Miranda R, Ray L, Blanchard A, et al. Effects of naltrexone on adolescent alcohol cue reactivity and sensitivity: an initial randomized trial. Addict Biol 2014;19(5): 941–54. Epub 2013 Mar 13. PMID: 23489253; PMCID: PMC3729253.

14. Leischow SJ, Muramoto ML, Matthews E, et al. Adolescent smoking cessation with bupropion: the role of adherence. Nicotine Tob Res 2016;18(5):1202–5. Epub 2015 Nov 13. PMID: 26567274; PMCID: PMC5896821.

15. Goldstein BI, Goldstein TR, Collinger KA, et al. Treatment development and feasibility study of family-focused treatment for adolescents with bipolar disorder and comorbid substance use disorders. J Psychiatr Pract 2014;20(3):237–48.

16. Danielson CK, Adams Z, McCart MR, et al. Safety and efficacy of exposure-based risk reduction through family therapy for Co-occurring substance use problems and posttraumatic stress disorder symptoms among adolescents: a randomized clinical trial. JAMA Psychiatry 2020;77(6):574–86.

17. Esposito-Smythers C, Spirito A, Kahler CW, et al. Treatment of co-occurring substance abuse and suicidality among adolescents: a randomized trial. J Consult Clin Psychol 2011;79(6):728–39. Epub 2011 Oct 17. PMID: 22004303; PMCID: PMC3226923.

18. Godley MD, Godley SH, Dennis ML, et al. A randomized trial of assertive continuing care and contingency management for adolescents with substance use disorders. J Consult Clin Psychol 2014;82(1):40–51. Epub 2013 Dec 2. PMID: 24294838; PMCID: PMC3938115.

19. Fadus MC, Squeglia LM, Valadez EA, et al. Adolescent substance use disorder treatment: an update on evidence-based strategies. Curr Psychiatry Rep 2019; 21:96. https://doi.org/10.1007/s11920-019-1086-0.

20. Goti J, Diaz R, Serrano L, et al. Brief intervention in substance-use among adolescent psychiatric patients: a randomized controlled trial. Eur Child Adolesc Psychiatry 2010;19(6):503–11. Epub 2009 Sep 25. PMID: 19779855.

21. Winters KC, Lee S, Botzet A, et al. One-year outcomes and mediators of a brief intervention for drug abusing adolescents. Psychol Addict Behav 2014;28(2): 464–74.

22. Kelly JF, Yeterian JD, Cristello JV, et al. Developing and testing twelve-step facilitation for adolescents with substance use disorder: manual development and preliminary outcomes. Subst Abuse 2016. https://doi.org/10.4137/SART.S39635.

23. Colby SM, Nargiso J, Tevyaw TO, et al. Enhanced motivational interviewing versus brief advice for adolescent smoking cessation: results from a randomized clinical trial. Addict Behav 2012;37(7):817–23. Epub 2012 Mar 16. PMID: 22472523; PMCID: PMC3356495.

24. Roberts-Wolfe D, Kalivas PW. Glutamate transporter GLT-1 as a therapeutic target for substance use disorders. CNS Neurol Disord Drug Targets 2015;14(6): 745–56.

25. Rhodes K, Braakhuis A. Performance and side effects of supplementation with N-acetylcysteine: a systematic review and meta-analysis. Sports Med 2017; 47(8):1619–36.

26. Gray KM, Carpenter MJ, Baker NL, et al. A double-blind randomized controlled trial of N-acetylcysteine in cannabis-dependent adolescents. Am J Psychiatry 2012;169(8):805–12. Erratum in: Am J Psychiatry. 2012 Aug 1;169(8):869. PMID: 22706327; PMCID: PMC3410961.

27. LaRowe SD, Kalivas PW, Nicholas JS, et al. A double blind placebo controlled trial of N-acetylcysteine in the treatment of cocaine dependence. Am J Addict 2013;22(5):443–52.
28. Mousavi SG, Sharbafchi MR, Salehi M, et al. The efficacy of N-acetylcysteine in the treatment of methamphetamine dependence: a double-blind controlled, crossover study. Arch Iran Med 2015;18(1):28–33.
29. Prado E, Maes M, Piccoli LG, et al. N-acetylcysteine for therapy-resistant tobacco use disorder: a pilot study. Redox Rep 2015;20(5):215–22.
30. Squeglia LM, Baker NL, McClure EA, et al. Alcohol use during a trial of N-acetylcysteine for adolescent marijuana cessation. Addict Behav 2016;63:172–7.
31. Doosti F, Dashti S, Tabatabai SM, et al. Traditional Chinese and Indian medicine in the treatment of opioid-dependence: a review. Avicenna J Phytomed 2013;3(3):205–15. PMID: 25050276; PMCID: PMC4075718.
32. Hao W, Zhao M. A comparative clinical study of the effect of WeiniCom, a Chinese herbal compound, on alleviation of withdrawal symptoms and craving for heroin in detoxification treatment. J Psychoactive Drugs 2000;32(3):277–84.
33. Lu H, Wang G, Lan S, et al. Clinial study of "qingjunyin" detoxification for the treatment of heroin addicts. Zhong Yao Cai 1997;20:319–21.
34. Wu J, Liu YQ, Chen KJ. Experimental study on the effect of abstinence with herbal preparation composite dong yuan gao. Zhongguo Zhong Xi Yi Jie He Za Zhi 1995;15:541–3.
35. Wang Z. Asafetida extract as medicine for abstinence of drugs. Google Patents 2007.
36. Kulkarni SK, Verma A. Prevention of development of tolerance and dependence to opiate in mice by BR-16A (Mentat), a herbal psychotropic preparation. Indian J Exp Biol 1992;30:885–8.
37. Tiwari P, Ramarao P, Ghosal S. Effects of shilajit on the development of tolerance to morphine in mice. Phytother Res 2001;15:177–9.
38. Bansal P, Banerjee S. Effect of withinia somnifera and shilajit on alcohol addiction in mice. Pharmacogn Mag 2016;12(Suppl 2):S121–8.
39. Marathe PA, Satam SD, Raut SB, et al. Effect of Withania somnifera (L.) Dunal aqueous root extract on reinstatement using conditioned place preference and brain GABA and dopamine levels in alcohol dependent animals. J Ethnopharmacol 2021;274:113304. PMID: 32920131.
40. Yang MMP, Yuen RCF, Kok SH. Experimental studies on the effects of certain Chinese herbs on morphine withdrawal syndrome in rats. J Amer Coll Trad Chin Med 1983;2:3–24.
41. Mee-Lee D, Shulman GD, Fishman M, et al. The ASAM criteria: treatment for addictive, substance-related and co-occurring conditions. American Society of Addiction Medicine: MD,USA; 2013.
42. Lu L, Liu Y, Zhu W, et al. Traditional medicine in the treatment of drug addiction. Am J Drug Alcohol Abuse 2009;35(1):1–11.
43. Albaugh BJ, Anderson PO. Peyote in the treatment of alcoholism among American Indians. Am J Psychiatry 1974 Nov;131(11):1247–50.
44. Caputi FF, Acquas E, Kasture S, et al. The standardized Withania somnifera Dunal root extract alters basal and morphine-induced opioid receptor gene expression changes in neuroblastoma cells. BMC Complement Altern Med 2018;18(1):9.
45. Garland EL, Howard MO. Mindfulness-based treatment of addiction: current state of the field and envisioning the next wave of research. Addict Sci Clin Pract 2018;2018:13–4.

46. Bowen Neha S, Witkiewitz K. Mindfulness-based relapse prevention for addictive behaviors. Second Edition. Mindfulness-based treatment approaches. Academic Press; 2014. p. 141–57.

47. Anicha CL, Ode S, Moeller SK, et al. Toward a cognitive view of trait mindfulness: distinct cognitive skills predict its observing and nonreactivity Facets. J Pers 2012;80(2):255–85.

48. Karyadi KA, VanderVeen JD, Cyders MA. A meta-analysis of the relationship between trait mindfulness and substance use behaviors. Drug Alcohol Depend 2014;143(Supplement C):1–10.

49. Garland EL, Roberts-Lewis A, Kelley K, et al. Cognitive and affective mechanisms linking trait mindfulness to craving among individuals in addiction recovery. Subst Use Misuse 2014;49(5):525–35.

50. Chaplin TM, Mauro KL, Curby TW, et al. Effects of A Parenting-Focused mindfulness intervention on adolescent substance use and psychopathology: a randomized controlled trial. Res Child Adolesc Psychopathol 2021;49(7):861–75. Epub 2021 Feb 23. PMID: 33620662; PMCID: PMC8159911.

51. Russell BS, Hutchison M, Fusco A. Emotion regulation outcomes and preliminary feasibility evidence from a mindfulness intervention for adolescent substance use. J Child Adolesc Substance Abuse 2019;28(1):21–31.

52. Alizadehgoradel J, Imani S, Nejati V, et al. Mindfulness-based substance abuse treatment (MBSAT) improves executive functions in adolescents with substance use disorders. Neurol Psychiatry Brain Res 2019;34:13–21. ISSN 0941-9500.

53. Bowen S, Witkiewitz K, Clifasefi SL, et al. Relative efficacy of mindfulness-based relapse prevention, standard relapse prevention, and treatment as usual for substance use disorders: a randomized clinical trial. JAMA Psychiatry 2014;71(5): 547–56. PMCID: PMC4489711.

54. Li W, Howard MO, Garland EL, et al. Mindfulness treatment for substance misuse: a systematic review and meta-analysis. J Subst Abuse Treat 2017;75:62–96. Epub 2017 Jan 31. PMID: 28153483.

55. Hawkins MA. Effectiveness of the Transcendental Meditation program in criminal rehabilitation and substance abuse recovery: a review of the research. J Offender Rehabil 2003;36:47–65.

56. Myers TI, Eisner EJ. An experimental evaluation of the effects of karate and meditation. Final report for the U.S. Army institute for the behavioral and social sciences, social processes technical area. Washington, DC, USA: American Institutes for Research; 1974.

57. Haaga DA, Grosswald S, Gaylord-King C, et al. Effects of the transcendental meditation program on substance use among university students. Cardiol Res Pract 2011;2011:537101.

58. Kishore C, Verma SK, Dhar PL. Psychological effects of vipassana on tihar jail inmates: research report. New Delhi: All India Institute of Medical Sciences; 2019.

59. Parks GA, Marlatt GA, Bowen SW, et al. The university of washinton vipassana meditation research project at the north rehabilitation facility. Am Jails Mag 2003;17:13–7.

60. Emavardhana T, Tori CD. Changes in self-concept, ego defense mechanisms, and religiosity following seven-day Vipassana meditation retreats. J Scientific Study Religion 1997;36(2):194–206.

61. Kochupillai V, Kumar P, Singh D, et al. Effect of rhythmic breathing (Sudarshan Kriya and Pranayam) on immune functions and tobacco addiction. Ann N Y Acad Sci 2005;1056:242–52.

62. Shahab L, Sarkar BK, West R. The acute effects of yogic breathing exercises on craving and withdrawal symptoms in abstaining smokers. Psychopharmacology (Berl) 2013;225:875–82.

63. Sidhu AK, Sussman S, Tewari A, et al. Project EX-India: a classroom-based to-bacco use prevention and cessation intervention program. Addict Behav 2016; 53:53–7.

64. Butzer B, LoRusso A, Shin SH, et al. Evaluation of yoga for preventing adolescent substance use risk factors in a middle school setting: a preliminary group-randomized controlled trial. J Youth Adolesc 2017;46(3):603–32. Epub 2016 May 31. PMID: 27246653; PMCID: PMC5133199.

65. McDaniel, Joseph Antonio, "Assessing the Impact of Yoga as a Moderator on Sub-stance Abuse Treatment Effectiveness" (2016). Walden Dissertations and Doctoral Studies.2993. https://scholarworks.waldenu.edu/dissertations/2993. Accessed 29 September 2022.

66. Vedamurthachar A, Janakiramaiah N, Hegde JM, et al. Antidepressant efficacy and hormonal effects of Sudarshana Kriya Yoga (SKY) in alcohol dependent in-dividuals. J Affect Disord 2006;94:249–53.

67. Reddy S, Dick AM, Gerber MR, et al. The effect of a yoga intervention on alcohol and drug abuse risk in veteran and civilian women with posttraumatic stress dis-order. J Altern Complement Med 2014;20(10):750–6. Epub 2014 Sep 11. PMID: 25211372; PMCID: PMC4195227.

68. Szuhany KL, Bugatti M, Otto MW. A meta-analytic review of the effects of exercise on brain-derived neurotrophic factor. J Psychiatr Res 2015;60:56–64. Epub 2014 Oct 12. PMID: 25455510; PMCID: PMC4314337.

69. Wang D, Wang Y, Wang Y, et al. Impact of physical exercise on substance use disorders: a meta-analysis. PLoS One 2014;9(10):e110728.

70. More A, Jackson B, Dimmock JA, et al. Exercise in the treatment of youth sub-stance use disorders: review and Recommendations. Front Psychol 2017;8:1839.

71. Wittenauer J, Ascher M, Briggie A, et al. The role of complementary and alterna-tive medicine in adolescent substance use disorders. Adolesc Psychiatry 2015; 5(2):96–104.

72. Zhao RJ, Yoon SS, Lee BH, et al. Acupuncture normalizes the release of accum-bal dopamine during the withdrawal period and after the ethanol challenge in chronic ethanol-treated rats. Neurosci Lett 2006;395(1):28–32. Epub 2005 Nov 10. PMID: 16289320.

73. Kim MR, Kim SJ, Lyu YS, et al. Effect of acupuncture on behavioral hyperactivity and dopaminerelease in the nucleus accumbens in rats sensitized to morphine. Neurosci Lett 2005;387(1):17.

74. Walton MA, Resko S, Barry KL, et al. A randomized controlled trial testing the ef-ficacy of a brief cannabis universal prevention program among adolescents in primary care. Addiction 2014;109(5):786–97.

75. Doumas DM. Web-based personalized feedback: is this an appropriate approach for reducing drinking among high school students? J Subst Abuse Treat 2015;50:76–80. Epub 2014 Sep 28. PMID: 25448614.

76. Trujillo KC, Kuo GT, Hull ML, et al. Engaging adolescents: animal assisted therapy for adolescents with psychiatric and substance use disorders. J Child Fam Stud 2020;29:307–14.

Complementary and Integrative Approaches to Sleep Disorders in Children

Swapna N. Deshpande, MD[a],*, Deborah R. Simkin, MD, DFAACAP[b]

KEYWORDS

- Child • Adolescent • Sleep disorders • Intensive lifestyle intervention • Melatonin
- Autism • L-theanine • Gabadone • Omega 3 fatty acids • L-5-HTP

KEY POINTS

- Melatonin use was found to be safe and effective in health and children with neurodevelopmental disorders.
- Melatonin, sleep hygiene, and parent education are interventions with the most impact with the least risk of harm in children.
- Adjunctive interventions that address low ferritin levels, iron deficiency (associated with restless leg syndrome and other sleep disorder movement disorders), and vitamin D3 deficiency are helpful in children and adolescents.
- The addition of L-5-hydroxytryptophan, gabadone, L-theanine, ashwagandha, omega 3 fatty acids, probiotics, meditation, exercise, and changing from a high-fat diet to a Mediterranean diet may be helpful adjunctive interventions.
- Actigraphy data should be collected in future sleep studies because subjective data may not reflect the true nature of sleep problems or the complete effect of the intervention.

INTRODUCTION

The International Classification for Sleep Disorders, third edition (ICSD-3) classifies 6 types of sleep disorders (SDs). The categories included are as follows: insomnia, sleep-related breathing disorders, central disorders of hypersomnolence, circadian rhythm sleep–wake disorders, parasomnias, and sleep-related movement disorders.[1] Sleep is a critical part of a child's physical and emotional development. It can significantly affect the child's overall functioning, and optimal sleep may help with improved regulation of mood and behaviors.[2] In typical preschool and school-aged children, the prevalence of sleep problems is around 25%.[3] SDs are frequently associated with various child and adolescent psychiatric conditions. Sleep quality can be affected by

[a] Department of Psychiatry and Behavioral Sciences, Oklahoma State University, 5310 East 31st Street, Tulsa, OK 74135, USA; [b] Department of Psychiatry, Emory University School of Medicine, 8955 Highway 98 West, Suite 204, Miramar Beach, FL 32550, USA
* Corresponding author.
E-mail address: Swapna.deshpande@okstate.edu

Child Adolesc Psychiatric Clin N Am 32 (2023) 243–272
https://doi.org/10.1016/j.chc.2022.08.008
1056-4993/23/© 2022 Elsevier Inc. All rights reserved.

mood and developmental disorders and vice-versa. They are one of the most frequent symptoms in child and adolescent psychiatry.[2]

Not only does poor sleep affects a child's quality of life but it also affects the whole family's functioning, and parents often seek help to address sleep difficulties in their child.[4]

Sleep difficulties can present in many ways, including difficulty initiating sleep, maintaining sleep, and waking up early, as well as other abnormal sleep-related behaviors or parasomnias. Sleep–wake cycles are controlled by endogenous circadian processes and exogenous environmental influences. Circadian rhythm abnormalities may play a role in SDs originating from complex biological and social factors.[2] Environmental and social influences are especially crucial in adolescence, with the increasing use of light-emitting devices at night and the rampant use of social media in this age group. Thus, finding safe and effective ways to address sleep issues in children is critical for their well-being and development. In addition, interventions targeting sleep could potentially be an essential therapeutic avenue to improve children's psychiatric disorders and psychosocial outcomes.[2] However, there are many concerns about long-term pharmacologic treatment of sleep difficulties, including dependence, tolerance, and adverse effects. One of the most frequently used pharmacologic treatments of SDs is melatonin, an endogenous hormone.[4]

Types of Sleep Disturbances in Children and Adolescents

ICSD-3 denotes behavioral insomnia of childhood as a distinct subtype of insomnia to emphasize its pathophysiology in children.[5] ICSD-3 has incorporated pediatric insomnia into a single entity, under the term "chronic insomnia disorder." Pediatric insomnia, the most common type of insomnia in children, is still described as "behavioral insomnia of childhood" divided into the classic 3 subtypes. The first is the Sleep-Onset Association Type, which includes children who refuse to sleep because they need a specific object or person to fall asleep or get back to sleep. The latter is common in younger infants where the children wake up several times a night. The second is the Limit-Setting Type, which occurs when parents lose control of the child's behavior at bedtime or awakening from sleep. This is often observed in older children, who tend to oppose their parents, especially at bedtime. The third is Combined Type, which is characterized by mixed symptoms of the 2 previous subtypes.[1,6]

Other ICSD-3 insomnia subtypes include psychophysiological, idiopathic (associated with excessive daytime sleepiness even though adequate sleep has occurred), paradoxic insomnias (associated with people who think they did not sleep even though they have), and inadequate sleep hygiene. Less common is psychophysiological insomnia characterized by heightened arousal, learned sleep prevention, and circadian rhythm abnormalities. An example of circadian rhythm abnormalities is delayed sleep–wake phase disorder (which is particularly observed in adolescents and is characterized by a tendency to go to bed late and difficulties in waking up). Another example is often seen in children with developmental disorders, which includes a tendency to go to bed late and difficulties in waking up. Learned sleep prevention and hyperarousal can be associated with electronic devices, caffeine, irregular bedtimes, and a lack of physical exercise, all of which may overlap with biological causes such as anxiety. Alcohol can also be a type of psycho-physiological insomnia that is not associated with hyperarousal.[7]

There may be biological reasons for the high incidence of hyperarousal in children with developmental disabilities, such as autism. Biological reasons include dysregulation of neurotransmitters such as gamma-aminobutyric acid (GABA), melatonin, and serotonin. In fact, melatonin is closely associated with the serotonin-N-acetylserotonin (NAS)-melatonin pathway, which is often disrupted in individuals with autism spectrum disorders (ASDs). Recent findings suggest that the low melatonin levels in patients with ASD may be the result of reduced enzyme activity used in producing melatonin. The pathway to producing melatonin involves the conversion of tryptophan to 5-hydroxytryptophan (5-HTP) by tryptophan hydroxylase. Then the enzyme aromatic amino acid decarboxylase converts 5-HTP to serotonin. Then arylalkylamine I-acetyltransferase (AANAT) converts serotonin to NAS. Finally, NAS is converted to melatonin by acetylserotonin methyltransferase (ASMT), also known as hydroxyindole-O-methyltransferase. Both AANAT and ASMT enzyme activity have been found to be reduced in children with autism, thus decreasing the production of serotonin and melatonin in the pineal gland, gut, and platelets (**Fig. 1**).[8]

Finally, medical reasons for sleep disturbances include gastrointestinal and pain-related diseases, pulmonary diseases such as asthma or chronic cough, upper airway pathologic conditions, especially snoring and obstructive sleep apnea, and inflammatory diseases that disturb sleep secondary to itching (atopic dermatitis). Other medical reasons include neurologic disease states, such as headache, restless leg syndrome (RLS), and seizures. Of course, psychiatric disorders such as anxiety, post traumatic stress disorder (PTSD), depression, attention-deficit hyperactivity disorder (ADHD), and bipolar disorder (BD) can cause sleep disruption. Obviously, clinicians should be able to differentiate these types of insomnias and sleep disturbances in order to decide on the proper intervention.[7]

Simple management measures, as suggested by Arns,[2] that target such factors include sleep hygiene and psychoeducation for patients and their caregivers, increasing exposure to morning light by simple means such as change of transport to school to walking or cycling, and reducing exposure to blue light in the evening with blue light–blocking features in devices or with blue light–blocking glasses. If these measures do not work, complementary integrative medicine (CIM) interventions such as the use of melatonin, bright light therapy, L-theanine, massage therapy, or L-5-HTP may be helpful and are discussed in this article. CIM interventions that address the microbiome and sleep will also be discussed.

However, when interventions fail, especially in very young children, there may be other reasons for these failures, which also can be addressed from a CIM/Functional Medicine perspective. Recent efforts have been made to assess the characteristics of insomnia in children, together with family sleep-related history in children who are resistant to behavioral and drug approaches. Family history can give the clinician clues as to what other entities may be contributing to problems with sleep. A structured parent interview was conducted in 338 children (mean age 21.29 months). Three categories were distinguished. The study found that 17% (n = 58) of children constituted the first class, characterized by difficulties in falling asleep, restlessness, nocturnal restlessness, and awakenings during the night; the second class, characterized by early morning awakenings, comprised 21% (n = 71) of children; 62% (n = 209) of children constituted the third class because of their high frequency of nocturnal awakenings and difficulties in falling asleep. The first class reported longer sleep latency (SL) and the presence of restless legs syndrome and anemia in the family history; depression and/or mood disorders were more frequent in class 2 and allergies and/or food intolerance were more frequent in class 3.[9] Class 2 would be familiar to child psychiatrists. However, class 3

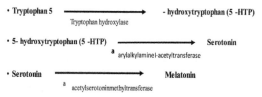

Fig. 1. Conversion of tryptophan to melatonin. [a]Indicates enzymes that may have reduced activity in autistics

is important because the National Institute for Health and Care Excellence gastroesoph-ageal reflux (GER)-guidelines suggest a greater likelihood of cow's milk allergy in the presence of regurgitation associated with chronic diarrhea or blood in the stool, other atopic manifestations (eczema) or a positive family history of allergy. In the European Society for Pediatric Gastroenterology, Hepatology, and Nutrition guidelines, detection of milk allergies may be difficult due to difficulty in obtaining a positive IgE response in infants. A milk elimination diet may be more appropriate.[10] Referral to a pediatric gastro-enterologist is appropriate for a suspected milk allergy. Class 1 may be related to an iron deficiency (ID) and RLS, which will be discussed later.

Complementary Integrative Medicine Pharmacologic Interventions

Melatonin

Melatonin is an indoleamine secreted by the pineal gland, which influences the circadian rhythm and is found in the suprachiasmatic nucleus (SCN) and cerebrospinal fluid. It is also a powerful antioxidant involved in immune function and neuroplasticity. Emerging evidence suggests that it can play an anti-inflammatory, antioxidant, and crucial role in neuroplasticity.[11] Melatonin is widely used in the child population and is readily available over the counter. Among various dietary supplements, the American Academy of Family Physicians considers melatonin as first-line pharmacologic therapy for the treatment of insomnia.[12] Melatonin can be used as a hypnotic agent to help reduce the time to fall asleep and as a chronobiotic to set the sleep–wake cycle and supplement the body's naturally occurring surge with dim light onset to help with sleep. Timing and dose of mela-tonin can be varied from 0.5 mg taken 9 to 11 hours before sleep midpoint to a much higher dose of 3 to 10 mg taken at bedtime. The exact timing, and not the dose, is crucial when it comes to chronobiotic use of melatonin, as reviewed in much greater detail by Arns. He recommends that melatonin dosing and timing be implemented appropriately, with preferably a low, nonsedating dose of melatonin 4 to 6 hours before the desired sleep time.[2] Thus, educating parents on the proper use of melatonin might be essential to ensure a successful trial of melatonin.

Of interest is the effect of melatonin early on in the development of the brain. Mela-tonin concentrations are very low during the first 3 months of life and then abruptly in-crease, probably, because the melatonin in human milk has a clear circadian curve and contributes to consolidating the sleep–wake rhythm of infants until their own circadian system matures.[13] Therefore, children who are not breastfed may have much difficulty with sleep in the first few months due to low-melatonin levels.

The interplay between melatonin and circadian rhythm is important to SDs. Light travels from the eye to the SCN in the ventral hypothalamus. Two genes are activated. The first is the Circadian locomotor output cycles kaput (CLOCK) gene and the other is the brain-and-muscle arnt-like protein 1(Bmal 1) gene. The activation of these genes pro-motes the transcription of Period 1 (Per1), Per2, Cryptochrome 1 (Cry1), and Cry2. These proteins act as negative feedback to CLOCK and Bmal 1. The inhibition of CLOCK and Bmal 1 is slowly relieved as these Cry and Per proteins degrade and a new cycle be-gins.[13] Synthesis of melatonin (N-acetyl-5-methoxytryptamine) within the pineal gland is induced at night, directly regulated by the suprachiasmatic nucleus (SCN). Two mela-tonin receptors are found in the SCN. MT1 inhibits neuronal activity and increases sleep onset and MT2 influences phase shift circadian firing rhythms in the SCN. MT_1 and MT_2 exert beneficial actions in sleep and circadian abnormality, mood disorders, learning and memory, neuroprotection, drug abuse, and cancer.[14] Melatonin not only acts by increasing the expression of Bmal 1 (thereby inhibiting its expression), both melatonin and Bmal 1 increase cellular survival after oxygen-glucose deprivation. Therefore, mela-tonin and Bmal 1 expression are neuroprotective.[15]

Long-Term Melatonin in Healthy Children

The Danish study by Von Geijlswijk sheds light on the safety of long-term use in a healthy pediatric population and its impact on pubertal development, sleep quality, and mental health development. This study demonstrated that long-term melatonin administration of a mean dose of 2.6 mg during 3 years did not negatively affect sleep quality, pubertal development, or mental health scores compared with age-matched controls.[16] Fifty-one healthy children aged between 6 and 12 years with sleep onset insomnia for more than 4 nights a week for more than 1 year were studied. Six of the 11 children who stopped melatonin did so due to improvement in sleep. There was no rebound insomnia after it was stopped.

Melatonin and Neurodevelopmental Disorders

Melatonin in Autism Spectrum Disorders

Sleep disturbances are common in children with neurodevelopmental disorders and children with ASD. ASD is a group of chronic neurodevelopmental disorders in 1% of the population. Low-melatonin levels are found in ASD and are inversely correlated with the severity of autism. Reasons for these lower levels have been studied. A highly significant decrease in ASMT activity ($P = 2 \times 10^{-12}$) and melatonin level ($P = 3 \times 10^{-11}$) has been found in individuals with ASD. These results indicate that a low-melatonin level, caused by a primary deficit in ASMT activity, is a risk factor for ASD. These results also support ASMT as a susceptibility gene for ASD and highlight the crucial role of melatonin in human cognition and behavior. SDs are pervasive in autistic children and can be as high as 67% to 89%. Circadian rhythms are very closely correlated with melatonin, and circadian melatonin supplementation could be an effective treatment of autism-related SDs.[11]

In a meta-synthesis sleep improved with melatonin treatment at doses between 0.75 mg and 10 mg in the short term in autistic children. Behavioral interventions that seemed effective were scheduled extinction for cosleeping and night waking.[17] When compared with clonidine, melatonin seemed to be more effective. Clonidine leads to reduced REM sleep in adults but there are no data yet about this in children. One randomized controlled crossover trial demonstrated that 3 months of nightly melatonin administration of up to 10 mg significantly improved SL and total sleep in children with ASD compared with placebo.[18]

In another randomized placebo-controlled trial of young children with ASD, active treatment with controlled released melatonin and cognitive behavior therapy (CBT), melatonin alone or CBT alone all demonstrated improvement in sleep quality measures compared with placebo. The study suggested melatonin may be more helpful for middle insomnia symptoms, whereas CBT may be more helpful for initial insomnia. However, the CBT with the melatonin group outperformed the other active treatment groups.[19]

Recently, in a randomized placebo-controlled trial, prolonged-release melatonin minitablet (PedPRM) was evaluated for insomnia. The study included children and adolescents with ASD, with or without ADHD comorbidity and neurogenetic disorders (NGD). Results demonstrated that PedPRM (once daily 2-mg or 5-mg dose) increased total sleep time (TST), reduced SL, and improved uninterrupted continuous sleep period throughout 13 weeks of treatment. No effects on seizures were reported, although mild adverse events, such as somnolence, headache, and fatigue, were recorded. No evidence of tolerance development was noted.[20]

In a double-blind RCT (DBRCT) by Gringas and colleagues, 2017, the efficacy of PedPRMs versus placebo for insomnia in children and adolescents with ASD, with or without ADHD comorbidity, and NGD was assessed. The study included 125 children and adolescents (aged 2–17.5 years; 96.8% ASD, 3.2% Smith-Magenis syndrome).

The active treatment group received PedPRM (2 mg escalated to 5 mg) or placebo for 13 weeks. Sleep measures included the validated caregivers' Sleep and Nap Diary and Composite Sleep Disturbance Index. Participants slept on average 57.5 minutes longer at night with PedPRM compared with 9.14 minutes with placebo (adjusted mean treatment difference PedPRM-placebo −32.43 minutes; $P = .034$). SL decreased by 39.6 minutes on average with PedPRM and 12.5 minutes with placebo (adjusted mean treatment difference −25.30 minutes; $P = .011$) without causing an earlier wake-up time. The rate of participants attaining clinically meaningful responses in TST and/or SL was significantly higher with PedPRM than with placebo (68.9% vs 39.3% respectively; $P = .001$).[21]

In another 4-week double-blind, randomized controlled crossover design study, 18 children with parent-reported sleep problems were studied. Participants were diagnosed with either Fragile X Syndrome (4 children), Autism and Fragile X syndrome (8 children), or both (4 children) or with premutation of the FMRI gene (2 children). The FMRI gene is related to fragile X syndrome. Participants in the study had to wear an actigraphy watch and maintain sleep diaries. Only 12 out of the 18 participants had data that could be analyzed. The results suggest that nightly administration of melatonin 3 mg for 2 weeks improved SL and TST and promoted earlier sleep compared with controls. Significant improvement was found in total sleep duration and initiation.[4] In fact, according to a recent review of literature, melatonin in ASD not only improves sleep but also improves behavior with fewer emotional outbursts during the day.[3]

Melatonin in Attention-Deficit/Hyperactivity Disorder

Approximately 28% of medication-free ADHD patients have difficulties initiating sleep. Authors note that children with ADHD who report difficulty falling asleep have delayed dim light melatonin onset behavior. In children with ADHD, good sleep hygiene should be the first intervention, followed by pharmacotherapy with melatonin.[22]

Melatonin in the Treatment of Persistent Post Concussion Syndromes

A study using functional-MRI revealed a significant reduction in the interconnections in the default mode network (DMN) between the medial prefrontal cortex (MPFC) and other regions during deep sleep. Although significant correlations were seen between MPFC and posterior cingulate cortex (PCC; $r = 0.36$, $P < .001$) and the MPFC and right inferior parietal cortices/angular gyri (IPC/AG) ($r = 0.38$, $P < .04$) during the wake state, both of these connections became nonsignificant during deep sleep.[23] Melatonin can attenuate the DMN. In addition, melatonin can repair connectivity caused by a concussion in the DMN. In a DBRCT (n = 62, aged 8–18 years), children with persistent post concussion syndrome (PPCS) were given 3 or 10 mg of melatonin. Increased frontal connectivity (FC) of the posterior DMN regions with visual, somatosensory, and dorsal networks were detected in the melatonin groups over time. FC increases also corresponded with reduced wake periods ($r = −0.27$, $P = .01$). Children who did not recover (n = 39) demonstrated significant FC increases within anterior DMN and limbic regions compared with those that did recover. In those individuals, the Post-Concussion Symptom Inventory scores returned to preinjury level (n = 23) over time ($P = .026$). Increases in GM volume within the PCC were found to correlate with reduced wakefulness after sleep onset ($r = −0.32$, $P = .001$) and sleep symptom improvement ($r = 0.29$, $P = .02$).[24]

A secondary follow-up analysis included 64 individuals who were followed-up for 4 to 6 weeks after injury. Actigraphy analysis demonstrated sleep-related problems decreased across all groups over time with a significant effect of melatonin 3 mg (3.7; 95% confidence interval [CI]: 2.1, 5.4) compared with placebo (7.4; 95% CI: 4.2, 10.6) and melatonin 10 mg (6.4; 95% CI: 3.6, 9.2). Sleep duration increased in the melatonin 3 mg (43 min; 95% CI: 6, 93) and melatonin 10 mg groups (55 min; 95% CI: 5, 104) compared with placebo. Sleep efficiency (SE) improved in the melatonin 10 mg group (P = .029). No serious adverse events were reported. Depressive symptoms significantly decreased with melatonin 3 mg (−4.7; 95% CI: −9.2, −.2) but not with melatonin 10 mg (−1.4, 95% CI: −5.9, 3.2) treatment compared with placebo.[25] In these two studies, the repair of connectivity that led to improved sleep may be related to melatonin's ability to act as an anti-inflammatory and/or increase cellular survival after oxygen-glucose deprivation.[15]

Other Complementary Integrative Medicine Supplements

ʟ-5-hydroxytryptophan for night terrors

An open pharmacologic trial of ʟ-5-HTP compared a group of children with sleep terrors to a group of children with the same disorder but without ʟ-5-HTP. The trial included 45 children (34 boys and 11 girls; age range 3.2–10.6 years). All subjects underwent a complete medical and sleep history, a neurologic examination, an electroencephalogram (EEG) recording while awake and sleeping. ʟ-5-HTP was administered (2 mg/kg/d) at bedtime to 31 randomly selected patients for a single period of 20 consecutive days. A structured sleep diary was recorded for 2 months. After 1 month, all subjects were examined again and the EEG was repeated. Then after 6 months, a structured interview was done in order to evaluate the clinical outcome. After 1 month of treatment, 29/31 (93.5%) of patients showed a positive response. In the comparison group without drug therapy, the episodes disappeared only in 4 children (28.6%), whereas 10 children (71.4%) showed the persistence of episodes with the same frequency as before. After 6 months, 26/31 (83.9%) of children treated with ʟ-5-HTP were sleep terror-free, whereas in 5 children (16.1%) sleep terror episodes persisted. Of the children in the comparison group, 10 (71.4%) continued to show sleep terrors at 6-month follow-up.[26] Further study is warranted on the use of 5-HTP for night terrors in children.

Gabadone

In an randomized double blind placebo control trial (RDBPCT), 18 patients (aged 19 years or older) with SDs were randomized to either placebo or an active treatment group, which included an amino acid preparation called Gabadone. SL and duration of sleep were measured by daily questionnaires. Sleep quality was measured using a visual analog scale. Autonomic nervous system function was measured by heart rate variability analysis using 24-hour electrocardiographic recordings. In the active group, the baseline time to fall asleep was 32.3 minutes, which was reduced to 19.1 after Gabadone administration (P = .01, n = 9). In the placebo group, the baseline latency time was 34.8 minutes compared with 33.1 minutes after the placebo (P = nonsignificant, n = 9). The difference was statistically significant (P = .02). In the active group, the baseline duration of sleep was 5.0 hours (mean), whereas, after Gabadone, the duration of sleep increased to 6.83 (P = .01, n = 9). In the placebo group, the baseline sleep duration was 7.17 ± 7.6 compared with 7.11 ± 3.67 after placebo (P = nonsignificant, n = 9). The difference between the active and placebo groups was significant (P = .01). Ease of falling asleep, awakenings, and morning grogginess improved. Objective measurement of parasympathetic function as measured by 24-hour heart rate variability improved in the active group compared with placebo.[27]

Phytoceuticals or Natural Plant-Based Products

Ashwagandha

In a double blind placebo control trial (DBPCT), 60 individuals (aged 18–60 years) were given a proprietary root-only extract (300 mg) of Ashwagandha (*Withania somnifera* Dunal) twice a day for 10 weeks. Ashwagandha is considered a phytoceutical, which is a natural plant-based product. Sleep actigraphy (Respironics Philips) was used for the assessment of sleep onset latency (SOL), TST, SE, and wake after sleep onset (WASO). SOL is the period from full wakefulness to light sleep. It includes the initial stage of nonrapid eye movement sleep (N-REMS). TST is the total of REMS and N-REMS in an entire sleep period. WASO is the time a person is awake before sleep onset. SE refers to the actual time spent sleeping in comparison to the overall time spent in bed. Other assessments were total time in bed (sleep log), mental alertness on rising, sleep quality, Pittsburgh Sleep Quality Index (PSQI), and Hamilton Anxiety Rating Scale (HAM-A) scales. The SOL was improved in both test and placebo at 5 and 10 weeks. However, the SOL was significantly shorter ($P = .019$) after 10 weeks with the test [29.00 (7.14)] compared with the placebo [33.94 (7.65)]. Moreover, significant improvement in SE scores was observed with Ashwagandha, which was 75.63 (2.70) for the test at the baseline and increased to 83.48 (2.83) after 10 weeks, whereas for placebo the SE scores changed from 75.14 (3.73) at baseline to 79.68 (3.59) after 10 weeks. Similarly, significant improvement in sleep quality was observed with the test compared with placebo ($P = .002$). Significant improvement was observed in all other sleep parameters, that is, SOL, SE, PSQI, and anxiety (HAM-A scores) with Ashwagandha root extract treatment of 10 weeks.[28]

In another DBPCT using Ashwagandha, 60 participants aged between 18 and 60 years, diagnosed with insomnia based on the Diagnostic and Statistical Manual-IV were included in the study. Forty individuals were in the experimental group and 20 were in the control group. Patients were included when their body mass index was between 16.5 and 30 kg/m^2. Only those patients were considered who take more than 30 minutes to fall asleep and who reported subjective TST of 6.5 hours or less per night. Participants were instructed to take one Ashwagandha root extract capsule (300 mg) twice daily with milk or water for a period of 10 weeks. Participants were evaluated at the screening, baseline, fifth week, and tenth week with the outcome measures. The SOL was improved in both test and placebo at 5 and 10 weeks. However, the SOL was significantly shorter ($P = .019$) after 10 weeks with the experimental group [29.00 (7.14)] compared with the placebo group [33.94 (7.65)]. Moreover, a significant improvement in SE scores was observed with Ashwagandha. SE was (75.63 (2.70) at baseline and increased to 83.48 (2.83) after 10 weeks, whereas for placebo the SE scores changed from 75.14 (3.73) at baseline to 79.68 (3.59) after 10 weeks. Similarly, significant improvement in sleep quality was observed with the experimental group compared with placebo group $P = .002$). Significant improvement was observed in all other sleep parameters, that is, SOL, SE, PSQI, and anxiety (HAM-A scores) with Ashwagandha root extract treatment of 10 weeks.[29]

These 2 studies demonstrate the effectiveness of Ashwagandha not only in regard to sleep but in regard to anxiety in young adults, as well. Therefore, Ashwagandha may be a more appropriate choice for individuals with anxiety and sleep difficulties. However, the effects may not be seen until after 10 weeks of treatment and further additional research should be done on children in the future with Ashwagandha.

L-theanine in ADHD boys

Green tea is known to be a rich source of flavonoid antioxidants. However, green tea also contains a unique amino acid, L-theanine. In an RCT,[30] EEG was measured in healthy, young participants at baseline and 45, 60, 75, 90, and 105 minutes after ingestion of 50 mg L-theanine (n = 16) or placebo (n = 19). Participants were recorded with their eyes closed during EEG recording. There was a greater increase in alpha activity across time in the L-theanine condition (relative to placebo ($P < .05$). A DBPCT using L-theanine was conducted involving 98 boys, aged 8 to 12 years, previously diagnosed with ADHD. Participants were randomized based on the current use of stimulant medication to ensure an equal distribution of stimulant/nonstimulant-treated subjects into active and placebo-treated groups. Participants consumed 2 chewable tablets twice daily (at breakfast and after school), with each tablet containing 100 mg of L-theanine (total of 400 mg daily Suntheanine) for 6 weeks. The children were evaluated for 5 consecutive nights using wrist actigraphy at baseline, and again at the end of the 6-week treatment period. The Pediatric Sleep Questionnaire (PSQ) was completed by parents at baseline and at the end of the treatment period. Boys who consumed L-theanine obtained significantly higher sleep percentage and SE scores, along with a nonsignificant trend for less activity during sleep (defined as less time WASO) compared with those in the placebo group. SL and other sleep parameters were unchanged. The PSQ data did not correlate significantly to the objective data gathered from actigraphy, suggesting that parents were not particularly aware of their children's sleep quality. L-theanine at relatively high doses was well tolerated with no significant adverse events.[31]

Nutraceuticals or Natural Nutrient-Based Products

Low-ferritin levels and iron supplementation

Low-ferritin levels and iron supplementation A review of the literature investigated associations of iron deficiency (ID) with the type and severity of SDs and whether iron supplementation improves sleep-related symptoms. Ninety-three articles met the inclusion criteria. Iron supplementation was beneficial in restless leg syndrome (RLS) and Periodic limb movement of sleep (PLMS) (including 5 RCTs), SD breathing (SDB), and general SDs (GSDs) treatment studies in young adults and adults. Iron supplementation was also beneficial in RLS (including 2 RCTs), GSD (RCT), and restless SD (RSD) studies identified in the ad hoc search. In pediatric populations, 1 RLS, 1 SDB, 2 PLMs, 2 GSD, and 1ADHD-SDs study found positive associations, and 6 RLS and 2 GSD studies demonstrated a benefit with iron supplementation.

Studies in pediatric populations

For RLS, 1 pediatric association study found a positive association of RLS with ID. Six out of 6 pediatric treatment studies demonstrated the benefit of iron supplementation, including 3 case series and 3 case reports. Participants in these studies ranged from age 2 and 16 years. In the case series, one case series included 17 children and adolescents who were treated with iron supplementation and 10 had improvement of RLS, 2 had no effect and 4 were lost to treatment. In another case series, 30 children were treated for ID, and 17 had a significant effect on RLS, 10 had a moderate effect, and 3 had no effect. In the last case series, 97 children were treated for ID and 80% had improvement for RLS. Additionally, an association with ID was found in adults with childhood-onset RLS, and one treatment study showed benefit of iron supplementation in early-onset RLS in infants and toddlers.

Of importance, in the treatment study in infants, giving 30 mg of elemental iron 2 times per day, showed not only better sleep patterns and a decrease in daytime irritability but also fewer illnesses. Infants were given 30 mg elemental iron twice a day for ID. In the study, 329 (55%) children completed the program until age 1 year, and 279 (46%) until 18 months of age. Of this latter group, 246 children were followed for an additional 6 months. This last group, called the "completed" group, was analyzed in detail. In the "completed" group 132 children had received the iron supplement and 114 the placebo. There was a significant improvement in RLS and sleep in the experimental group and ID. One 8-week open-label pilot study of treatment of low ferritin in children with autism was done. Thirty-three children completed the study. Seventy-seven percent had restless sleep at baseline, which improved significantly with iron therapy.

These studies confirm an association between ID and RLS-triggered insomnia and that iron supplementation is beneficial for patients with RLS.[32]

A case study of RLS in a 2-year-old and another case series study of infants aged 0 to 40 months are worth mentioning to help clinicians be aware of looking for low ferritin or

ID as a cause for sleep difficulty that may be early signs of RLS in toddlers that might otherwise be missed. Al-Shawwa and colleagues described a 2-year-old with similar symptoms of restless sleep, bedtime resistance, and daytime sleepiness who was found to have an underlying ID without anemia that was treated successfully with iron infusion.[33] In another study of children aged between 0 and 40 months, 22 children with a ferritin level less than 50 ng/mL were treated with oral iron. Fourteen were examined by polysomnography as well, and periodic limb movement index during sleep (PLMSI) was calculated. The symptoms included children exhibiting difficulties in falling asleep, rolling and kicking the covers off the bed, and night awakenings followed by screaming, crying, kicking, and slapping the legs. Relief of symptoms was recorded by the parents and correlated with ferritin levels and PLMSI. Oral iron supplementation had a positive ferritin-concentration-dependent clinical effect.[34] Another case study involved a 5-year-old preschooler with RLS, who presented with an uncomfortable sensation in his toes before bedtime and insomnia. Blood tests showed reduced iron stores (serum ferritin, 15.9 ng/mL). The subjective symptoms and a maternal history of RLS were consistent with pediatric RLS. Iron supplement therapy resulted in improvement in the uncomfortable leg sensation and subjective daytime alertness.[35]

A pilot study confirmed the association between low ferritin and RLS and RSD, as well. Fifteen children with RLS (mean age 11.9), 15 children with a RSD (mean age 9.5) and 37 controls (mean age 10.6) were studied. Parents reported body movements involving the head, limbs, and trunk. They also reported restless sleep without nighttime awakenings. All of the children with RSD and RLS had low-ferritin levels (mean 20). Polysomnographic data revealed decreased SE similar to the RLS group but not prolonged SL. This study implied a new diagnostic category of RSD is also associated with low-ferritin levels.[36] Gold hypothesized that iron treatment might act by correcting a dopaminergic dysfunction that is reported as a major pathogenetic factor in several SDs such as RLS, periodic limb movements of sleep, and RSD but also ADHD.[37]

Therefore, these studies provide good evidence that ID and low-ferritin levels may be linked to RLD, RSD, and other disordered sleep problems in children and young adults. In addition, treatment of the ID seems to improve these sleep problems even in infants. More research is needed.

Omega 3 fatty acids

In a meta-analysis, RCTs, or clinical trials that included a control group, and longitudinal studies that investigated the impact of omega-3 long chain- polysaturated fatty acids (LC-PUFA) or diet rich in omega-3 LC-PUFA on sleep-related outcomes in humans were included. Twelve RCTs and 8 cohort studies were included. The intervention or exposure for infants and toddlers involved omega-3 LC-PUFA–intake by pregnant women) and interventions directly targeting infants themselves (ie, daily intake of docosapentaenoic acid [DHA] and arachidonic acid [AA] supplementation). Children and adults received capsules that contained various compositions of LC-PUFA supplementation (DHA, or DHA plus AA, or DHA plus eicosapentaenoic acid [EPA] or meals rich in omega-3 LC-PUFA). It reduced the percentage of infants' active sleep (weighted mean difference [WMD] = −8.40%; 95%CI, −14.50 to −2.29), sleep–wake transition (WMD = −1.15%; 95%CI, −2.09 to −0.20), and enhanced the percentage of wakefulness (WMD = 9.06%; 95%CI, 1.53–16.59) but had no effect on quiet sleep. Omega-3 reduced children's total sleep disturbance score for those with clinical-level sleep problems (WMD = −1.81; 95%CI, −3.38 to −0.23) but had no effect on healthy children's total sleep duration, SL, or SE. No effectiveness was found in adults' total sleep duration, SL, SE, sleep quality, or insomnia severity.[38] This study did not use a higher EPA to DHA ratio in the infant and child studies.

Vitamin D

In a meta-analysis of vitamin D and SDs, 9 studies were included with 9397 participants (aged 16 years and older). By comparing the lowest verse highest levels of serum vitamin D, participants with vitamin D deficiency (VDD) had a significantly increased risk of SDs (odds ratio [OR]: 1.50, 95% CI: 1.31, 1.72). Subgroup analysis showed that VDD also was associated with poor sleep quality (OR: 1.59, 95% CI: 1.23, 2.05), short sleep duration (OR: 1.74, 95% CI: 1.30, 2.32), and sleepiness (OR: 1.36, 95% CI: 1.12, 1.65). Subgroup analyses further indicated that serum 25(OH)D less than 20 ng/mL could significantly increase the risk of unhealthy sleep.[39]

A retrospective cohort study included a total of 39 patients (mean age, 6.6 years; 46% women). Twenty (51%) patients had VDD (25-hydroxy vitamin D level < 30 ng/mL). Children with VDD had less TST (470.3 minutes ± 35.6 vs 420.3 minutes ± 61.7; P = .004) and poorer SE (91.9% ± 5.6% vs 84.5% ± 9.5%; P = .015) compared with children with sufficient vitamin D. In addition, children with VDD had later weekday bedtimes (21:02 PM ± 1:01 vs 20:19 PM ± 0:55; P = .037) and later weekend bedtimes (21:42 PM ± 0:59 vs 20:47 PM ± 1:08; P = .016) than children with sufficient vitamin D, with a tendency for later wake time that did not reach statistical significance.[40]

Probiotics

Microbiome effects on sleep

A review of the literature has shown that the gut microbiome is capable of altering sleep by changes in the gut microbiome leading to dysbiosis (the change in healthy gut microbes to unhealthy gut microbes). This dysbiosis is caused by high-fat diets, a lowering of short-chain fatty acids normally produced by healthy gut microbes, lipopolysaccharides (LPS) produced by pathologic bacteria, which causes inflammation followed by vagal afferent excitation in response to these enteric LPS, regulation of serotonin production, and inflammatory cytokine regulation. All of these processes reset the clock genes, which control circadian rhythm. For decades, bacterial metabolites have been known to increase and induce sleepiness in response to sleep loss. However, recent studies have shown that probiotic supplementation can improve sleep quality, which may be due to their anti-inflammatory properties. Probiotics use in sleep may lead to prebiotic or probiotic interventions to upregulate serotonin (needed for the production of melatonin) or decrease LPS production. In contrast, sleep loss is capable of altering the gut microbiota composition through increased hunger and decreased physical activity, immunomodulation, or hypothalamic-pituatary- adrenal axis (HPA) axis activation and subsequent intestinal barrier disruption.[41]

Further research has identified a reason why changes in the microbiome may influence sleep. A UK study with 91,105 study participants was published in the LANCET Psychiatry. Multiple clock gene variants predispose to psychiatric disorders such as major depressive disorder, BD, ADHD, schizophrenia, and delirium.[42] Group 3 innate lymphoid cells (ILC3s) are immune cells that respond rapidly to damage, inflammation, and infection and are crucial mediators of circadian brain–gut signaling. ILC3s express high levels of circadian clock genes and inversion of light–dark cycles lead to major circadian oscillations of ILC3s. This effect depends on the presence of Bmal 1 and CLOCK, the clock genes in the central nervous system, and the SCN of the hypothalamus and is furthermore associated with changes in gut microbiome composition, especially alterations in Proteobacteria and Bacteroidetes abundance.[43]

Microbiome and bipolar disorder

A review of the literature[44] yielded 2 cross-sectional studies analyzing sleep and gut microbiome in 154 individuals with BD and one interventional study analyzing the effect of fecal microbiota transplantation in 17 individuals with irritable bowel syndrome (IBS) on sleep (aged 18 years and older). In patients with BD, *Faecalibacterium* was significantly associated with improved sleep quality scores, and there was a significant correlation between *Lactobacillus* counts and sleep. In one study involving BD, a negative relationship between *Faecalibacterium* and sleep quality on the PSQI at the subscale level ($\beta = -0.329$; $P = .001$; $d = -1.357$; $r = -0.5$). In the other study of BD, there was a negative correlation between *Lactobacillus* counts and sleep ($P = -0.45$, $P = .01$; $d = 0.885$; $r = 0.405$). In the interventional study of fecal microbiota transplantation in individuals with IBS, significant improvement in HAM-D total and sleep-subscale scores occurred. Baseline Shannon index (which measures lower diversity in the microbiome) in patients with HAM-D ≥ 8 showed significantly lower microbiota diversity compared with patients HAM-D < 8. ($P = .005$, FDR $= 0.007$).

Microbiome (Lactobacillus reuteri) and colic
In a meta-analysis, 6 RCTs of 423 infants with colic were included. Of these subjects, 213 were in the *L reuteri* group, and 210 were in the placebo group. *L reuteri* increased colic treatment effectiveness at 2 weeks (relative risk [RR] $= 2.84$; 95% CI: 1.24–6.50; $P = .014$) and 3 weeks (RR $= 2.33$; 95% CI: 1.38 to 3.93; $P = .002$) but not at 4 weeks (RR $= 1.41$; 95% CI: 0.52–3.82; $P = .498$). *L reuteri* decreased crying time (min/d) at 2 weeks (WMD $= -42.89$; 95% CI: -60.50 to -25.29; $P = 0$) and 3 weeks (WMD $= -45.83$; 95% CI: -59.45 to -32.21; $P = 0$). In addition, *L reuteri* did not influence infants' weight, length, or head circumference and was not associated with serious adverse events.[45]

Nutrition and Diet

High-fat diet
Higher fat intake is associated with disordered sleep, whereas the Mediterranean diet is associated with fewer sleeping problems. Additionally, skipping breakfast, irregular eating habits, low intake of vegetables and fish, and high intake of simple carbohydrates (such as sweets and noodles) have been associated with poor sleep quality in Japanese women.[46] Therefore, high-fat diets that change the microbiome can influence clock genes in the SCN and, hence influence sleep.

Nonpharmacological and Nonbehavioral Approaches for Sleep Disorders

Sleep hygiene and parent education
Sleep hygiene is a set of behavioral, environmental, or cognitive modifications to improve sleep.[47] These include changes to[1] bedtime and bedtime routines,[2] restriction of electronic media use,[3] restriction of caffeine use,[4] exposure to natural or bright light in the morning, and[5] modification of exercise timings, and[6] modification to the bedroom and sleeping environment.[11] Sleep hygiene and behavioral interventions are recommended as the first-line treatment when addressing children's sleep issues. Often these are parent-directed interventions that include several components. They are low-cost, tend to improve structure and routine in daily activity in a child's life, and can potentially help target more than sleep disturbance.

Sleep hygiene and ADHD
Parker reviewed the literature on children aged 5 to 18 years with ADHD on the effectiveness of sleep hygiene in treating sleep problems that are very common in children with ADHD, compared with no intervention or alternative intervention. The review included 16 studies with 1469 children with ADHD, with a mean age of 9.6 years across 6 countries. Fifteen studies found that sleep hygiene interventions were effective in improving sleep. Current evidence favors sleep hygiene's effectiveness. The authors grade their current evidence as B and note that the number of studies is limited, heterogeneity of the

interventions, and high risk of bias make it difficult to draw definite conclusions. The limited number of studies makes a case for the need for more high-level evidence.[4]

Massage therapy and vitamin supplementation

Mc Lay and colleagues examined the literature for evidence of nonpharmacological and nonbehavioral approaches. They found positive outcomes for massage therapy and vitamin supplementation but not for aromatherapy. Although the results are positive for massage therapy, the authors suggest that the studies reviewed had methodical issues making it difficult to rule out an alternative explanation for the positive treatment effect. For example, attention to a sleep routine and more structured bedtime, and not massage could be why sleep improved.[48]

Mindfulness/meditation

A preliminary study, 32 children with ADHD aged 7 to 11 years were randomly assigned to the mindfulness-oriented meditation group (MOM G), which underwent 8 weeks of mindfulness training or joined the active control condition group (ACC G), which entered an 8-week emotional awareness and recognition program. Participants were assessed at baseline (T0) and postprogram (T1) for objective (actigraphy) and subjective measures (the Sleep Disturbance Scale for Children) for sleep. The following actigraphy measures were studied: SL, TST, WASO, number of awakenings and duration of awakenings, motility, sleep fragmentation, and SE. The Sleep Disturbance Scale for Children (SDSC) contains 6 subscales representing the most common areas of SDs in childhood and adolescence: disorders of initiating and maintaining sleep; sleep breathing disorders; disorders of arousal (DA) such as sleepwalking, sleep terrors, nightmares; sleep–wake transition disorders as hypnic jerks, rhythmic movement disorders, hypnagogic hallucinations, nocturnal hyperkinesia, bruxism; disorders of excessive somnolence (DOES); and sleep hyperhidrosis. Behavioral measures included the Child Behavior Checklist for Ages 6 to 18 years (CBCL 6–18) and 2 global index subscales for ADHD of the Conners' Parent Rating Scales Long Version Revised (CPRS-R: L) for the Restless-Impulsive subscale (Clinical Global Impression [CGI] Restless-Impulsive) and for the Total (CGI Total) were used. Accounting for the potential effects of confounding variables in interpreting results of MOM program, children with ADHD with psychiatric comorbidity and under psychostimulant therapy were excluded from the study. The 7 SDSC scales were analyzed. The DA scale groups differed at T0 ($P = .004$) and at T1 ($P = .016$) with fewer disorders of arousal for MOM G than for ACC G. Concerning the DOES subscale, groups differed at T0 ($P = .03$), with MOM G showing higher scores than ACC G (even if in the normal range) but not at T1 ($P = .16$). About behavioral measures, only the MOM G had significantly lower T scores at T1 than at T0. At postprogram, analyses on frequency confirmed that the number of children in the MOM G having clinical scores was significantly lower than that of ACC G in 3 subscales (ie, Attention Problems subscale of the CBCL 6–18, the CGI Restless-Impulsive subscale, and the CGI Total of the CPRS-R: L). In the MOM G, also the average score of 3 out of 4 behavioral measures decreased from a clinical level at T0 to a borderline range. However, the groups did not differ [$F^{1,23} = 0.53, P = .47, \eta p^2 = 0.02$] after the programs for the considered actigraphy measure. The results, although they are preliminary, suggest that mindfulness meditation practices may promote specific positive changes in sleep indices and behavioral measures in children with ADHD.[49]

Exercise and screen time

A systematic review examined the association between screen time/movement behaviors (sedentary behavior, physical activity) and sleep outcomes in infants (aged 0–1 years); toddlers (aged 1–2 years); and preschoolers (aged 3–4 years). Thirty-one articles were included. A systemic review indicated that screen time is associated with poorer sleep outcomes in infants, toddlers, and preschoolers. A meta-analysis confirmed these unfavorable associations in infants and toddlers but not preschoolers. For movement behaviors, results were mixed, although physical activity and outdoor play, in particular, were favorably associated with most sleep outcomes in toddlers and preschoolers. Overall, the quality of evidence was very low for exercise but there was strong evidence for daily/evening screen time use in toddlers and preschoolers. Although high-quality experimental evidence is required, the findings should prompt parents, clinicians, and educators to encourage sleep-promoting behaviors (eg, less evening screen time) in the less than 5-year range.[50]

Across all types of screens, 90% of published studies show a significant adverse association with at least one of the measured sleep outcomes. Computer use (94% of studies), unspecified screen time (91% of studies), video games (86%), and mobile devices (83%) were most consistently observed to be associated with adverse sleep outcomes. The screen category that was least likely to have an adverse association with sleep outcomes was television use (76%).

A systemic review was done to examine the effects of screen time on sleep in children and adolescents aged from 5 to 17 years. Sixty-seven studies were included that investigated the association between any type of screen time and any of the following sleep outcomes: sleep timing, sleep duration, sleep quality, SOL, subjective assessment of daytime tiredness or daytime sleepiness, or other reported outcomes including subjective assessment of insomnia symptoms. Studies were divided into types of media including (eg, television, computer, mobile phone, and video gaming devices. Screen time is adversely associated with sleep outcomes (primarily shortened duration and delayed timing) in 90% of studies. Computer use (94% of studies), unspecified screen time (91% of studies), video games (86%), and mobile devices (83%) were most consistently observed to be associated with adverse sleep outcomes. The screen category that was least likely to have an adverse association with sleep outcomes was television use (76% of studies). However, limitations of the current studies: (1) causal association not confirmed, (2) measurement error (of both screen time exposure and sleep measures), and (3) limited data on the simultaneous use of multiple screens, characteristics and content of screens used.[51] Children and adolescents should limit screen time before bed.

Continuous noise

In a systematic review of all studies examining the relationship between continuous noise and sleep, the quality of evidence for continuous noise was very low. The results had wide variability, with some studies showing it helps sleep onset and quality, whereas others suggested it might disrupt sleep. Results from the review suggest that additional research is needed to elucidate the effects of continuous noise on sleep among human subjects. The evidence's low quality and contradictory nature is a stark contrast to the widespread use of white noise machines for sleep, particularly considering they may negatively affect sleep and hearing.[52]

A summary of these studies can be found in (**Table 1**) using the United States Preventative Services Task Force ratings for the strength of the recommendation and level of certainty for each study (See **Table 1**).

SUMMARY

Melatonin has been proven safe with both short[16] and prolonged release[53] from up to 3 years. In a study of prolonged melatonin[53] at 2 mg, 5 mg, or 10 mg, the most frequent adverse events were fatigue (6.3%) somnolence (6.3%), and mood swings (4.2%). No observed detrimental effects on children's growth and pubertal development and no withdrawal or safety issues related to the use or discontinuation of the drug occurred.

Table 1
Strength of Recommendations based on benefit and safety

Treatment	Level of Certainty by USPTF Definitions	Strength of recommendation based on Benefit and Safety	Evidence Base in Youth	Personal Recommendations Of the Reviewer
I. Pharmacologic (Children and Adolescents)				
A. Melatonin				
1. Melatonin therapy, pharmacologic treatments other than melatonin, behavioral interventions, parent education/education programs, and alternative therapies n = 1808, aged 0–18 y, Dx autism and insomnia, (Cuomo et al, 2017[17])	Moderate	C, but safe	Meta-synthesis = 8 systemic reviews (5 DBPCTs)	Melatonin, behavioral interventions, and parent education seem the most effective but no single interventions addresses all sleep problems. Melatonin seemed to work best with autism. Safe, effective, low-risk Recommend Passes SECS
2. Melatonin, long-term safety n = 679, 13 trials, aged 1–13 y, Dx neuro-developmental disorders, (Parker et al, 2019[4])	Low	C, but safe	Systematic review and meta-analyses-no RCTs	Benefit and safety of melatonin higher than placebo Recommend as adjunct Passes SECS
3. Melatonin, long-term treatment (avg 3 y, avg dose 2.69 mg), n = 51, aged 6–12 y Dx Chronic sleep onset insomnia (Van Geijlswijk et al, 2011[16])	Low	C	Follow-up study of prior placebo-controlled trial	Long-term treatment with melatonin in children was not found to affect sleep quality, puberty development, or mental health scores compared with controls Recommend as adjunct Passes SECS

(continued on next page)

Table 1
(continued)

Treatment	Level of Certainty by USPTF Definitions	Strength of recommendation based on Benefit and Safety	Evidence Base in Youth	Personal Recommendations Of the Reviewer
4. Melatonin dose up to 10 mg/night for 3 mo, n = 17, Dx Autism Spectrum Disorder with severe dysomnias (Wright et al, 2011[18])	Low	C	Randomized placebo controlled crossover trial	In children with ASD who have not responded to behavioral management for dysomnias, melatonin significantly improved SL and total sleep compared with placebo. Number of nighttime awakenings was not affected Recommend as adjunct Passes SECS
5. Melatonin 3 mg for 2 wk vs Placebo n = 18, aged 2–15 y, ASD and/or Fragile X Syndrome individuals with parent reported sleep problems (Wirojanan et al, 2009[3])	Low	C	Double-blind, randomized controlled, crossover design	In children with ASD and/or Fragile X Syndrome, melatonin administration improved TST, decreased SL, and promoted earlier sleep timing compared with those without melatonin in the same population Recommend as adjunct Passes SECS
6. Melatonin and CBT n = 186, Children aged 4–10 y ASD with initial and middle insomnia, 4 arms: melatonin and CBT, CBT only, Melatonin only and placebo	Low	C	Randomized placebo-controlled trial	In children with ASD, all active treatment groups demonstrated improvement in SL, TST, decreased wakefulness after sleep onset, and reduced number of awakenings compared

Over a 12-wk period (Cortesi et al, 2012[19])				with placebo. CBT with the melatonin group outperformed the other active treatment groups, especially for initial insomnia. Recommend as adjunct. Passes SECS
Prolonged-Release 7. Melatonin mini tablets (PedPRM), n = 125, aged 2–17.5 y, 13 wk, Dx Insomnia in ASD, (Gringas et al, 2017[21])	Low	C	Randomized placebo-controlled trial	PedPRM was efficacious and safe for treatment of insomnia in children and adolescents with ASD with/without ADHD and NGD. Safe, efficacious, low risk, may not be cheap. Recommend as adjunct. Passes SECS
8. 3 or 10 mg of Melatonin for recovery of PPCS in a pediatric population, n = 62, aged 8-18 y. (Iyer et al, 2020[24])	Low	C	DBPCT	Children with PPCS who reported better sleep and reduced wake periods following sleep onset had a net increase in the gray matter within the PCC. Gray matter changes corresponded to increases in functional connectivity between posterior DMN nodes and visual, somatosensory, and dorsal brain networks in those that recovered vs increased functional connectivity between anterior DMN and limbic network regions in those that did not. Recommended as an adjunct in PPCS. Passes SECS

(continued on next page)

Table 1
(continued)

Treatment	Level of Certainty by USPTF Definitions	Strength of recommendation based on Benefit and Safety	Evidence Base in Youth	Personal Recommendations Of the Reviewer
9. Follow-up of Iyer study. n = 64, aged 8-18 y (Barlow et al, 2020[25])	Low	C	RCT	Sleep duration improved in 3 and 10 mg groups. Sleep efficacy improved in the 10 mg group. Depressive symptoms improved in the 3 mg group. No adverse effects Recommended as an adjunct for PPCS Passes SECS
10. Sleep, Growth, and Puberty After 2 Years of Prolonged-Release Melatonin in Children With Autism Spectrum Disorder 2-17.5 years of age (Malow et al, 2019[53])	Low	C	DBPCT	2 mg, 5 mg, or 10 mg PedPRM nightly up to 104 weeks, followed by a 2-week placebo period to assess withdrawal effects. The most frequent treatment-related adverse events were fatigue (6.3% somnolence (6.3%), and mood swings (4.2%). No observed detrimental effects on children's growth and pubertal development and no withdrawal or safety issues related to the use or discontinuation of the drug.

B. Other Pharmacological Treatments

1. L-5-HTP for night terrors, n = 45, aged 3.2–10.6 y, Dx night terrors, (Bruni et al, 2004[26])	Low	C	Open trial	After 6 mo of treatment, 83.9% of children were night terror free vs 29.6% in comparison group L-5-HTP could be considered as a treatment option in children with persistent night terrors Intervention is safe, cheap, low risk but more research is needed Recommend as adjunct when no intervention works for night terrors Passes SECS
2. Omega-3 LC-PUFA, 20 studies, (5 studies on infants and 5 on children, 10 on adults), Dx not specified, (Dai et al, 2021[38])	Low	C, but safe	Meta-analysis = no RCTs	Omega-3 LC-PUFA may benefit certain aspects of sleep health throughout childhood. Maternal intake or exposure to omega-3 LC-PUFA during pregnancy improve infants' sleep maturity and organization Omega-3 reduced children's total sleep disturbance score for those with clinical-level

(continued on next page)

Table 1
(continued)

Treatment	Level of Certainty by USPTF Definitions	Strength of recommendation based on Benefit and Safety	Evidence Base in Youth	Personal Recommendations Of the Reviewer
				sleep problems but had no effect on healthy children. Although the study was a meta-analysis, it did not have any RCTs in children. Recommend as adjunct. Passes SECS
3. L-theanine, 400 mg twice daily for 6 wk, n = 98 boys, Dx ADHD, (Lyon et al, 2011[31])	Low	C	double-blind placebo-controlled trial	Active group had significantly higher sleep percentage and SE scores, along with a nonsignificant trend for less activity during sleep. L-theanine at relatively high doses was well tolerated with no significant adverse events. L-theanine may be a safe effective adjunctive treatment in boys with ADHD. Recommend as adjunct. Passes SECS
4. Iron deficiency (ID) (ages birth to 16, 3 case series, 3 case studies, n = 144, one pilot study in infants with IDID and RLS, n = 356, 132	Low-no RCTs	C	Review with 2 pilot studies, 3 case series, 3 case studies	Proved a definite link between ID and RLS. Treatment improved RLS significantly. Clinicians should be aware of early signs of RLS in infants

treatment and 114 placebo) and one pilot study of low ferritin in autistic children, N = 52, 15 treatment and 37 control Total N = 503) (Leung et al, 2020[32])				and children with ID. More research is needed but can be used as an adjunctive treatment of SDs that includes RLS. Very few side effects Monitor ferritin, iron, sed rate, and TIBC levels Passes SECS
5. Low ferritin and RLS Case study 2 y old, (El Shawa et al, 2022[33]) Case series (Tima et al, 2013[35]), aged 0–40 mo, n = 14 Case study 5 y old, (Banno et al, 2009[36])	Low	C	1 case series, and 2 case studies	Low ferritin treatment decreased RLS. However, studies are insufficient in number May be used adjunctively in children with RLS and low ferritin. Monitor ferritin, iron, sed rate, and TIBC levels Passes SECS
II Pharmacologic (Young Adults)				
A. Association between screen time/movement behaviors (sedentary behavior, physical activity) and sleep outcomes in infants (0–1 y old); toddlers (1–2 y); and preschoolers (3–4 y old) (Janssen et al, 2019[50])	Low for screen time Low for physical activity	C for screen time C for exercise	Systemic reviews and meta-analysis-No RCTs	A meta-analysis confirmed these unfavorable associations in evening screen time for infants and toddlers but not preschoolers. Systemic review revealed association for infants, toddlers, and preschoolers Mixed results for exercise. There were no RCTs included Recommend as adjunctive treatment of SDs in infants, toddlers and *(continued on next page)*

Table 1
(continued)

Treatment	Level of Certainty by USPTF Definitions	Strength of recommendation based on Benefit and Safety	Evidence Base in Youth	Personal Recommendations Of the Reviewer
				preschoolers should include limited screen time Passes SECS
B. Association between screen time and sleep disturbance in 5-18y olds, 67 published studies. (Hale et al, 2015[51])	Low	C	Systemic review	Screen time is adversely associated with sleep outcomes (primarily shortened duration and delayed timing) in 90% of studies. However, limitations of the current studies: (1) causal association not confirmed; (2) measurement error (of both screen time exposure and sleep measures); (3) limited data on simultaneous use of multiple screens, characteristics, and content of screens used. Children and adolescents should limit screen time before bedtime Passes SECS

C. White Noise as sleep aid, 38 studies, n = 313 participants, ages infancy to adult, in various settings, 0–18 y, n = 13, (Riedy et al, 2012[52])	Low	C, but safe	Systemic review	Studies focused on children were few. Continuous noise may improve SL and sleep fragmentation. It might also disrupt sleep Intervention is safe, cheap, low risk but more research is needed before it can be recommended This challenges the widespread belief that white noise may improve sleep quality Passes SECS
D. Mindfulness for 8 wk or active control, n = 32, ages 7–11, Dx ADHD, (Zaccari et al, 2022[49])	Low	C	RCT	The preliminary results suggest that mindfulness meditation practices may promote specific positive changes in sleep indices and behavioral measures in children with ADHD. However, no change in actigraphic measures It is safe to recommend as an adjunct Passes SECS
E. Sleep hygiene for improving sleep in ADHD, n = 1469, mean age 9.6 y, DX insomnia and ADHD (Parker et al, 2019[4])	Low	C	Review 13 RCTs but only one had low risk of bias	15 out of the 16 studies reviewed found sleep hygiene interventions improved sleep quality in children with ADHD Recommend Passes SECS

(continued on next page)

Table 1
(continued)

II. Non- Pharmacological Interventions

F. Sleep Hygiene in ADHD N=1469, ages 5-18, DX insomnia and ADHD, (Nikles et al, 2020[54])	Low	C	Systematic Review	4 RCTs; 2 =no bias, 2 did not report One RCT favored an extended over a brief intervention to reduce caregiver-reported sleep problems. Three RCTs showed improvement in sleep difficulties on the Children's Sleep Habits Questionnaire (CSHQ) with behavioral management plans incorporating SH measures (setting bedtime, bedtime routines and media-free bedroom). Some studies demonstrated methodological weaknesses. All studies in the future should have standardization of sleep measurements and include actigraphy or polysomnography.

B. Other pharmacological treatments

6. Non traditional treatments for autism interventions, 8 studies, n = 346 participants, Dx autism and insomnia, (Mclay et al, 2016[48])	Low vitamins Low Massage	C vitamins C massage	Review 4 studies used a randomized between group study, 1 study was a DBPCT (n=141, ages 5-16)	Massage therapy and vitamin supplements had positive outcomes Vitamins/Minerals and Massage passes SECS

III. Nonpharmacologic interventions

A. Vitamin D, n = 9397, aged 16 y and older, Dx low vitamin D levels, (Gao et al, 2018[39])	Low	C in those 16 and above	Meta-analysis-no RCTs but no bias 9 studies	Vitamin D Deficiency had a 60% risk of poor sleep quality, especially <20 ng/mL. It may be important to test Vitamin D levels and replenish for optimal sleep. Recommended in young adults and adolescents as adjunct. Monitor Vitamin D. Passes SECS
B. Gabadone, n = 18, aged 19 y or older, Dx SDs, (Shell et al, 2010[27])	Low	C in young adults; C more studies in children needed	Randomized double-blind placebo-controlled trial	An amino acid preparation containing both GABA and 5-HTP reduced time to fall asleep, decreased SL, increased the duration of sleep, and improved quality of sleep. All of the ingredients included in GABA done are classified as generally recognized as safe by the United States Food and Drug Administration. More research needed in children, Recommended in young adults. Passes SECS
C. Ashwagandha stress-relieving and pharmacologic actions (300 mg twice daily X 10 wk) (Lopresti et al, 2019[28])	Low	C in young adults; C safety in children not established	DBPCT	Sleep onset latency, Sleep efficacy, Sleep quality and improvements on the PSQI and Anxiety on the HAM-A all significantly improved

(continued on next page)

Table 1
(continued)

| D. Ashwagandha 300 mg twice daily X 10 wk for insomnia, aged 18–60 y, n = 60, (40 test, 20 placebo), Dx insomnia (Langade et al, 2019[29]) | Low | C in young adults C, safety in children not established | DBPCT | Sleep onset, SE, anxiety, and sleep quality significantly improved in active treatment group after 10 wk, especially in those with comorbid anxiety Passes SECS |
| | | | | after 10 wk Aswagandha may be useful in those with anxiety and sleep problems Recommended in young adults. More studies need to be done in children Passes SCES) |

Abbreviation: TIBC, total iorn binding capacity.

Strength of Recommendations based on benefit and safety:

A=Recommend Strongly. There is a high certainty that the net benefit is substantial **and safe.**

B=Recommend. There is a high certainty that the net benefit is moderate or there is moderate certainty that the net benefit is moderate to substantial **and safe.**

C=Neutral (offer or provide this service for selected patients depending on individual circumstances, based on professional judgment and patient preferences). There is at least moderate certainty that the net benefit is small.

D=Discourage. There is moderate or high certainty that the service has no net benefit or that the harms outweigh the benefits.

I = Insufficient (if the service is offered, patients should understand the uncertainty about the balance of benefits and harms) Current evidence is insufficient to assess the balance of benefits and harms of the service. Evidence is lacking, of poor quality, or conflicting, and the balance of benefits cannot be determined.)

Level of certainty regarding quality:

HIGHLevel of Evidence with robust positive data meta-analyses or meta-reviews involving 2 or more RCTs of excellent, robust quality. The available evidence usually includes consistent results from well-designed, well-conducted RCTs in representative child, adolescent or young adult (18-24 years old) populations, assessing the effects on mental health outcomes.

MODERATE Level of Evidence with robust positive data involving 2 or more RCTs of excellent, robust quality. The available evidence usually includes consistent results from well-designed, well-conducted RCTs in representative child, adolescent or young adult (18-24 years old) populations, assessing the effects on mental health outcomes.

LOW Level of evidence with less than 2 RCTs with good or average quality. The available evidence is insufficient to assess the effects on mental health outcomes.

SECS Criteria:

A guide to clinical decisions is that interventions that are Safe, Easy, Cheap, **and** Sensible (SECS) require less evidence to justify individual trials than those that are Risky, Unrealistic, Difficult, **or** Expensive (RUDE). Because some of the treatments do not have much solid, compelling evidence but would be reasonable to try with a lower bar of evidence, this criterion is also taken into account. Being risky, unrealistic, difficult **OR** expensive (RUDE) disqualifies from SECS. The bolded conjunc-

Sleep disruption in children is a significant clinical problem affecting children and families and is a critical child psychiatric intervention target given its broad impact. Sleep hygiene, parent education, and melatonin remain the cornerstones of effective intervention strategies. Behavioral interventions, including cognitive-behavioral therapy, are essential nonpharmacological interventions to address sleep difficulties in children. Melatonin treatment is widely researched, has minimal side effects, and is considered first-line pharmacologic treatment. However, improper dose and timing of melatonin may lead to perceived failure and underline the importance of educating parents on how to optimize melatonin administration for proper results.

Most studies note that there were methodological issues in the literature, and better-designed larger scale trials are needed in the future to understand better what interventions are helpful for SDs in children with psychiatric disorders. In fact, in the DBPCT involving ADHD boys, aged 8 to 12 years, with L-theanine (Suntheanine), parents did not feel the L-theanine produced any changes in sleep on the PSQ. In contrast, actigraphy watch data findings indicated that boys who consumed L-theanine obtained significantly higher sleep percentage and SE scores, along with a nonsignificant trend for less activity during sleep (defined as less time WASO) compared with those in the placebo group. This study indicates that parents were not particularly aware of their children's sleep quality. Therefore, future studies should include actigraphy data.[25]

Overall, melatonin, sleep hygiene, and parent education have emerged as the more effective, low-risk, and cheapest interventions among children with psychiatric disorders. In addition, endogenous melatonin may be abnormal in children with ASD making a solid case for its use in this population. Adjunctive interventions are helpful in children that address low-ferritin levels and vitamin D3 deficiency. ID may be an early sign of RLS in children and children and infants treated for ID improved sleep. Moreover, the addition of L-5-HTP for night terrors, L-theanine for insomnia and ADHD, and Ashwagandha for anxiety and insomnia may be good adjunctive treatments. Gabadone and omega-3 fatty acids may be helpful for insomnia in all children and adolescents. Probiotics in individuals with BD and IBS, and in children with colic (specifically *L reuteri*) may decrease problems with sleep in these individuals. Finally, meditation, combination vitamins/minerals, exercise, and changing from a high-fat diet to a Mediterranean diet may also be useful as adjunctive therapies.

DISCLOSURE

The author has no conflicts to report.

REFERENCES

1. American Academy of Sleep Medicine. International classification of sleep disorders. 3rd edition. Darien, IL: American Academy of Sleep Medicine; 2014.

2. Arns M, Kooij JS, Coogan AN. Identification and management of circadian rhythm sleep disorders as a transdiagnostic feature in child and adolescent psychiatry. J Am Acad Child Adolesc Psychiatry 2021;60(9):1085–95.

3. Wirojanan J, Jacquemont S, Diaz R, et al. The efficacy of melatonin for sleep problems in children with autism, fragile X syndrome, or autism and fragile X syndrome. J Clin Sleep Med 2009;5(2):145–50.

4. Parker A, Beresford B, Dawson V, et al. Oral melatonin for non-respiratory sleep disturbance in children with neurodisabilities: systematic review and meta-analyses. Dev Med Child Neurol 2019;61(8):880–90.

5. Sateia MJ. International classification of sleep disorders-third edition: highlights and modifications. Chest 2014;146(5):1387–94. PMID: 25367475.

6. Bruni O, DelRosso L, Mogavero MP, et al. Is behavioral insomnia "purely behavioral." J Clin Sleep Med 2022;18(5):1475–6. PMID: 35172920; PMCID: PMC9059583.

7. Esposito S, Laino D, D'Alonzo R, et al. Pediatric sleep disturbances and treatment with melatonin. J Transl Med 2019;17(1):77.

8. Pagan C, Goubran-Botros H, Delrome R, et al. Disruption of melatonin synthesis is associated with impaired 14-3-3 and miR-451 levels in patients with autism spectrum disorders. Sci Rep 2017;7:2096.

9. Bruni O, Sette S, Angriman M, et al. Clinically oriented subtyping of chronic insomnia of childhood. J Pediatr 2018;196:194–200.e1. Epub 2018 Mar 15. PMID: 29550236.

10. Rosen R, Vandenplas Y, Singendonk M, et al. Pediatric gastroesophageal reflux clinical practice guidelines, joint Recommendations of the north American society for pediatric Gastroenterology, Hepatology, and nutrition (NASPGHAN) and the European society for pediatric Gastroenterology, Hepatology, and nutrition (ESPGHAN). J Pediatr Gastroenterol Nutr 2018;66:516–54.

11. Melke J, Goubran Botros P, Chaste P, et al. Abnormal melatonin synthesis in autism spectrum disorders. Mol Psychiatry 2008;13:90–8.

12. Ferlazzo N, Andolina G, Cannata A, et al. Is melatonin the cornucopia of the 21st century? Antioxidants 2020;9(11):1088.

13. Bolsius YG, Zurbriggen MD, Kim JK, et al. The role of clock genes in sleep, stress and memory. Biochem Pharmacol 2021;191:114493. Epub 2021 Feb 27. PMID: 33647263.

14. Liu J, Clough SJ, Hutchinson AJ, et al. MT1 and MT2 melatonin receptors: a therapeutic perspective. Annu Rev Pharmacol Toxicol 2016;56:361–83. Epub 2015 Oct 23. PMID: 26514204; PMCID: PMC5091650.

15. Beker MC, Caglayan B, Caglayan AB, et al. Interaction of melatonin and Bmal1 in the regulation of PI3K/AKT pathway components and cellular survival. Sci Rep 2019;9(1):19082. PMCID: PMC6910929.

16. Van Geijlswijk IM, Mol RH, Egberts TC, et al. Evaluation of sleep, puberty and mental health in children with long-term melatonin treatment for chronic idiopathic childhood sleep onset insomnia. Psychopharmacology 2011;216(1):111–20.

17. Cuomo BM, Vaz S, Lee EA, et al. Effectiveness of sleep-based interventions for children with autism spectrum disorder: a meta-synthesis. Pharmacother J Hum Pharmacol Drug Ther 2017;37(5):555–78.

18. Wright B, Sims D, Smart S, et al. Melatonin versus placebo in children with autism spectrum conditions and severe sleep problems not amenable to behavior management strategies: a randomized controlled crossover trial. J autism Dev Disord 2011;41(2):175–84.

19. Cortesi F, Giannotti F, Sebastiani T, et al. Controlled-release melatonin, singly and combined with cognitive behavioral therapy, for persistent insomnia in children with autism spectrum disorders: a randomized placebo-controlled trial. J Sleep Res 2012;21(6):700–9.

20. Schroder CM, Malow BA, Maras A, et al. Pediatric prolonged-release melatonin for sleep in children with autism spectrum disorder: impact on child behavior and caregiver's quality of life. J Autism Dev Disord 2019;49(8):3218–30. PMID: 31079275; PMCID: PMC6647439.

21. Gringras P, Nir T, Breddy J, et al. Efficacy and safety of pediatric prolonged-release melatonin for insomnia in children with autism spectrum disorder. J Am

Acad Child Adolesc Psychiatry 2017;56(11):948–57.e4. Epub 2017 Sep 19. PMID: 29096777.

22. Rzepka-Migut B, Paprocka J. Efficacy and safety of melatonin treatment in children with autism spectrum disorder and Attention-Deficit/Hyperactivity Disorder—a review of the literature. Brain Sci 2020;10(4):219.

23. Horovitz SG, Braun AR, Carr WS, et al. Decoupling of the brain's default mode network during deep sleep. Proc Natl Acad Sci U S A 2009;106(27):11376–81. Epub 2009 Jun 19. PMID: 19549821; PMCID: PMC2708777.

24. Iyer KK, Zalesky A, Cocchi L, et al. Neural correlates of sleep recovery following melatonin treatment for pediatric concussion: a randomized controlled trial. J Neurotrauma 2020;37(24):2647–55. PMID: 32772826.

25. Barlow KM, Kirk V, Brooks B, et al. Efficacy of melatonin for sleep disturbance in children with persistent post-concussion symptoms: secondary analysis of a randomized controlled trial. J Neurotrauma 2021;38(8):950–9. PMID: 32988292.

26. Bruni O, Ferri R, Miano S, et al. L-5-Hydroxytryptophan treatment of sleep terrors in children. Eur J Pediatr 2004;163(7):402–7. Epub 2004 May 14. PMID: 15146330.

27. Shell W, Bullias D, Charuvastra E, et al. A randomized, placebo-controlled trial of an amino acid preparation on timing and quality of sleep. Am J Ther 2010;17(2):133–9. PMID: 19417589.

28. Lopresti AL, Smith SJ, Malvi H, et al. An investigation into the stress-relieving and pharmacological actions of an ashwagandha (Withania somnifera) extract: a randomized, double-blind, placebo-controlled study. Medicine (Baltimore) 2019;98(37):e17186. PMID: 31517876; PMCID: PMC6750292.

29. Langade D, Kanchi S, Salve J, et al. Efficacy and safety of ashwagandha (Withania somnifera) root extract in insomnia and anxiety: a double-blind, randomized, placebo-controlled study. Cureus 2019;11(9):e5797. PMID: 31728244; PMCID: PMC6827862.

30. Nobre AC, Rao A, Owen GN. L-theanine, a natural constituent in tea, and its effect on mental state. Asia Pac J Clin Nutr 2008;17(Suppl 1):167–8. PMID: 18296328.

31. Lyon MR, Kapoor MP, Juneja LR. The effects of L-theanine (Suntheanine®) on objective sleep quality in boys with attention deficit hyperactivity disorder (ADHD): a randomized, double-blind, placebo-controlled clinical trial. Altern Med Rev 2011;16(4):348–54. PMID: 22214254.

32. Leung W, Singh I, McWilliams S, et al. Iron deficiency and sleep - a scoping review. Sleep Med Rev 2020;51:101274. Epub 2020 Feb 8. PMID: 32224451.

33. Al-Shawwa B, Sharma M, Ingram DG. Terrible twos: intravenous iron ameliorates a toddler's iron deficiency and sleep disturbance. J Clin Sleep Med 2022;18(2):677–80.

34. Tilma J, Tilma K, Norregaard O, et al. Early childhood-onset restless legs syndrome: symptoms and effect of oral iron treatment. Acta Paediatr 2013;102(5):e221–6. Epub 2013 Mar 6. PMID: 23360128.

35. Banno K, Koike S, Yamamoto K. Restless legs syndrome in a 5-year-old boy with low body stores of iron. Sleep Biol Rhythms 2009;7:52–4.

36. DelRosso LM, Bruni O, Ferri R. Restless sleep disorder in children: a pilot study on a tentative new diagnostic category. Sleep 2018;41(8).

37. Gold MS, Blum K, Oscar-Berman M, et al. Low dopamine function in attention deficit/hyperactivity disorder: should genotyping signify early diagnosis in children? Postgrad Med 2014;126(1):153–77.

38. Dai Y, Liu J. Omega-3 long-chain polyunsaturated fatty acid and sleep: a systematic review and meta-analysis of randomized controlled trials and longitudinal studies. Nutr Rev 2021;79(8):847–68. PMID: 33382879; PMCID: PMC8262633.

39. Gao T, Kou B, Zhuang B, et al. The association between vitamin D deficiency and sleep disorders: a systematic review and meta-analysis. Nutrients 2018;10(10):1395.

40. Al-Shawwa B, Ehsan Z, Ingram DG. Vitamin D and sleep in children. J Clin Sleep Med 2020;16(7):1119–23. PMID: 32672533; PMCID: PMC7954071.

41. Matenchuk BJ, Mandhane PJ, Kozyrskyj AL. Sleep, circadian rhythm, and gut microbiota. Sleep Med Rev 2020;53:101340. ISSN 1087-0792.

42. Yall LM, Wyse CA, Graham N, et al. Association of disrupted circadian rhythmicity with mood disorders, subjective wellbeing, and cognitive function: a cross-sectional study of 91 105 participants from the UK biobank. Lancet Psychiatry 2018;5:507–14.

43. Godinho-Silva C, Domingues RG, Rendas M, et al. Light-entrained and brain-tuned circadian circuits regulate ILC3s and gut homeostasis. Nature 2019;574:254–8.

44. Wagner-Skacel J, Dalkner N, Moerkl S, et al. Sleep and microbiome in psychiatric diseases. Nutrients 2020;12(8):2198. PMID: 32718072; PMCID: PMC7468877.

45. Xu M, Wang J, Wang N, et al. The efficacy and safety of the probiotic bacterium Lactobacillus reuteri DSM 17938 for infantile colic: a meta-analysis of randomized controlled trials. PLoS One 2015;10(10):e0141445. PMID: 26509502; PMCID: PMC4624960.

46. Pot GK. Sleep and dietary habits in the urban environment: the role of chrono-nutrition. Proc Nutr Soc 2018;77:189–98.

47. Nikles J, Mitchell GK, de Miranda Araújo R, et al. A systematic review of the effectiveness of sleep hygiene in children with ADHD. Psychol Health Med 2020;25(4):497–518.

48. McLay LLK, France K. Empirical research evaluating non-traditional approaches to managing sleep problems in children with autism. Developmental Neurorehabil 2016;19(2):123–34.

49. Zaccari V, Santonastaso O, Mandolesi L, et al. Clinical application of mindfulness-oriented meditation in children with ADHD: a preliminary study on sleep and behavioral problems. Psychol Health 2022;37(5):563–79. Epub 2021 Mar 7. PMID: 33678073.

50. Janssen X, Martin A, Hughes AR, et al. Associations of screen time, sedentary time and physical activity with sleep in under 5s: a systematic review and meta-analysis. Sleep Med Rev 2020;49:101226. Epub 2019 Nov 1. PMID: 31778942; PMCID: PMC7034412.

51. Hale L, Guan S. Screen time and sleep among school-aged children and adolescents: a systematic literature review. Sleep Med Rev 2015;21:50–8. Epub 2014 Aug 12. PMID: 25193149; PMCID: PMC4437561.f studies).

52. Riedy SM, Smith MG, Rocha S, et al. Noise as a sleep aid: a systematic review. Sleep Med Rev 2012;55:101385.

53. Malow BA, Findling RL, Schroder CM. Sleep, Growth, and Puberty After 2 Years of Prolonged-Release Melatonin in Children With Autism Spectrum Disorder. J Am Acad Child Adolesc Psychiatry 2021;60(2):252–61.e3. https://doi.org/10.1016/j.jaac.2019.12.007. Epub 2020 Jan 23. PMID: 31982581; PMCID: PMC8084705.

54. Nikles J, Mitchell GK, de Miranda Araújo R, Harris T, Heussler HS, Punja S, Vohra S, Senior HEJ. A systematic review of the effectiveness of sleep hygiene in children with ADHD. Psychol Health Med 2020;25(4):497–518. https://doi.org/10.1080/13548506.2020.1732431. Epub 2020 Mar 24. PMID: 32204604.

Complementary/Integrative Medicine Treatment and Prevention of Youth Psychosis

Vinod S. Bhatara, MD, MS, MSHS[a],*,
Jeremy Daniel, PharmD, BCPS, BCPP[b], Carol Whitman, MD[c],
Tamara Vik, MD[c], Bettina Bernstein, DO[d,e],
Deborah R. Simkin, MD, DFAACAP[f]

KEYWORDS

- Complementary and integrative treatments • First-episode psychosis
- Prodromal stage • Omega-3 fatty acids • N-acetyl cysteine

KEY POINTS

- The rationale for CIM treatments in youth psychoses is to optimize treatment by targeting symptoms not resolved by antipsychotics, such as negative symptoms (significant drivers of disability, decresed quality of life, and poor outcomes).
- Adjunctive omega-3 fatty acids (ω-3 FA), N-acetyl cystine (NAC usage for > 24-week) or weekly moderate/vigorous exercise can potentially reduce negative symptoms and improve function in youth with psychosis.
- Cultural sensitivity regarding the trauma-psychosis link for Native Americans is needed for equity of care.
- Early identification and treatment of early stages:ultra-high risk (UHR) and First Episode Psychosis (FEP) in youth is necessary required for the prevention of progression of psychosis.
- A trial of omega-3 fatty acids (ω3FA) in UHR is supported by the Vienna High-Risk study and biomarker studies on ω3FA-symptom/function correlation. Awaiting better research, the clinical use of ω3FA in UHR is a safe and effective treatment.

[a] Department of Psychiatry and Pediatrics, University of South Dakota, Sanford School of Medicine, 2601 W Nicole Drive, Sioux Falls, SD 57105-3329, USA; [b] South Dakota State University, College of Pharmacy and Allied Health Professions, Avera Behavioral Health; [c] University of South Dakota Sanford School of Medicine, Sioux Falls, SD, USA; [d] Philadelphia College of Osteopathic Medicine, Philadelphia, PA, USA; [e] Clinical Affiliate Department of Child and Adolescent Psychiatry, The Children's Hospital of Philadelphia, Philadelphia, PA, USA; [f] Department of Psychiatry, Emory University School of Medicine, 8955 Highway 98 West, Suite 204, Miramar Beach, FL 32550, USA
* Corresponding author. 2601 W Nicole Drive, Sioux Falls, SD 57105-3329
E-mail address: vsbhatara@gmail.com

Child Adolesc Psychiatric Clin N Am 32 (2023) 273–296
https://doi.org/10.1016/j.chc.2022.08.009
1056-4993/23/© 2022 Elsevier Inc. All rights reserved.

Abbreviations and definitions	
Abbreviations	**Expansions**
AOS	Adult-onset schizophrenia starts at or after age 18
AI	American Indian/Alaska Native
APs	Antipsychotics
BIPOC	Black Indigenous People of Color
BPRS	Brief Psychiatric Rating Scale
COS, EOS	Childhood-onset schizophrenia starts before the age of 13 years, early-onset schizophrenia starts before age 18
CIM	Complementary and integrative medicine
DUP	Duration of untreated psychosis
FEP, OP	First-episode psychosis, of poverty
PANSS	Positive and Negative Syndrome Scale
RDBPCTs/ PDBRCTs/ PDRBCTs	Placebo-Controlled, Double-Blind Randomized Controlled Trials
SSD	Schizophrenia-spectrum disorders and other psychoses
UHR	Ultra-high risk
USPSTF	U.S. Preventive Services Task Force
Youth	Person younger than 27 years old

INTRODUCTION

This article reviews the evidence-base for complementary and integrative medicine (CIM) treatments in youth and includes interventions that have at least one randomized controlled trial (RCT) supporting their use. Youth with psychosis are underserved by currently used interventions for prevention and treatment, and CIM treatments can potentially optimize their care. Cultural and trauma awareness is necessary: there is an intersection of psychosis with current/historical discrimination/trauma for people living in the United States who identify as American Indian (AI),[1] Black Indigenous People of Color (BIPOC), of poverty, and other minorities.[2] This article discusses experiences based on AI youth in South Dakota.

UNMET NEEDS FOR PREVENTION AND TREATMENT IN EARLY-ONSET SCHIZOPHRENIA

Dissatisfaction with the effectiveness of antipsychotics (APs) in improving negative symptoms, cognition, and social/occupational functioning in early-onset schizophrenia (EOS) has led to a search for alternatives. Relative to adults, children, and adolescents are more likely to experience sedation, extrapyramidal symptoms, elevated prolactin, weight gain, and metabolic changes with AP treatment.[3,4]

CIM treatments are needed in EOS as adolescence is a neurodevelopmentally sensitive period with expectant neuronal plasticity for a variety of neurocognitive and emotional functions.[5]

EOS can predict poor outcomes; thus, early identification potentially decreases morbidity, prevents cumulative disability, and reduces the individual and societal burden. Substantial differences occurred especially when comparing participants with duration of untreated psychosis (DUP) ≤ 74 weeks to greater than 74 weeks: effect size 0.54 versus 0.07 effect sizes per Quality of Life Scale and 0.42 versus 0.13 for the Positive and Negative Syndrome Scale (PANSS) scores.[6]

In view of several lines of evidence supporting a role for neurodevelopmental processes in schizophrenia, there are opportunities for early intervention, and treatment from childhood and adolescence all the way to the stage of disease onset. Because currently used standard treatments are not meeting the needs of youth EOS, evidence-based CIM treatments in EOS are urgently needed.

DISCUSSION

Trauma-informed care is needed to reduce disparities in care.[2] AI youth resembles veterans returning from Afghanistan in rates of experiencing trauma estimated at 22%, triple the rates of the general population, suggesting a high-psychosis risk.[7] A trauma-psychosis association was also found in Jewish Holocaust survivors with childhood trauma[8] and in the general population.[9] Research studies on CIM interventions that are safe, easy, cheap, and sensible may be especially needed in AI children and adolescents because of difficult differential diagnosis in early schizophrenia-spectrum disorders (SSD) due to the overlap between SSD and trauma/cultural factors.

Caring for the Mental Health of American Indian: The South Dakota Experience

AI youth living in the rural state of South Dakota experience many barriers to treatment: stigma, lack of psychiatric services, lack of mental health awareness, and the disparate treatments of traditional indigenous approaches versus Western medicine. Differential diagnoses are broader when evaluating AI youth due to the need to address cultural factors, spiritual beliefs, and unique trauma responses. Many AI youth in South Dakota experience longer DUP. Comparisons of longer versus shorter DUP data showed an association between longer DUP and worse outcomes at 6 months regarding total symptoms, overall functioning, positive symptoms, and quality of life (QOL).[10] Symptom remission was less likely with longer DUP. Prevention strategies to lower DUP require an appreciation of symptoms in the AI spiritual/cultural context. Plains AI, while resembling the general population in the prevalence of SSD, may differ regarding higher rates of transient psychotic experiences, often occurring during positive sacred/spiritual experiences that originate from a loving place.[11] During the third rite (Wanagi Wicagluha or spirit keeping), the Lakota believe that the spirit is still present for up to 1 year, allowing youth to see their (deceased) relative and participate in the sacred experience. Hallucinations in SSD among nonindigenous people may be derogatory, distressing, and disabling. Health professionals and community education are needed for early referral of youth suspected to have first-episode psychosis (FEP).[12,13]

Early Detection of Psychosis

To detect individuals at high and imminent risk of developing FEP, (ultra-high-risk) UHR criteria to identify youth at high risk for developing psychosis were developed.[14] UHR was found to facilitate early detection and research of prevention strategies for patients with unfavorable prognosis and functional impairment[15]; advancements in adolescent UHR populations are less established, but still useful.[16] It was noticed[17] that UHR youth had an elevated risk of developing psychosis of about 20% within 2 years as well as a significant risk for nonpsychotic disorders.

AP treatment currently is not recommended for persons with UHR as they may not all have psychotic disorders; this can be related to the pleiotropic nature of UHR found in heterogenous samples.[15] Given the possibility of false-positive psychoses, it is best to avoid a high-risk treatment (APs): consider close monitoring and treatments with lower side effect burden such as omega-3 fatty acids (ω3FA), unless FEP has occurred.

Staged Effectiveness of Omega-3 Fatty Acids Supplementation in Schizophrenia-Spectrum Disorders

Ultra-high risk: Prevention of transition to first-episode psychosis

Two systematic reviews focusing exclusively on UHR suggested the effectiveness of ω3FA in preventing UHR-to-FEP conversion. One was based on a review of the Cochrane database, reporting evidence supporting the lowering of transition rates to psychosis by ω3FA.[18] The other[19] was based on a review of four primary UHR studies, including two placebo-controlled, double-blind randomized controlled trials (PDRBCTs) (Vienna High-Risk study [VHR,[20,21]] and NEUROPRO[22]) and two non-RCT studies: Program of Rehabilitation and Therapy[23]), North American Prodrome Longitudinal Study.[24]

Interventional studies

VHR study[20,21] (n= 81, 13-25 years old UHR youth) found that after 12-week treatment with 1.2 g/daily of ω-3FA, UHR-to-FEP progression rates were 4.9% in the ω3FA group versus 27.5% in controls, suggesting strong effects, which sustained at 6.7 years postintervention. Supporting the effectiveness of ω3FA and in a post hoc data analysis of RDBPCT in UHR youth (mean age 16.2 years) with borderline personality, ω3FA significantly improved functioning and reduced psychiatric symptoms.[25] VHR results were not replicated by NEUROPRO22, which was a large, 6-month, multisite, PDBRCT involving 304, 12-to-40 year old UHR youth (153 given 1.4 g/d of w3FA and 151 received paraffin oil). Both groups also received up to 20 sessions of cognitive-behavioral case management (CBCM) during 6-month intervention period and on as needed basis from months 6 to 12. Antidepressants were given to nearly 62% of controls.[26]. This study22 found no w3FA effects (but both groups had, lower conversion to psychosis, and 57% nonadherence rate).[26,27] VHR needs to be replicated in a larger sample despite the challenges faced by prevention trials, such as conversions rates to psychosis have declined.[27]

Omega-3 fatty acids biomarker studies

A recent systematic review of UHR studies[19] noted that review of cross-sectional data of 19 articles (n = 560, age range 12–40) found a positive correlation between dietary ω3FA/red blood cell (RBC) membrane EPA and functional status. Note the limitations of RCT methodology, Amminger and colleagues[28] analyzed ω3FA biomarkers in 218 participants with longitudinal biomarker data from NEUROPRO cohort. They found that higher baseline erythrocyte membrane ω3 and increases of the ω3 index, eicosapentaenoic acid (EPA), and docosahexaenoic acid (DHA) predicted low symptoms and better function at 6 and −12 months, suggesting that ω3FA can exert therapeutic effects in UHR patients. The findings support a safe and effective use of ω3FA supplements in clinical settings. Based on data from 285 patients in NEUROPRO cohort, Berger and colleagues[29] found that the baseline ω3index (sum of EPA and DHA as percent of total RBC FA) was negatively correlated with the severity of general psychopathology, psychotic symptoms, depressive symptoms, and manic symptoms in UHR subjects.

Mechanism of action of omega-3 fatty acids in early schizophrenia-spectrum disorders

The detailed pathophysiology of SSD remains relatively unknown.[30] As noted by biomarker studies,[28,29] deficits/dysregulation of membrane ω3FA play a role in pathogenesis, at least in a subgroup of SSD, as shown by the negative correlation of phospholipid membrane ω3 (ω3-index) with the severity of psychopathology in UHR subjects. The rationale for using ω3FA is based on membrane phospholipid hypothesis by Horrobin,[31] according to which ω3FA deficiency in the neuronal cell membrane, resulting from elevated intracellular phospholipase A2 activity (inPLA$_2$), the main enzymes regulating phospholipid metabolism cause progressive deterioration of key brain circuits and SSD in susceptible individuals. A mechanistic RCT of UHR youth from the VHR cohort found that ω3FA supplementation significantly decreased inPLA$_2$ activity and changed membrane FA profiles, supporting the role of ω3FA and ω6FA in neuroprogression of psychosis.[32] These findings suggested that ω3FA supplementation may act by normalizing inPLA$_2$ activity and ω3/ω6FA metabolism.

A systematic review of 13 RCTs by Hsu and colleagues[33] discussed possible mechanisms underlying the beneficial effects of ω3FA in SSD. They also reviewed the evidence supporting the association of ω3FA deficiency in plasma and erythrocyte cell membranes[34] and SSD and summarized causes of ω3FA deficiency in neuronal phospholipid membrane, including inefficient conversion of alpha-linolenic acid to DHA in humans (requiring ingestion of essential ω3FA), high ω6/ω3 diet, low synthesis due to abnormal metabolic enzymes, or low absorption due to mutated FA binding protein and elevated inPLA$_2$ activity. They emphasized that baseline ω3FA is important because patients with low baseline ω3FA index and DHA may be more responsive to the ω3FA intervention.

The FEP typically occurs in late adolescence or early adulthood, during the ongoing process of brain maturation. Efficacy of ω3FA augmentation in patients with FEP can be explained by the restoration of physiological levels of ω3FA. The target of treatment is the normalization of neuronal membrane FA levels thought to be important for neuronal integrity and prevention of progression to psychosis, which may be associated with a chronic deterioration of key brain circuits, mediated by oxidative stress, inflammation, decreased neurotrophic growth factors, apoptosis, mitochondrial dysfunction, and impaired neuroplasticity.[32,33] Frajerman and colleagues[30] reviewed the shared effects of ω3FAs and APs and proposed the following mechanism: ω3FAs provide neuroprotection, modify the properties of the cell membrane, reduce oxidative stress, and inflammation, improve myelination, influence glutamate, and dopamine signaling pathways. The neuroprotective effects of ω3FA may be more pronounced in adolescence when brain maturation takes place possibly due to a time window for optimum effects.[33]

First-episode psychosis and omega-3 fatty acids augmentation of antipsychotics

A 2021 meta-analysis by Goh and colleagues,[35] involving 1494 SSD patients on ω3FA augmentation, found that both FEP and chronic SSD showed similar reductions in total and positive symptoms. Subgroup analysis comparing participants' responses in the three SSD stages (FEP [n = 139, ages: 15–48 years] vs UHR vs chronic SSD) found that FEP stood out as the only SSD stage showing decreased primary negative symptoms, known to be significant drivers of long-term disability, deteriorating QOL, and poor outcomes.[36] Primary negative symptoms are intrinsic to the underlying pathophysiology of SSD, occurring in up to 60% of cases, and are still an unmet treatment need in SSD due to their inadequate response to APs. By contrast, secondary negative symptoms are related to psychiatric or medical comorbidities, adverse effects, or environmental factors.[36] Goh and colleagues[35] concluded that ω3FA augmentation was particularly recommended for FEP. They confirmed the safety and tolerability of ω3FA and found that ω3FA lowered triglycerides levels.

In 2021, Hsu and colleagues[37] published a systematic review of ω3FA augmentation effects in SSD by developmental stages. Based on their overall review of trials in FEP subjects that included three studies from two independent PBDRCTs in FEP,[38–40] they concluded that longer duration augmentation (16–24 weeks) can improve function and reduce negative symptoms, neuronal oxidative damages, and peripheral lipid peroxidation/oxidative stress. ω3FA add-on treatment was associated with earlier treatment response, decreased negative symptoms and depression, lower AP dosages, more patients reaching greater than 50% improvement, fewer extra-pyramidal symptoms (EPS), and better tolerability (less extrapyramidal and sexual side effects), but no benefit to prevent relapse in FEP off APs.[37,41] The effectiveness of ω3FA augmentation is modulated by age, DUP, baseline ω3FA levels, and status of antioxidant capacity of patients.[37]

Chronic schizophrenia-spectrum disorders and omega-3 fatty acids augmentation

A recent meta-analysis of 15 PDBRCTs in chronic SSD[35] reported that ω3FA augmentation improved general psychopathology/positive symptoms but not negative symptoms, and only in patients who were severely ill. Results showed that ω3FA augmentation is a useful treatment option, particularly in those who are severely ill.

N-Acetyl cysteine augmentation by developmental stages of schizophrenia-spectrum disorders

No published RCTs of N-acetyl cysteine (NAC) in UHR were found.

Adjunctive N-acetyl cysteine in first-episode psychosis

The effectiveness of NAC supplementation in FEP is supported by a systematic review[42] of three PDBRCTs (n = 265. age 20–40 years) with divergent findings. One small study[43] found that NAC significantly reduced PANSS scores (negative, positive, general, and total). Another small study[44] demonstrated a significant superiority of 52-week NAC treatment versus placebo in decreasing PANSS total, negative, and disorganized thought factor symptom scores. NAC had no effects on positive symptom.

In a larger PDBRCT,[45] NAC-augmentation (2700 mg/day) for 6 months did not improve PANSS scores, but processing speed significantly improved in the NAC group. A subgroup of the participants from this study were scanned for a follow-up multimodal MR imaging study and was found to show improvements in white matter integrity.[46]

Overall, these findings suggest that NAC has the potential for improving negative symptoms in FEP, complementing and augmenting AP effects. Treatment of negative symptoms is an unmet need and is especially important in FEP, not only for disability reduction but perhaps for improving the outcome of FEP. Early treatment of FEP emphasizes prevention and the case for using NAC is based on its potential for reducing primary negative symptoms, and through its antioxidant, anti-inflammatory, and glutamate modulation activity.[42] NAC as an add-on treatment may be a safe and effective way to protect white matter integrity in early psychosis patients. There is currently a large RCT being conducted into NACs effect in FEP.[47]

Chronic schizophrenia-spectrum disorders and N-acetyl cysteine augmentation of antipsychotics

The use of NAC in established SSD is supported by a robust pairwise meta-analysis by Yolland and colleagues,[48] a net-work meta-analysis by Xu and colleagues,[49] and updates to Yolland meta-analysis by a systematic review by Bradlow.[42] The meta-analysis[48] was based on a review of seven studies (n = 220 on NAC and 220 on placebo), and it found that longer term (>24 weeks) NAC treatment reduced PANSS negative and total scores and improved working memory. It[48] included a total of five out of eight blinded RCTs of NAC augmentation, one was excluded due to missing data and two had not yet been published.[42] One of the newer studies not included in Yolland's[48] meta-analysis) reported no effects of NAC on PANSS[50] and the other[51] showed a significant decrease in negative PANSS and total PANSS relative to placebo. These findings support that NAC augmentation is an evidence-based and useful adjunct to standard treatment for the improvement of negative and total scores, and possibly for the cognitive domain of working memory. Treatment effects were observed at a later time point ($\geq$24 weeks), suggesting that longer interventions are required for the success of NAC treatment.

NAC usage is also supported by a recent systematic review and network meta-analysis[49] of 17 RCTs (including those of supplementation by NAC, ω3 FA, folic acid, and B12). It was found that NAC add-on treatment was significantly more efficacious than folic acid, vitamin B12, and ω3FA in terms of PANSS score changes.[49] Based on their ranking probabilities and PANSS scores, NAC was considered to be among the most effective nutritional supplementations in patients with SSD.[49]

Mechanism of action

It has been hypothesized that redox dysregulation may be central to the pathophysiology of SSD.[42,48] Oxidative stress is shown by decreased concentrations of the antioxidant glutathione (GSH) in the brain,[52] and NAC is a precursor to GSH. As the acetylated form of cysteine, NAC is bioavailable and able to cross the blood–brain barrier. Cysteine is the rate-limiting component in the production of the antioxidant GSH. Several animal studies have shown evidence of increased brain GSH following oral administration of NAC accompanied by reduced oxidative stress.[42,53] NAC also has neurobiological effects on inflammation, glutamate signaling, mitochondrial energy generation, and apoptosis, all pathways additionally dysregulated in schizophrenia inflammation.[42,53,54]

Exercise. A meta-review in the European Psychiatric Association (EPA)[55] found aerobic exercise or physical activity (PA) improved outcomes for FEP and SSD. Ninety minutes of moderate-to-vigorous PA (MVPA) weekly reduced total psychiatric symptoms (standardized mean difference [SMD]: 0.72, 95% CI -1.14 to -0.29), positive symptoms (SMDs -0.54, and 95% CI -0.95 to -0.13), negative symptoms (SMD -0.44, 95% CI -0.78 to -0.09), and improved QOL and cognition as reflected in improved scores on the Matrix Consensus Cognitive Body executive functioning ($g = 0.33$, 95%CI $= 0.13$–0.53, $P = .001$).

In 2007, Cotman and colleagues[56] found that exercise improves psychosis through the hypothesized reversal of putative changes associated with the onset of psychosis; aggressive synaptic pruning may underlie the onset of psychosis in some cases as well as brain neurotrophic alterations, neuronal dysregulation, and degeneration, decreased brain volumes (lost neurons/dendritic spines, loss of brain plasticity, reduced supporting glial cells, loss of neuronal connectivity). They[56] also found that people in early psychosis are particularly sensitive to the deleterious impact of AP and may benefit from using exercise to maintain physical fitness, prevent weight gain and insulin, glucose, and lipid dysregulation to reduce the impact of AP treatment causing the cardiometabolic dysregulation that overrides the genetic linkage between schizophrenia and anthropomorphic markers of thinness.

The disruption of myelination has been proposed as a mechanism of psychosis that is revered by exercise-induced neuroprotective reduced neuroinflammation, upregulation of neurotrophic growth effects (decreased oxidative stress), and potentiation of remyelination.[55,57]

Indirect comparisons of PA to cognitive remediation[57] recommended a multidisciplinary treatment to include PA; Grade B quality of evidence (good and consistent evidence consistent that is generalizable to the target populations); and evidence level -1 (indicating high bias risk). To improve symptoms, cognition, and QOL in SSD,

EPA supported using MVPA two to three times a week/150 minutes per week for optimal results; light exercise or less frequent exercise is still beneficial. EPA emphasized that PA should be integrated into real-life treatments for SSD; culturally relevant research should identify motivational frameworks to determine optimal uptake, maintenance, and use of PA in real-world settings.

Exercise in FEP A 12-week multicenter, open-label supervised exercise intervention (N = 90) and found moderate postintervention improvements in persons with FEP for processing speed, visual learning, and visual attention.[58] A systematic review of five studies in FEP found group-based exercise to be effective in reducing psychiatric symptoms, improving function, cognition, and QOL.[59]

In a systematic review and meta-analysis of 59 RCT studies including FEP improvement of diet and PA in non-affective psychosis patients, postintervention benefit for psychotic symptoms severity was found to persist after follow-up for several cognitive domains, physical/global functioning, and QOL.[60] Improvement was generally larger for interventions including exercise, especially moderate/vigorous aerobic exercise.

Comparing effects of 12-week moderate-intensity aerobic exercises, hatha yoga, and waitlisting on cortical grey matter (based structural MRI), an RCT in 51 young women (mean age by group range 21–22) with early psychosis found increased cortical volume/thickness in the medial temporal cortical regions (primarily in the fusiform cortical region) only in the aerobic arm.[61] These findings suggest that exercise-induced neuroplasticity in medial temporal cortical regions may be associated with improvements in psychosis symptom severity.

Exercise and UHR In a DBRCT (n=32) ,[62] 17 were randomized to either 17 high-intensity exercise twice weekly for 3 weeks or waitlist (n=15). The exercising UHR group showed excellent adherence and significant improvement in measures of fitness, cognitive performance, and positive symptoms compared with the waitlist group. Exercising individuals showed stable hippocampal volumes; waitlist CHR-p individuals showed 3.57% decreased hippocampal subfield volume. The findings suggested that high-intensity exercise can be a beneficial intervention in UHR. A possible mechanism may be that exercise generates hippocampal neurogenesis that may improve hippocampal abnormalities and related cognitive/clinical symptoms.

Vitamin D

In the DFEND trial,[63] no association was found between vitamin D supplementation and mental health or metabolic outcomes at 6 months, providing strong evidence that vitamin D deficiency does not worsen or cause FEP with psychosis.

Folate/Folic acid/L-methyl folate

In a meta-analysis of 7 DBPCT's, (5 with folate and 2 with L-methyl folate) pooled (folate/methyl folate) FA + antipsychotics (AP) treatments were more effective than placebo + AP for negative symptoms (N = 5, n = 281; SMD = −0.25, 95% CI = −0.49, −0.01, P = .04, I 2 = 0%)[64]. A more detailed analysis of these studies may help to understand the mechanisms involved. One of the studies showed the addition of folate had a greater effect on serum folate levels when the patients with a methylenetetrahydrofolate reductase (MTHFR) gene had an MTHFR 677 C/T or MTHFR 677 T/T genotype but no significant change in negative symptoms.[65] MTHFR is partly responsible for converting folate to active form of L-methyl folate (see **Fig. 1**). In another study, supplementation of antipsychotic medications with folate and B12 improved negative symptoms of schizophrenia, but only when a mutation of the

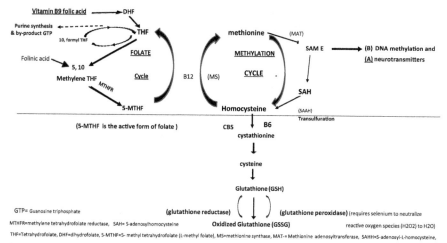

Fig. 1. Role of MTHFR, Vitamin B9, B6, B12, methionine, and glutathione in oxidative stress and MTHFR.

484C > T variant of folate hydrolase 1 (FOLH1-rs202676) was present. This gene may be associated with impaired intestinal absorption of dietary folates, resulting in low blood folate levels and consequent hyperhomocysteinemia. Methylcobalamin (methyl B12) and folate (after conversion to its active form L-methylfolate) are used to combine with homocysteine to form methionine.[66] Another study in the meta-analysis[67] demonstrated that I-methyl folate was associated with convergent changes in ventromedial prefrontal physiology, including increased task-induced deactivation, altered limbic connectivity, and increased cortical thickness. Since folate conversion to L-methyl folate is dependent on MTHFR and the MTHFR 677 T/C and T/T decreases the production of L-methyl folate, the use of I-methyl folate in the latter study was not dependent on the MTHFR genotypes 677 C/T or 677 T/T for improving negative symptoms because L-methylfolate corrected the defect in MTHFR. PANSS Total and General Psychopathology changes were influenced by the genotype methionine synthase (MS). MS is the enzyme responsible for using L-methyl folate and activated vitamin B12 (methylcobalamin) to re-methylate homocysteine back to methionine. Hyperhomocysteinemia has been associated with schizophrenia.[68] More larger studies are needed to elucidate the relationship between MTHFR, homocysteine levels and the positive and negative effects of schizophrenia. In a study to determine the risk for developing schizophrenia in childhood, pediatric patients with schizophrenia (n = 97) as well as age- and sex-matched controls (n = 92) were enrolled. The study included disease onset age, duration, the Positive and Negative Syndrome Scale (PANSS), Personal and Social Performance Scale (PSP), and Clinical Global Impression (CGI). Interestingly, three major MTHFR genotypes (G1793A, C677T, and A1298C) were examined in all subjects. The G1793A polymorphism and the total number of MTHFR risk alleles were associated with an increased risk of schizophrenia in children. The A1298C polymorphism contributed to prolonging the duration time of schizophrenia. Although the MTHFR C677T alleles are associated with adult schizophrenia, this study suggests the MTHFR alleles associated with schizophrenia may differ in childhood.[69]

There are still some patients who do not respond to folate even without the MTHFR C/T or T/T alleles. This may be due to a folate antibody that prevents folate from entering the blood-brain barrier. Auto-antibodies against folate receptor alpha (FRα) can bind to the receptor preventing the influx of folate into the brain. Therefore, folate

1. <u>Guanosine triphosphate (GTP) is used to produce tetrahydrobiopterin (BH4),</u>
2. <u>BH 4 is a co-factor used to form serotonin, dopamine, and nitric oxide (NO), by way of the enzymes Tryptophan Hydroxylase(TRH), Tyrosine Hydroxylase (TH), and Nitric Oxide Synthetase (NOS)</u>
3. <u>If BH 4 is unavailable, BH 2 will form reactive oxygen species (ROS) like superoxides and hydrogen peroxides using NOS, thereby increasing oxidative stress and less serotonin and dopamine would be produced.</u>

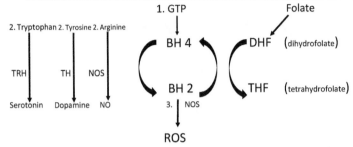

Fig. 2. When 10, formyl THF is formed from THF to produce purines for DNA synthesis, a by product is GTP.

could not be converted to l-methyl folate and hyperhomocysteinemia, associated with schizophrenia may occur (See **Fig. 1**).

In the pathway to form L-methyl folate, normally folate becomes dihydrofolate (DHF) and DHF is then converted to tetrahydrofolate (THF) which in turn becomes 5,10 methylene THF. 5, 10 methylene THF is then converted to L-methyl folate (MTHF) by MTHFR. However, 5,10 methylene THF can also be utilized to produce purines. A by-product produced when purines are formed is called guanosine derivative tetrahydrobiopterin (GTP). GTP is converted to Tetrahydrobiopterin (BH4) which acts as a common co-factor for the enzymes producing dopamine, serotonin, and nitric oxide. If folate cannot enter the brain, then CSF MTHF, BH4 levels, and CSF dopamine and serotonin metabolites would be low. In addition, low nitric acid would increase oxidized stress (see **Fig. 2**). A form of folate called folinic acid can pass through the blood-brain barrier which can then be used to form 5, 10 methylene THF (see **Fig. 1**). In a study of schizophrenics who were unresponsive to treatment, in those that had FRα antibody titers, high doses of folinic acid (between 0.3 and 1.0 mg/kg/d) were administered to 8 patients (ages 11–50). Seven of the 8 participants had clinical improvement.[70,71] Due to the interaction of the auto-antibodies against the FRα receptor, it may be wise to screen infants for the antibody who have a family history of schizophrenia. More research is needed.

In children with auto-antibodies against the FRα receptor, it may also be wise to restrict their intake of dairy, especially milk. One study demonstrated that an Intervention with a milk-free diet lowered FRa antibody titers.[71]

Microbiome

In a study of first-episode psychosis, drug-naïve adult patients compared to healthy controls,[72] had increased abundance of harmful bacterial (Proteobacteria) and decreased short-chain fatty acid (SCFA)-producing bacteria (important to gut integrity), such as the *Faecalibacterium and Lachnospiraceae* genera. The gut mycobiota were characterized by a relative reduction in diversity and altered composition. Most notably, the schizophrenia (SC) group had a higher level of *Chaetomium* and a lower level of *Trichoderma* than the healthy control (HC) group. The drug naïve group also demonstrated changes in the bacteria–fungi correlation network. Although the relative abundance of Candida was comparable between the two groups in the present study, another study[73] demonstrated that an antibody against *C. albicans* is a

Table 1
Complementary/integrative prevention & treatments for youth psychoses

Population Schizophrenia Spectrum Disorder (SSD) Stage and Treatment	Recommendation Strength	Certainty (USPTF)	Evidence Base in Youth	Evidence Based or Meets SECS Criteria	Reviewer Recommendations
UHR (Ultra High-Risk Prodrome) and Omega-3 fatty acids (ω-3 FA): Prevention of UHR-to- First Episode Psychosis (FEP) conversion					
ω-3 FA (Susai et al, 2021[19], N = 560, ages 12-40) (Bosnjak-Kuharic et al, 2019[18], N = 2151, ages >12 y) (Amminger et al, 2020[28], N = 218, UHR ages 13-40) (Berger et al, 2020[29], N = 285, UHR ages 13-40)	B	Moderate	2 Systematic Reviews 4 primary studies, including 2 DBPCRCTs: Vienna High Risk (VHR) and NEUROPRO and 2 non-RCT studies. Three ω3FA Biomarker studies	Evidence based	Recommended: Well-established safety VHR: ω-3 lowered progression to FEP, symptomatic/functional improvement, lasting 7 y. NEUROPRO found no ω-3 effects (but both groups had cognitive management, lower conversion to psychosis & ~57% non-adherence rate. Antidepressants given to ~ 62% of controls). Higher baseline erythrocyte ω-3 and increase in ω-3 predicted low symptoms & high function at 6-8-12 mo. Positive correlation between functional improvement and

(continued on next page)

Table 1
(continued)

Population Schizophrenia Spectrum Disorder (SSD) Stage and Treatment	Recommendation Strength	Certainty (USPTF)	Evidence Base in Youth	Evidence Based or Meets SECS Criteria	Reviewer Recommendations
					frequency of ω-3 FA dietary intake. Definitive studies needed due to inconsistency of findings.
Damme et al, 2022[62] n = 32 (17 high intensity exercise twice weekly for 3 mo vs 15 waitlisted)	C	Low	1 small DBRCT	SECS	Exercising individuals showed stable hippocampal volumes and improved symptoms. Preliminary suggestion that moderate to high-intensity exercise can be beneficial in the psychosis risk period.
FEP: ω-3FA augmentation of antipsychotics (APs)					
ω-3FA: Hsu et al, 2021[37], n = 195, ages 15–48 y	B	Moderate	1 Meta-Analyses 1 Systematic review 3 DBPCRCTs	Evidenced based For FEP SECS For chronic SSD	Likely effectiveness of adjunctive ω-3FA in FEP > chronic SSD and recommended in FEP despite inconsistent findings. Longer duration (16–24 wk) augmentation can improve function

& reduce: negative symptoms (significant drivers of disability-representing unmet need in SSD due to limited response of primary negative symptoms to antipsychotics), neuronal oxidative damage & peripheral lipid peroxidation/oxidative stress. ω-3FA augmentation yielded earlier treatment response, decreased negative symptoms & depression, lower AP dosages, more patients reaching >50% improvement, less EPS, ω-3FAs alone without antipsychotics do not prevent relapse. Augmentation was safe, well-tolerated & reduced triglyceride levels.

(continued on next page)

Table 1
(continued)

Population Schizophrenia Spectrum Disorder (SSD) Stage and Treatment	Recommendation Strength	Certainty (USPTF)	Evidence Base in Youth	Evidence Based or Meets SECS Criteria	Reviewer Recommendations
Chronic Schizophrenia Spectrum Disorder (SSD) and ω-3FA augmentation					
Goh et al, 2021[35], N = 1494, mean age = 30 y	B	Moderate	1 meta-analysis 15 DBPCRCTs	SECS	ω-3FA augmentation reduced triglyceride levels, improved general psychopathology/positive symptoms but not negative symptoms, and only in patients who were severally ill. Results showed ω-3FA augmentation is a useful treatment option, particularly in those who are severely ill.
N-Acetyl Cysteine (NAC) effects by developmental stages of SSD: no published RCTs in UHR					
FEP and NAC augmentation of APs					
Adjunctive NAC: Bradlow et al, 2022[42], n = 265, age 20–40 y	B	Moderate	1 Systematic Review 3 DBPCRCTs	Evidence based	Pending more RCTs, use NAC in FEP for neuroprotection, negative symptoms & possible improved cognition. Improvement in negative symptoms (significant driver of poor outcome &

disability, compliments APs inability to adequately improve negative symptoms and providing neuroprotection.

Chronic SSD and NAC augmentation of APs

Study	Grade				
Adjunctive NAC: Yolland et al, 2020[48]. n = 220 NAC, 220 placebo. Age: adults; Xu 2022, n = 1165, age adults	B	Moderate	1 Meta-analysis of 7 PDBRCTs 1 Net-work meta-analysis of 17 RCTs including those of supplementation by NAC, ω-3 FA, folic acid and B12	Evidence based	Meta-analysis found longer term (>24 wk) NAC improved working memory, total symptoms, & negative symptoms. In a net-work meta-analysis, adjunctive NAC was significantly more efficacious than folic acid or vitamin B12 & ω-3 FA supplementation in PANSS score changes. If used, needs to be long-term. Although it is evidenced based, more n are urgently needed to determine if the effect size is clinically significant.

(continued on next page)

Table 1
(continued)

Population Schizophrenia Spectrum Disorder (SSD) Stage and Treatment	Recommendation Strength	Certainty (USPTF)	Evidence Base in Youth	Evidence Based or Meets SECS Criteria	Reviewer Recommendations
SSD and 90-min of moderate-to-vigorous physical activity (MVPA) per week or aerobic exercise					
Exercise: Stubbs et al, 2019[55], n = 659 adults with SSD	B	Moderate	1 Meta-analysis 7 RCTs	SECS	Consider, given low risk of harm and many documented benefits of exercise. 90-min MVPA was associated with reduced positive and negative symptoms.
Folate/Folic acid/L-methyl folate add-on to antipsychotics with MTHFR C/T or T/T for SSD					
Sakuma et al, 2018[64] N = 436, folate/ folic acid/ methyl-folate add-on to antipsychotics (FA + AP), N = ≥18	B	Moderate	Meta-analysis (7 DBPCRCTs), (5 = folic acid DBPCRCTs, N = 340, and 2 methyl-folate DBPCRCTs, N = 96)		FA + AP for negative symptoms were more effective than placebo (N = 5, n = 281; SMD = −0.25, 95% CI = −0.49, −0.01, P = .04, I2 = 0%), but not other outcomes. The genotypic variations MTHFR genotypes (G1793A, C677T, and A1298C), MTR and FOLH1 may predict positive response to negative and positive symptoms and need more investigation.

Strength of Recommendations based on benefit and safety

A = Recommend Strongly. There is a high certainty that the net benefit is substantial and safe.

B = Recommend. There is a high certainty that the net benefit is moderate or there is moderate certainty that the net benefit is moderate to substantial and safe.

C = Neutral (offer or provide this service for selected patients depending on individual circumstances, based on professional judgment and patient preferences). There is at least moderate certainty that the net benefit is small.

D = Discourage. There is moderate or high certainty that the service has no net benefit or that the harms outweigh the benefits.

I = Insufficient (if the service is offered, patients should understand the uncertainty about the balance of benefits and harms). Current evidence is insufficient to assess the balance of benefits and harms of the service. Evidence is lacking, of poor quality, or conflicting, and the balance of benefits cannot be determined.

Level of certainty regarding quality

HIGH: Level of evidence with robust positive data meta-analyses or meta-reviews involving two or more RCTs of excellent, robust quality. The available evidence usually includes consistent results from well-designed, well-conducted RCTs in representative child, adolescent, or young adult (18–24 years old) populations, assessing the effects on mental health outcomes.

MODERATE: Level of evidence with robust positive data involving two or more RCTs of excellent, robust quality. The available evidence usually includes consistent results from well-designed, well-conducted RCTs in representative child, adolescent, or young adult (18–24 years old) populations, assessing the effects on mental health outcomes.

LOW: Level of evidence with less than two RCTs with good or average quality. The available evidence is insufficient to assess the effects on mental health outcomes.

SECS criteria

A guide to clinical decisions is that interventions that are Safe, Easy, Cheap, and Sensible (SECS) require less evidence to justify individual trials than those that are Risky, Unrealistic, Difficult, or Expensive (RUDE). Because some of the treatments do not have much solid, compelling evidence but would be reasonable to try with a lower bar of evidence, this criterion is also taken into account. Being risky, unrealistic, difficult OR expensive (RUDE) disqualifies from SECS. The bolded conjunctions are essential in applying this guide.

discriminating biomarker for SC and is associated with worse psychiatric symptom. In males, C. albicans seropositivity conferred increased odds for a schizophrenia diagnosis (OR 2.04–9.53, $P \leq .0001$). In females, *C. albicans* seropositivity conferred increased odds for lower cognitive scores on Repeatable Battery for the Assessment of Neuropsychological Status (RBANS) in schizophrenia (OR 1.12, $P \leq .004$), with significant decreases on memory modules for both disorders ($P \leq .0007–.03$).

Drug naïve, first-episode, normal-weight schizophrenia patients treated after 24-weeks of risperidone treatment were compared to healthy controls. There were significant increases in body weight, BMI, fasting blood-glucose, triglycerides, LDL, hs-CRP, anti-oxidant superoxide dismutase (SOD) and the homeostasis model of assessment of insulin resistance (HOMA-IR) ($P < .001$) in the risperidone treated group. Only the changes in fecal *Bifidobacterium* spp. significantly correlated with the changes in weight (unstandardized coefficient B = 4.413, R^2 change = 0.167, $P = .009$) and BMI (B = 1.639, R^2 change = 0.172, $P = .008$) after 24-week treatment as compared to healthy controls.[74]

One study investigated gut microbiome composition in 50 individuals, including 25 persons with chronic schizophrenia and 25 demographically-matched non-psychiatric comparison subjects (NCs). Within individuals with schizophrenia, abundance of Ruminococcaceae was correlated with lower severity of negative symptoms; Bacteroides were associated with worse depressive symptoms; and Coprococcus was related to greater risk for developing coronary heart disease.[75]

Many of these studies are small, but more research is needed in regard to the microbiome to determine the relationship to first time psychosis, chronic schizophrenia and medication effect.

Guideline-recommended treatments and barriers to their dissemination

It is important to note that a recent literature review provided support for using CBT and family interventions[76–78] in the prevention and psychosocial treatment for early psychosis despite the lack of access in some places. A British systematic review on the implementation of CBT and family interventions (FI) found rates of implementation varied from 4% to 100% for CBT and 0% to 53% for FI. Studies at Exeter University in the UK have found a manualized program (TEMPO) to be helpful to improve communication barriers that exist for psychiatrists (as well as other healthcare providers) with persons experiencing psychosis.[79] Collaboration at all levels of healthcare is needed for effective implementation of guideline-based treatment.

A summary of these studies are found in (**Table 1**) using the United States Preventative Services Task Force ratings for the strength of the recommendation and level of certainty for each study (See **Table 1**).

SUMMARY

Cultural sensitivity regarding the trauma-psychosis link for AIs is needed for equity of care. The prevention of progression of SSD by early identification of UHR and FEP is necessary to improve outcomes. The trial of ω3FA in UHR is supported by the VHR study and biomarker studies on ω3FA-symptom/function correlation. Awaiting better research, the clinical use of ω3FA in UHR is a safe and effective treatment, especially when cognitive-behavior therapy (psychosis) (CBTp) is not feasible. Early identification of FEP is necessary. A longer DUP is associated with worse outcomes. In FEP, the adjunctive use of ω-3FA or NAC may potentially complement AP effects by reducing primary negative symptoms (significant drivers of long-term disability, decreased QOL, and poor outcomes). If NAC is to be used, then a long-term (>24-week treatment) is needed to demonstrate clinical effects, such as improvement in negative symptoms (that respond inadequately to APs). Accumulating evidence is supportive of adjunctive NAC to be a useful and evidence-based treatment for SSD. NAC is also safe, widely available, well tolerated and lacks abuse potential. Exercise in SSD can reduce psychotics symptoms and improves various subdomains of cardiorespiratory fitness. More studies are needed regarding the Microbiome, the MTHFR genotypes and the FRa antibodies and their role in schizophrenia.

CLINICS CARE POINTS

- In youth at ultra-high risk prodrome, recommend ω-3FA in indicated prevention of first-episode psychosis and psychosocial disability in youth with ultra-high risk prodrome. Although CBT and family intervention (FI) have been recommended by guidelines, rates of implementation for CBT and FI have been unsatisfactory. Unlike antipsychotics, ω-3FA are almost completely devoid of serious side effects.

- In first episode psychosis, early identification and intervention is necessary because duration of untreated psychosis is associated with worse outcomes.

- Antipsychotics do not resolve primary negative symptoms of SSD, which are significant drivers of disability, low quality-of-life and poor functional outcomes. Adjunctive ω-3FA, NAC and/or weekly moderate/vigorous aerobic exercise can potentially reduce negative symptoms and improve function, complimenting antipsychotic effects.

- If it is decided that NAC is to be used, then this agent must be used for > 24-week to demonstrate its beneficial and neuroprotective effects. Studies have shown that NAC is almost completely devoid of any serious side effects

DISCLOSURE

The authors have nothing to disclose.

REFERENCES

1. Brave Heart MY, Chase J, Elkins J, et al. Historical trauma among Indigenous Peoples of the Americas: concepts, research, and clinical considerations. J Psychoactive Drugs 2011;43(4):282–90.
2. Rafla-Yuan E, Moore S, Carvente-Martinez H, et al. Striving for equity in community mental health: opportunities and challenges for integrating care for BIPOC youth. Child Adolesc Psychiatr Clin N Am 2022;31(2):295–312.
3. Sikich L, Frazier JA, McClellan J, et al. Double-blind comparison of first- and second-generation antipsychotics in early-onset schizophrenia and schizoaffective disorder: findings from the treatment of early-onset schizophrenia spectrum disorders (TEOSS) study. Am J Psychiatry 2008;165(11):1420–31, published correction appears in Am J Psychiatry. 2008 Nov;165(11):1495.
4. Kendhari J, Shankar R, Young-Walker L. A review of childhood-onset schizophrenia. Focus (Am Psychiatr Publ). 2016;14(3):328–32.
5. Jaaro-Peled H, Sawa A. Neurodevelopmental factors in schizophrenia. Psychiatr Clin North Am 2020;43(2):263–74.
6. Kane JM, Robinson DG, Schooler NR, et al. 2-year outcomes from the NIMH RAISE early treatment program. Am J Psychiatry 2016;173(4):362–72.
7. Lechner A, Cavanaugh M, Blyler C. Addressing trauma in American Indian and Alaska native youth. report. 2016. https://aspe.hhs.gov/pdfreport/addressing-trauma-american-indian-and-alaska-native-youth (Accessed June 30, 2022).

8. Reulbach U, Bleich S, Biermann T, et al. Late-onset schizophrenia in child survivors of the holocaust. J Nerv Ment Dis 2007;195(4):315–9.

9. Popovic D, Schmitt A, Kaurani L, et al. Childhood trauma in schizophrenia: current findings and research perspectives. Front Neurosci 2019;13:274.

10. Marshall M, Lewis S, Lockwood A, et al. Association between duration of untreated psychosis and outcome in cohorts of first-episode patients: a systematic review. Arch Gen Psychiatry 2005;62(9):975–83.

11. Robin RW, Gottesman II, Albaugh B, et al. Schizophrenia and psychotic symptoms in families of two American Indian tribes. BMC Psychiatry 2007;7:30.

12. Bhatara VS, Fuller WC, Fogas BS. An educational perspective of reservation mental health service deficit: the South Dakota experience. Am Indian Alsk Native Ment Health Res 1995;6(3):56–68.

13. Novins DK, Green AE, Legha RK, et al. Dissemination and implementation of evidence-based practices for child and adolescent mental health: a systematic review. J Am Acad Child Adolesc Psychiatry 2014;53(3):382.

14. Yung AR, Yuen HP, McGorry PD, et al. Mapping the onset of psychosis: the comprehensive assessment of at-risk mental states. Aust N Z J Psychiatry 2005;39(11–12):964–71.

15. Mei C, van der Gaag M, Nelson B, et al. Preventive interventions for individuals at ultra-high risk for psychosis: an updated and extended meta-analysis. Clin Psychol Rev 2021;86:102005.

16. Catalan A, Salazar de Pablo G, Vaquerizo Serrano J, et al. Annual Research Review: prevention of psychosis in adolescents—systematic review and meta-analysis of advances in detection, prognosis and intervention. J Child Psychol Psychiatry 2021;62:657–73.

17. Lin A, Wood SJ, Nelson B, et al. Outcomes of nontransitioned cases in a sample at ultra-high risk for psychosis. Am J Psychiatry 2015;172(3):249–58.

18. Bosnjak Kuharic D, Kekin I, Hew J, et al. Interventions for prodromal stage of psychosis. Cochrane Database Syst Rev 2019;2019(11):CD012236.

19. Susai SR, Sabherwal S, Mongan D, et al. Omega-3 fatty acid in ultra-high-risk psychosis: a systematic review based on functional outcome. Early Intervention in Psychiatry 2022;16:3–16.

20. Amminger GP, Schäfer MR, Papageorgiou K, et al. Long-chain omega-3 fatty acids for indicated prevention of psychotic disorders: a randomized, placebo-controlled trial. Arch Gen Psychiatry 2010;67(2):146–54.

21. Amminger GP, Schäfer MR, Schlögelhofer M, et al. Longer-term outcome in the prevention of psychotic disorders by the Vienna omega-3 study. Nat Commun 2015;6:7934.

22. McGorry PD, Nelson B, Markulev C, et al. Effect of ω-3 polyunsaturated fatty acids in young people at ultrahigh risk for psychotic disorders: the NEURAPRO randomized clinical trial. JAMA Psychiatry 2017;74(1):19–27.

23. Kotlicka-Antczak M, Podgórski M, Oliver D, et al. Worldwide implementation of clinical services for the prevention of psychosis: the IEPA early intervention in mental health survey. Early Interv Psychiatry 2020;14(6):741–50.

24. Addington J, Cadenhead KS, Cannon TD, et al. North American Prodrome Longitudinal Study: a collaborative multisite approach to prodromal schizophrenia research. Schizophr Bull 2007;33(3):665–72.

25. Amminger GP, Chanen AM, Ohmann S, et al. Omega-3 fatty acid supplementation in adolescents with borderline personality disorder and ultra-high risk criteria for psychosis: a post hoc subgroup analysis of a double-blind, randomized controlled trial. Can J Psychiatry 2013;58(7):402–8.

26. Nelson B, Amminger GP, Yuen HP, et al. NEURAPRO: a multicentre RCT of omega-3 polyunsaturated fatty acids versus placebo in young people at ultra-high risk of psychotic disorders-medium-term follow-up and clinical course. NPJ Schizophr 2018;4(1):11.

27. Kane JM, Correll CU. ω-3 Polyunsaturated fatty acids to prevent psychosis: the importance of replication studies. JAMA Psychiatry 2017;74(1):11–2.

28. Amminger GP, Nelson B, Markulev C, et al. The NEURAPRO biomarker analysis: long-chain omega-3 fatty acids improve 6-month and 12-month outcomes in youths at ultra-high risk for psychosis. Biol Psychiatry 2020;87(3):243–52.

29. Berger M, Nelson B, Markulev C, et al. Relationship between polyunsaturated fatty acids and psychopathology in the NEURAPRO clinical trial. Front Psychiatry 2019;10:393, published correction appears in Front Psychiatry. 2020 Jun 10;11:514.

30. Frajerman A, Scoriels L, Kebir O, et al. Shared biological pathways between antipsychotics and omega-3 fatty acids: a key feature for schizophrenia preventive treatment? Int J Mol Sci 2021;22(13):6881.

31. Horrobin DF. The membrane phospholipid hypothesis as a biochemical basis for the neurodevelopmental concept of schizophrenia. Schizophr Res 1998;30: 193–208.

32. Smesny S, Milleit B, Hipler UC, et al. Omega-3 fatty acid supplementation changes intracellular phospholipase A2 activity and membrane fatty acid profiles in individuals at ultra-high risk for psychosis. Mol Psychiatry 2014;19(3):317–24.

33. Hsu MC, Huang YS, Ouyang WC. Beneficial effects of omega-3 fatty acid supplementation in schizophrenia: possible mechanisms. Lipids Health Dis 2020; 19(1):159.

34. McEvoy J, Baillie RA, Zhu H, et al. Lipidomics reveals early metabolic changes in subjects with schizophrenia: effects of atypical antipsychotics. PLoS One 2013; 8(7):e68717.

35. Goh KK, Chen CY, Chen CH, et al. Effects of omega-3 polyunsaturated fatty acids supplements on psychopathology and metabolic parameters in schizophrenia: a meta-analysis of randomized controlled trials. J Psychopharmacol 2021;35(3): 221–35.

36. Correll CU, Schooler NR. Negative symptoms in schizophrenia: a review and clinical guide for recognition, assessment, and treatment. Neuropsychiatr Dis Treat 2020;16:519–34.

37. Hsu MC, Ouyang WC. A systematic review of effectiveness of omega-3 fatty acid supplementation on symptoms, social functions, and neurobiological variables in schizophrenia. Biol Res Nurs 2021;23(4):723–37.

38. Pawełczyk T, Grancow-Grabka M, Kotlicka-Antczak M, et al. A randomized controlled study of the efficacy of six-month supplementation with concentrated fish oil rich in omega-3 polyunsaturated fatty acids in first episode schizophrenia. J Psychiatr Res 2016;73:34–44.

39. Pawełczyk T, Trafalska E, Pawełczyk A, et al. Differences in omega-3 and omega-6 polyunsaturated fatty acid consumption in people at ultra-high risk of psychosis, first-episode schizophrenia, and in healthy controls. Early Interv Psychiatry 2017;11(6):498–508.

40. Robinson D, Gallego J, John M, et al. A potential role for adjunctive omega-3 polyunsaturated fatty acids for depression and anxiety symptoms in recent onset psychosis: results from a 16 week randomized placebo-controlled trial for participants concurrently treated with risperidone. Schizophrenia Res 2019;204: 295–303.

41. Chen AT, Chibnall JT, Nasrallah HA. A meta-analysis of placebo-controlled trials of omega-3 fatty acid augmentation in schizophrenia: possible stage-specific effects. Ann Clin Psychiatry 2015;27(4):289–96.

42. Bradlow R, Berk M, Kalivas P, et al. The potential of N-Acetyl-L-Cysteine (NAC) in the treatment of psychiatric disorders. CNS Drugs 2022;36:451–82.

43. Zhang J, Chen B, Lu J. Treatment effect of risperidone alone and combined with N-acetyl-cysteine for first-episode schizophrenic patients. J Clin Psychiatry 2015; 1005:394–6.

44. Breier A, Liffick E, Hummer TA, et al. Effects of 12-month, double-blind N-acetyl cysteine on symptoms, cognition and brain morphology in early phase schizophrenia spectrum disorders. Schizophr Res 2018;199:395–402.

45. Conus P, Seidman LJ, Fournier M, et al. N-acetylcysteine in a double-blind randomized placebo-controlled trial: toward biomarker-guided treatment in early psychosis. Schizophr Bull 2018;44(2):317–27.

46. Klauser P, Xin L, Fournier M, et al. N-acetylcysteine add-on treatment leads to an improvement of fornix white matter integrity in early psychosis: a double-blind randomized placebo-controlled trial. Transl Psychiatry 2018;8(1):1.

47. Cotton SM, Berk M, Watson A, et al. ENACT: a protocol for a randomised placebo-controlled trial investigating the efficacy and mechanisms of action of adjunctive N-acetylcysteine for first-episode psychosis. Trials 2019;20(1):658.

48. Yolland CO, Hanratty D, Neill E, et al. Meta-analysis of randomised controlled trials with N-acetylcysteine in the treatment of schizophrenia. Aust N Z J Psychiatry 2020;54(5):453–66.

49. Xu X, Shao G, Zhang X, et al. The efficacy of nutritional supplements for the adjunctive treatment of schizophrenia in adults: a systematic review and network meta-analysis. Psychiatry Res 2022;311:114500.

50. Yang Y, Davis M, Wynn J, et al. N-acetylcysteine improves EEG measures of auditory deviance detection and neural synchronization in schizophrenia: a randomized, controlled pilot study. Schizophr Res 2019;208:479–80.

51. Pyatoykina AS, Zhilyaeva TV, Semennov IV, et al. The double-blind randomized placebo-controlled trial of N-acetylcysteine use in schizophrenia: preliminary results. Zh Nevrol Psikhiatr Im S S Korsakova 2020;120(9):66–71.

52. Yao JK, Leonard S, Reddy R. Altered glutathione redox state in schizophrenia. Dis markers 2006;22(1–2):83–93.

53. Dean O, Giorlando F, Berk M. N-acetylcyteine in psychiatry: current therapeutic evidence and potential mechanisms of action. J Psychiatry Neurosci 2011; 36(2):78–86.

54. Naguy A, Naguy C. N-acetyl-cysteine in schizophrenia—there is more than meets the eyes. CNS Spectrums 2021;26(5):446–7.

55. Stubbs B, Vancampfort D, Hallgren M, et al. EPA guidance on physical activity as a treatment for severe mental illness: a meta-review of the evidence and Position Statement from the European Psychiatric Association (EPA), supported by the International Organization of Physical Therapists in Mental Health (IOPTMH). Eur Psychiatry 2018;54:124–44.

56. Cotman CW, Berchtold NC, Christie L-A. Exercise builds brain health: key roles of growth factor cascades and inflammation. Trends. Neurosci 2007;30:464–72.

57. Noordsy DL, Burgess JD, Hardy KV, et al. Therapeutic potential of physical exercise in early psychosis. Am J Psychiatry 2018;175(3):209–14.

58. Hallgren M, Skott M, Ekblom Ö, et al. Exercise effects on cognitive functioning in young adults with first-episode psychosis: fit for Life. Psychol Med 2019;49(3): 431–9.

59. Shannon A, McGuire D, Brown E, et al. A systematic review of the effectiveness of group-based exercise interventions for individuals with first episode psychosis. Psychiatry Res 2020;293:113402.

60. Fernández-Abascal B, Suárez-Pinilla P, Cobo-Corrales C, et al. In- and outpatient lifestyle interventions on diet and exercise and their effect on physical and psychological health: a systematic review and meta-analysis of randomised controlledtrials in patients with schizophrenia spectrum disorders and first episode of psychosis. Neurosci Biobehav Rev 2021;125:535–68.

61. Woodward ML, Lin J, Gicas KM, et al. Medial temporal lobe cortical changes in response to exercise interventions in people with early psychosis: a randomized controlled trial. Schizophr Res 2020;223:87–95.

62. Damme KSF, Gupta T, Ristanovic I, et al. Exercise intervention in individuals at clinical high risk for psychosis: benefits to fitness, symptoms, hippocampal volumes, and functional connectivity. Schizophr Bull 2022;48(6):1394–405.

63. Gaughran F, Stringer D, Wojewodka G, et al. Effect of vitamin D supplementation on outcomes in people with early psychosis: the DFEND randomized clinical trial. JAMA Netw Open 2021;4(12):e2140858.

64. Sakuma K, Matsunaga S, Nomura I, et al. Folic acid/methylfolate for the treatment of psychopathology in schizophrenia: a systematic review and meta-analysis. Psychopharmacology (Berl) 2018;235(8):2303–14. Epub 2018 May 22. PMID: 29785555.

65. Hill M, Shannahan K, Jasinski S, et al. Folate supplementation in schizophrenia: a possible role for MTHFR genotype. Schizophr Res 2011;127(1–3):41–5 [PubMed: 21334854].

66. Roffman JL, Lamberti JS, Achtyes E, et al. Randomized multicenter investigation of folate plus vitamin B12 supplementation in schizophrenia. JAMA Psychiatr 2013;70:481–9.

67. Roffman JL, Petruzzi LJ, Tanner AS, et al. Biochemical, physiological and clinical effects of l-methylfolate in schizophrenia: a randomized controlled trial. Mol Psychiatry 2017;23(2):316–22.

68. Levine J, Stahl Z, Sela BA, et al. Homocysteine-reducing strategies improve symptoms in chronic schizophrenic patients with hyperhomocysteinemia. Biol Psychiatry 2006;60(3):265–9. Epub 2006 Jan 17. PMID: 16412989.

69. Wan L, Li Y, Zhou Y, et al. Age matters: an atypical association between polymorphism of MTHFR and clinical phenotypes in children with schizophrenia. J Mol Neurosci 2019;69(3):485–93. Epub 2019 Jul 13. PMID: 31302825.

70. Ramaekers VT, Thöny B, Sequeira JM, et al. Folinic acid treatment for schizophrenia associated with folate receptor autoantibodies. Mol Genet Metab 2014;113(4):307–14. Epub 2014 Oct 12. PMID: 25456743.

71. Ramaekers VT, Sequeira JM, Blau N, et al. A milk-free diet downregulates folate receptor autoimmunity in cerebral folate deficiency syndrome. Dev Med Child Neurol 2008;50(5):346–52. Epub 2008 Mar 19. PMID: 18355335; PMCID: PMC2715943.

72. Zhang X, Pan LY, Zhang Z, et al. Analysis of gut mycobiota in first-episode, drug-naïve Chinese patients with schizophrenia: A pilot study. Behav Brain Res 2020;379:112374. Epub 2019 Nov 20. PMID: 31759045.

73. Severance EG, Gressitt KL, Stallings CR, et al. Candida albicans exposures, sex specificity and cognitive deficits in schizophrenia and bipolar disorder. NPJ Schizophrenia 2016;2(1):1–7.

74. Yuan X, Zhang P, Wang Y, et al. Changes in metabolism and microbiota after 24-week risperidone treatment in drug naïve, normal weight patients with first

episode schizophrenia. Schizophrenia Research 2018;201:299–306. ISSN 0920-9964.

75. Nguyen TT, Kosciolek T, Maldonado Y, et al. Differences in gut microbiome composition between persons with chronic schizophrenia and healthy comparison subjects. Schizophr Res 2019;204:23–9. Epub 2018 Sep 26. PMID: 30268819; PMCID.

76. Galletly C, Castle D, Dark F, et al. Royal Australian and New Zealand College of Psychiatrists clinical practice guidelines for the management of schizophrenia and related disorders. Aust N Z Psychiatry 2016;50(5):410–72.

77. Lecomte T, Abidi S, Garcia-Ortega I, et al. Canadian treatment guidelines on psychosocial treatment of schizophrenia in children and youth. Can J Psychiatry 2017;62(9):648–55.

78. Ince P, Haddock G, Tai S. A systematic review of the implementation of recommended psychological interventions for schizophrenia: rates, barriers, and improvement strategies. Psychol Psychother 2016;89(3):324–50.

79. McCabe R, John P, Dooley J, et al. Training to enhance psychiatrist communication with patients with psychosis (TEMPO): cluster randomised controlled trial. Br J Psychiatry 2016;209(6):517–24.

FURTHER READINGS

Galletly C, Castle D, Dark F, Royal, et al. Australian and New Zealand College of Psychiatrists clinical practice guidelines for the management of schizophrenia and related disorders. Australian & New Zealand Journal of Psychiatry 2016;50(5): 410–72. https://doi.org/10.1177/0004867416641195.

Lecomte T, Abidi S, Garcia-Ortega I, et al. Canadian Treatment Guidelines on Psychosocial Treatment of Schizophrenia in Children and Youth. The Canadian Journal of Psychiatry 2017;62(9):648–55. https://doi.org/10.1177/0706743717720195.

Ince P, Haddock G, Tai S. A systematic review of the implementation of recommended psychological interventions for schizophrenia: Rates, barriers, and improvement strategies. Psychol Psychother 2016;89(3):324–50. https://doi.org/10.1111/papt. 12084.

Complementary and Integrative Treatments of Aggressiveness/Emotion Dysregulation: Associated with Disruptive Disorders and Disruptive Mood Dysregulation Disorder

Vinod S. Bhatara, MD, MS, MSHS[a,b],*, Bettina Bernstein, DO[c,d],
Sheeba Fazili, MA[e]

KEYWORDS

- Emotion dysregulation • Irritability • Disruptive disorders
- Complementary and integrative treatments

KEY POINTS

- The degree of impairing emotion dysregulation (ED) and aggressiveness associated with disruptive disorders and disruptive mood dysregulation disorder (highly comorbid with attention-deficit/hyperactivity disorder [ADHD]) and the disruption to family and school settings makes this one of the most frequent reasons for a psychiatric referral. This article covers CIM treatments that may be helpful.
- Broad spectrum micronutrients supplementation: Two blinded RCTs showed that this treatment reduced aggressiveness/ED in children (low-medium effects, $d = 0.16$ to $d = 1.1$; risk ratio 2.97; 97.5% CI 1.50, 5.90) and is safe (including height growth > placebo). Such supplementation has shown larger effects than those of adjunctive Ω-3 fatty acids ($d = 0.16–0.21$) and similar to those of psychosocial treatments.
- The small effect seen with Ω-3 fatty acids may be due to research design and may require using the Ω-3 index when using eicosapentaenoic acid and docosahexaenoic acid.

Continued

---

[a] Department of Psychiatry, University of South Dakota, Sanford School of Medicine, Sioux Falls, SD, USA; [b] Department of Pediatrics, University of South Dakota, Sanford School of Medicine, Sioux Falls, SD, USA; [c] Philadelphia College of Osteopathic Medicine, 4170 City Ave, Philadelphia, PA 19131, USA; [d] Department of Child and Adolescent Psychiatry, The Children's Hospital of Philadelphia, 3401 Civic Center Blvd, Philadelphia, PA 19104, USA; [e] University of South Dakota Sanford School of Medicine, 4400 West 69th street, suite 1500, Sioux Falls, SD 57104, USA
* Corresponding author. 2601 W Nicole Drive, Sioux Falls, SD 57105.
E-mail address: vsbhatara@gmail.com

Child Adolesc Psychiatric Clin N Am 32 (2023) 297–315
https://doi.org/10.1016/j.chc.2022.08.010
1056-4993/23/© 2022 Elsevier Inc. All rights reserved.

Continued

- Decreasing exposure to virtual violence: Several meta-analyses have found a small but consistent association between media violence exposure and aggressiveness. Parents should manage the media experience of youth.
- Increased exposure to green (foliage) and blue (water) space is associated with decreased ED.

INTRODUCTION

Impairing emotional outbursts (IEO) is defined by extreme anger or distress in response to relatively ordinary frustrations and disappointments, is a cross-cutting, neurodevelopmental, early-onset disabling problem of regulating emotions.[1] This article uses a broader term emotion dysregulation (ED) that is like IEO but has been more frequently used in the literature. ED/ aggressiveness is frequently comorbid with Disruptive Disorders (oppositional defiant disorder [ODD], conduct disorder [CD]) and disruptive mood dysregulation disorder [DMDD].[2] Disruptive Disorders associated with ED/ aggressiveness are major public health problems and are frequently comorbid with attention-deficit/hyperactivity disorder (ADHD). They are one of the most frequent reasons for psychiatric referral.[2–6] This article covers CIM treatments that may be helpful for ED/ aggressiveness associated with disruptive disorders (**Table 1**). Conventional treatments underserve youth with ED/irritability/aggression. Complementary and integrative (CIM) treatments can optimize their care.[7]

At least 40% of ADHD cases are also complicated by ED.[8–11] ED is a significant contributor to ADHD impairment. ED negatively predicts short-term response to methylphenidate in medication-naive youth with ADHD. Youth with ED/aggressiveness are clinically challenging, require multiple treatments, and are at risk for functional impairment and poor outcomes.[12]

DIFFERENTIAL DIAGNOSIS

ED is a cross-cutting, neurodevelopmental, early-onset disorder regulating emotions, co-morbid with a wide range of internalizing and externalizing disorders.[13] Differential diagnosis can be challenging.[1] Indeed, in two large community samples, DMDD was highly associated with ODD,[14,15] leading Freeman to highlight the need to clarify the difference.

Unlike ODD, DMDD must have duration of 1 year or more, be present in more than one setting, and require outburst frequency several times a week.[16] DMDD preempts the diagnosis of ODD or intermittent explosive disorder.[16] Also, 77% of youth with DMDD may have coexisting ADHD, CD,[15] and/or substance use disorder. Longitudinal follow-ups have shown that youth with DMDD have no increased risk of bipolar disorder as adults.[17,18] However, a wide range of diagnoses is associated with DMDD in older adolescents, including borderline personality disorder,[19] post-traumatic stress disorder (PTSD)/dissociative disorders,[20] and bipolar disorder[21] or major depressive disorder symptoms.

UNMET NEEDS: JUSTIFICATION FOR COMPLEMENTARY AND INTEGRATIVE TREATMENT

The need for CIM interventions in youth with ODD, CD, and DMDD who also have ED/aggressiveness is justified by dissatisfaction with the safety and effectiveness of

Table 1
Complementary and integrative treatments of aggressiveness/emotion dysregulation: Associated with disruptive disorders and disruptive mood dysregulation disorder

Treatment	Level of certainty based on benefit and quality of evidence	Strength of recommendation based on Benefit and Safety	Evidence of Base in Youth/ Basis for Recommendation	Personal Recommendations of the Reviewer/Passes SECS
I. Supplements and Diets				
Broad-spectrum micronutrients a. DBPCRCT (BSM, all-known vitamins + minerals with amino acids) (Johnstone et al, 2022[36], $N = 126$, 8-week) b. DBPCRCT Nonmedicated ADHD children 6–12 years with irritability (Rucklidge et al, 2014[27], 2018[32])	Moderate	B	A and b=2 DBPCRCTs	Showed that BSM decreased Irritability + inattention $d = 0.16$ -1.1 (RR 2.97; 97.5% CI 1.50–5.90) Safe and efficacious. Recommend, preferably before medication titration. (Passes SECS)
Omega (ω)-3 fatty acids a. 40 studies, youth and adults, but effect size (ES) did not vary with age, (Gajos et al, 2016[43], 73 ESs, $N = 7173$) b. 4 high-quality RCTs in children: $N = 1352$ (Cooper et al, 2016[44], 10 studies)	a. Low b. Moderate	a. C b. B	a. meta-analyses b. meta-analyses with 4 RCTs	Small effect size ($d \sim .20$) due to small-N + not using ω-3 Index Suggest adjunctive Omega (ω)-fatty acids, preferably foods rich in ω-3, but supplementation acceptable. (Passes SECS)
II. Interactive Interpersonal Activities				
Music-based interventions Ye et al, 2021[55] (10 trials in children age ≤16 years:, $N = 3465$)	Low	C	Meta-analysis of 10 trials no RCTs	Music therapy reduced aggression and improved self-control (standardized mean difference [SMD] = -1.79; 95% CI = -3.23) Recommended for use, awaiting better research, may have small but positive neurodevelopmental effects (Passes SECS, OK in schools)

(continued on next page)

Table 1
(continued)

Treatment	Level of certainty based on benefit and quality of evidence	Strength of recommendation based on Benefit and Safety	Evidence of Base in Youth/ Basis for Recommendation	Personal Recommendations of the Reviewer/Passes SECS
Martial arts Meta-analysis of 12 studies (4 experimental) on disruptive disorders and martial arts (Harwood et al, 2017[59], N = 507 children)	Low	C	Meta-analysis no RCTs	Martial arts training reduced aggressiveness Encourage youth participation in martial arts, need more research studies (Passes SECS)
III. External Factors				
Violent Video Games (VVG)				
Restriction of VVG: 1 meta-analysis in youth, mean age 13.5 years, range 8.9 to 23.1 years (Burkhardt et al, 2022[58]), 4 meta-analyses in adults (American Psychological Association Violent Videogame Task Force 2015[57])	High	B	One meta-analysis in youth with 30 effect sizes from 21 observational longitudinal studies (N = 15,836).	A significant and relevant positive effect of VVG exposure on subsequent physically aggressive behavior ($r = .21$), with a peak of effect sizes in early adolescence. VVG increase negative outcomes (aggressive behavior, cognitions, and affect) and decrease positive outcomes (prosocial behavior, empathy, and sensitivity to aggression). Parents should strictly enforce Entertainment Software Ratings Board age ratings, and manage VVG watching in youth < 16 years. (Restricting VVG in children and adolescents is evidence-based)

IV. Environmental Factors

a. Green space and blue space are protective. Used linear regression model to determine NDVI. (Madzia, 2019[69], n = 562, data collected at age 7)	a. Low	a. C	Data analyzed from the Cincinnati Childhood Allergy and Air Pollution Study, an ongoing prospective birth cohort study. No RCTs	a. Externalizing behaviors as measured on the BASC-2 at age 7 reduced for those living within 1/10 mile of green space. Passes SECS
b. Exposure used a linear regression model to calculate NVDI (Younan, 2016[70], n = 1,287)	b. Low	b. C	b. Data analyzed from a multi-ethnic cohort of twins and triplets born from 1990 to 1995. No RCTs	b. Adolescents' exposure to green space had a 0.36 to 0.41 reduction in aggressive behavior scores and there were earlier decreased conduct problem scores at age 7. Green space was equivalent to 2 to 2.5 years of behavioral maturation for adolescents. Passes SECS
c. Secondhand and thirdhand tobacco Smoke. Multivariable logistic regression analyses. (Mahabee-Gittens, 2022[73], n = 21,539 of 6- to 11-year-olds and n = 11,439 of youth aged 9 to 11 years old.)	c. Low	c. C	c. Secondary analysis of the 2018–2019 National Survey of Children's Health data	c. Among children aged 6 to 11 years old especially younger age children who lived with a smoker had increased odds of behavioral conduct problems and ADHD as well as other problems such as anxiety. Passes SECS
d. Systemic review Blue (water) space for well-being (Britton et al, 2020[72], n = 2073 of which 1468 were ages	d. Low	d. C for physical health and mental health	d. Systemic Review. No RCTs	d. Suggest that blue spaces can have a direct benefit on health, especially mental health and psychosocial well-being and suggest that blue spaces can have a direct benefit for health, especially mental health and psychosocial well-being. Inconsistent and mixed results across studies with very few findings for physical health. Green/outdoor spaces desirable.

(continued on next page)

Table 1
(continued)

Treatment	Level of certainty based on benefit and quality of evidence	Strength of recommendation based on Benefit and Safety	Evidence of Base in Youth/ Basis for Recommendation	Personal Recommendations of the Reviewer/Passes SECS
				Increased participation in physical activity may improve self-esteem, and parents of children with aggression should encourage physical activity outside. Recommend caregivers do not smoke tobacco-containing products at home and encourage smoke-free environments in all locations including public places. Passes SECS

Strength of Recommendations based on benefit and safety

A = Recommend Strongly. There is a high certainty that the net benefit is substantial *and safe.*

B = Recommend. There is a high certainty that the net benefit is moderate or there is moderate certainty that the net benefit is moderate to substantial *and safe.*

C = Neutral (offer or provide this service for selected patients depending on individual circumstances, based on professional judgment and patient preferences). There is at least moderate certainty that the net benefit is small.

D = Discourage. There is moderate or high certainty that the service has no net benefit or that the harms outweigh the benefits.

I = Insufficient (if the service is offered, patients should understand the uncertainty about the balance of benefits and harms). Current evidence is insufficient to assess the balance of benefits and harms of the service. Evidence is lacking, of poor quality, or conflicting, and the balance of benefits cannot be determined. Level of certainty regarding quality.

HIGH: Level of evidence with robust positive data meta-analyses or meta-reviews involving two or more RCTs of excellent, robust quality. The available evidence usually includes consistent results from well-designed, well-conducted RCTs in representative child, adolescent, or young adult (18–24 years old) populations, assessing the effects on mental health outcomes.

MODERATE: Level of evidence with robust positive data involving two or more RCTs of excellent, robust quality. The available evidence usually includes consistent results from well-designed, well-conducted RCTs in representative child, adolescent, or young adult (18–24 years old) populations, assessing the effects on mental health outcomes.

LOW: Level of evidence with less than two RCTs with good or average quality. The available evidence is insufficient to assess the effects on mental health outcomes.

SECS criteria: A guide to clinical decisions is that Interventions that are Safe, Easy, Cheap, and Sensible (SECS) require less evidence to justify individual trials than those that are Risky, Unrealistic, Difficult, or Expensive (RUDE). Because some of the treatments do not have much solid, compelling evidence but would be reasonable to try with a lower bar of evidence, this criterion is also taken into account. Being RUDE disqualifies from SECS. The bolded conjunctions are essential in applying this guide.

psychopharmacological treatments. In addition, psychosocial treatments that target underlying IEO are still developing.[5,12] An 8-week RCT[6] found aggression remitting in nearly three out of five children with rigorous optimization of stimulants; however, a significant minority of patients did not respond. Although stimulants and other medications can reduce symptoms, stimulants wear off at the end of the school day, failing to address evening needs. There are also concerns about the side effects of stimulants (such as height and appetite suppression, mood changes, daily withdrawal irritability, and decreased sleep).

When aggressiveness does not remit with stimulants, adjunctive medications such as risperidone have been used. However, the incremental improvement in children who needed adjunctive medication was slight compared with initial stimulant improvement.[5,22] In addition, adverse effects include the risk of metabolic syndrome, weight gain, abnormal lipids, and hyperglycemia. Therefore, adding antipsychotics may not be appropriate, given the side effects. In addition, clinicians need guidance about where to turn when significantly dysregulated children respond only partially to stimulants.[23]

Owing to the poor efficacy of pharmacological treatments and adverse side effects, youth with ED/aggressiveness coexisting with disruptive disorders and DMDD may benefit from CIM treatments.[7] Furthermore, as disruptive disorders and DMDD frequently have coexisting ADHD, it is not surprising that most CIM treatments reviewed in this article are also treatments for ADHD.[1]

NUTRITIONAL TREATMENTS

Nutritional intervention is one of the most evidence-based CIM treatments for ODD, CD, and DMDD with aggression/ED. The rationale is related to individual genetic and physiologic differences in absorption, metabolism, and distribution locally within the gut and systemic needs throughout the body. These interventions result in significant individual variability in need for various nutrients.[24] Because many micronutrients are involved in many biologic roles, optimal functioning requires adequate levels of all nutrients.[24] Supplementation with a single nutrient (eg, zinc, magnesium) has shown mixed and modest benefits in a few cases, but no single magic nutrient works in most cases.[25] Broad-spectrum micronutrient (BSM) supplementation is more consistent with physiological reality. BSM formulations (vitamins + minerals + amino acids) have demonstrated more robust effects than formulas with fewer ingredients[24] and effectiveness seem comparable to conventional non-psychopharmacological treatments in youth, with markedly fewer side effects and a more long-term stable course.[26]

EFFECTS OF BROAD-SPECTRUM MICRONUTRIENT IN ADHD + IRRITABILITY: IS THERE AN IRRITABLE SUBTYPE OF ADHD?

Based on the ratings from clinicians, parents, and teachers in a 10-week DBRCT in 7 to 12 years old medication-free children ($N = 93$) with ADHD[27] have highlighted that BSM was found to have low to medium effects in reducing IEO, irritability/aggressiveness, and function (ES 0.35–0.66). The direct benefit for core ADHD symptoms was modest (with mixed findings across raters) for improving attention, not hyperactivity. Results of this study led them to register a large, three-site North American DBRCT known as MADDY (Micronutrients for Attention-Deficit Disorder in Youths),[28] designed to investigate changes in behavioral and biological measures in children with ADHD and irritability using a commercially available BSM. Based on research suggesting an irritable ADHD subtype[29,30] and on the findings of the Rucklidge study,[27] MADDY focused on ADHD children who also had irritability.

BROAD-SPECTRUM MICRONUTRIENT INGREDIENTS

In their trial registration article for MADDY, Johnstone[28] described a 36-ingredient BSM formulation (14 vitamins, 16 minerals, 3 amino acids, and 3 antioxidants). This formula was initially developed by David Hardy and Tony Stephan.[31] The slightly modified versions of the original formula, marketed as EMPower plus by TrueHope, and as Daily Essential Nutrient, by Hardy Nutritionals, were used by the MADDY study[32] and two previous studies.[27,32] EMPower plus[25] has an established safety record for the relatively high dosages of micronutrients (above Recommended Daily Allowances/Dietary Reference Intakes [RDA/RDI] but below the tolerable upper limit) used in the MADDY study.[24,33] Because the brain has active metabolism and RDA levels have not been established for brain function (particularly for persons with psychiatric disorders), dosages higher than RDA/DRI (but not "megavitamin" doses) were used.[24]

Kaplan and Rucklidge[26] explain that BSM may enable several brain functions. First, feeding the brain with a steady supply of micronutrients to provide cofactors optimizes brain metabolism ("tuning up of brain metabolism"), enabling critical brain functions, homeostasis, and multiple biochemical reactions, such as synthesis and catabolism of neurotransmitters. The high need for nutrition by the brain may be gleaned from observations that cerebral metabolism requires 20% of the body's oxygen while representing only 2% of total body weight. To illustrate this point, the metabolism of dopamine (relevant for the pathophysiology of ADHD) is noted to require seven micronutrients: four minerals (iron, copper, zinc, and magnesium) and three vitamins (pyridoxine or B6, riboflavin or B2, and ascorbic acid).[34,35] Second, BSM may improve the production of adenosine triphosphate for energy by providing additional vitamins (C and E) and amino acid acetyl L-carnitine. Third, BSM may keep genes healthy by improving methylation balance. Fourth, BSM may help fight inflammation; inflammatory cytokines may play a role. Fifth, BSM may help with protection from toxins.

Micronutrients for ADHD in Youth (MADDY) Study

This study was a fully blinded, 3-site, 8-week randomized controlled trial in 126 children and evaluated the effectiveness of BSM supplementation in children with ADHD and disabling symptoms of irritability.[36] Participants were non-medicated (psychotropic medication-free for at least 2 weeks before participation). Randomization was to BSM capsules (gradually titrated up to 9–12/day in three doses) versus visually identical capsules containing cellulose filler and 0.1 mg of riboflavin per capsule to mimic the color of urine when supplemented. Using two primary outcome measures (the clinician-completed Clinical Global Impression [CGI]and the parent-completed Child and Adolescent Symptom Inventory 5 [CASI-5]), Johnstone and associates[32] found that[1] the percentage of CGI-I responders within the supplement group was significantly greater than with placebo (54% vs 18%),[2] height growth was significantly greater within the supplement group than placebo, and[3] parents reported improvement on CASI-5 scores in both groups without group differences. In addition, the intervention and placebo groups did not differ in the 18 core symptoms of ADHD on the CASI-5. This study replicated a similar fully blinded RCT in children by Rucklidge.[27] This replicated finding suggests that this treatment is helpful for 40% to 50% of ADHD children who also have ED. A DBRCT and an open trial in adults also found similar beneficial effects of BSM in adults.[33,37]

The effect sizes reported in MADDY (range, 0.16–1.14) matched or exceeded those of other non-pharmacological treatments, including elimination diets (SMD 0.21–0.46), omega-3 (Ω-3) fatty acids (SMD 0.16–0.21), and psychological treatment (SMD 0.40–0.64). Without head-to-head trials, it is premature to draw firm conclusions about the differential efficacy of BSM versus other interventions for ADHD + BD. Nonetheless, comments by Stevenson[7] in his editorial accompanying the MADDY publication are pertinent. Comparing relative risk ratios (RR) of the BSM formula (RR 2.97; 97.5% CI 1.50, 5.90) with methylphenidate (5.22 assuming 18% placebo response as in MADDY) and behavior therapy (RR 2.96),[38] Stevenson[7] concluded that the efficacy of BSM was equal to that of behavior therapy. However, methylphenidate was more efficacious than the two non-pharmacological treatments. From the perspective of ADHD children with ED, research studies on combined therapy with BSM + behavior therapy or parent training[39] were recommended as more benign interventions.

Adverse effects did not exceed placebo and previously reported safety of BSM was confirmed. Because the patients were not on any medications, no conclusions can be drawn about BSM–drug interactions. Popper[25] has reviewed safety data on BSM formulations, reporting them to be generally safe. Based on clinical experience, he reported a likely 3- to 5-fold potentiation of most psychotropics and 100-fold potentiation of lithium by BSM. These results mean that in youths on BSM, lithium should be avoided, and[2] dosages of most psychotropics may need to be carefully reduced (about 20%–30% in his experience) and even stopped. Such transitions from conventional medications to BSM are complex and may be complicated by withdrawal syndromes (from benzodiazepine or selective serotonin reuptake inhibitor [SSRI]) because BSM seems to potentiate the withdrawal reactions. He recommends careful supervision by a clinician with knowledge and experience in using BSM. Without previous experience, starting with a medication-naive patient is best to avoid BSM–drug interactions.

HOUSEHOLD FOOD INSECURITY–ED RELATIONSHIP

Using data from 134 children aged 6 to 12 years old enrolled in MADDY study, Hatsu[40] found food insecurity to be directly associated with more severe ED (β = 2.30; 95% CI = 0.87–3.73; P = 0.002), conduct problems (β = 1.15; 95% CI = 0.01–2.30; P = 0.049), and total difficulties scores (β = 4.59; 95% CI = 1.82–7.37; P = 0.001) after adjusting for covariates (child's sex, parent marital status, household income, parental anxiety, and other parental psychopathology). Discussing and addressing food insecurity may be appropriate initial steps for youths with ADHD and ED.[41]

ADJUNCTIVE OMEGA-3 FATTY ACIDS: EICOSAPENTAENOIC ACID AND DOCOSAHEXAENOIC ACID)

Systematic reviews support the clinical use of adjunctive Ω-3 in disruptive disorders with ED/aggressiveness, and meta-analyses have mostly (but not unanimously) supported a low ES (d ~ 0.20).[42] An exception is a meta-analysis by Gajos and Beaver[43] that found Ω-3 fatty acids to have a small to large ES in reducing aggressive behaviors in child and adult populations. Data from 40 studies (n = 7173) were meta-analyzed to calculate 73 ESs separately for two-group comparison studies (SMD = 0.20), pre–post contrast studies (ESsg = 0.62), and associational studies (r = −0.06), in the fixed-effect model. Findings from the random-effects model were similar (SMD = 0.24; ESsg = 0.82; r = −0.09). Based on the unsatisfactory findings from a meta-analysis of 10 trials, Cooper[44] focused on a subgroup analysis of four high-quality (better sample size + low bias risk) RCTs (n = 1352). They found that Ω-3 significantly reduced ED + oppositionality. However, due to factors such as low N, they concluded that Ω-3 might have a small effect on ED/aggressiveness.

The small ES seen with adjunctive Ω-3 may be due to the research design and may require using the Ω-3 Index, defined as the percentage of eicosapentaenoic acid (EPA) + docosahexaenoic acid (DHA) in the erythrocyte cell membrane as a measure (biomarker) of body Ω-3 status.[45] Because of interindividual differences in bioavailability of Ω-3 fatty acids, EPA/DHA erythrocyte levels correlate better with complex brain functions than reliance on drug dosages used in conventional trials. In addition, effect sizes are more significant in trials that have targeted the Ω-3 Index.[46] Compiling recent data supports the target range for the Ω-3 index of 8% to 11%,[47] suggesting that future trial designs of EPA/DHA be based on the targeted Ω-3 index as a better approach.

However, meanwhile a recent meta-analysis and review[46] recommended "ADHD: a combination of EPA + DHA ≥ 750 mg/d and a higher dose of EPA (1200 mg/d) for those with inflammation or allergic diseases for duration of 16 to 24 weeks." The latter may be more beneficial to children with ADHD due to the reduction of inflammation associated with Ω-3s.

OMEGA-3 INDEX AND PREGNANCY

To prevent premature childbirth and maternal and child health issues in pregnancy, Von Schacky[47] recommends (based on the indirect evidence of the poor correlation between dosage and Ω-3 Index) that the target range for the erythrocyte Ω-3 Index of 8% to 11% during pregnancy and in lactation period, rather than relying on the recommended increased dose of Ω-3 by 200 mg daily.

SAFETY DATA

Ω-3 fatty acids have been extensively studied, and they have been found to be well tolerated. Based on their systematic review of safety data from 21 RCTs ($n = 24,460$: 12,750 intervention group and 11,710 controls) on marketed Ω-3 (EPA and DHA) products[48] reported that they found no severe side effects and general good tolerability. The most frequently reported side effects were nausea and a fishy aftertaste, but they were mild and rarely induced discontinuation. Compared with controls, intervention group also had significantly more skin abnormalities (eruption, itching, exanthema, or eczema). An important precaution to note is that Ω-3 fatty acids, depending on the preferences of an anesthesiologist, may need to be stopped 2 weeks before surgery.

MECHANISM OF ACTION

Ω-3 fatty acids are essential fatty acids because they cannot be efficiently synthesized by the human body and have to be ingested.[49] Although mechanism of action of Ω-3 fatty acids in ED/aggressiveness associated with disruptive disorders is unclear, several lines of evidence support that Ω-3 fatty acids (particularly EPA and DHA) improve brain function in neurodevelopmental disorders such as ADHD perhaps because youth with ADHD have greater severity of insufficient Ω-3 fatty acids.[49–51] DHA and EPA also have an anti-inflammatory action via inhibition of free radical generation and oxidized stress and have also been shown to regulate neurotransmitter and immune functions. Ω-3 fatty acids play a part in the production of phospholipids in neuronal membranes in the central nervous system. They are responsible for fluidity and permeability of the neuronal membrane.[52,53] Ω-3 fatty acids can alter serotonin (5-HT) and dopamine neurotransmission.[54] The effectiveness of Ω-3 in conditions characterized by high levels of aggression may be partly due to the effect of these compounds in enhancing the serotonin system that is implicated in inhibiting impulsive aggression[54] and optimization of dopamine system that has multiple effects, including those on the reward system. The modulatory role of 5-HT in aggression is strongly supported by studies of acute manipulations of 5-HTergic availability in humans.[55] Most likely, 5-HT influences aggression through neural networks involving the amygdala, ventromedial prefrontal regions, and the striatum. The neural basis of the complex relationship between 5-HT and aggression likely involves neural circuits that are modulated by 5-HT. However, these pathways are also involved in the various facets of appraisal and response to social threat-stimuli. Thus, deficiencies in serotonergic innervation of these regions could be expected to result in disinhibited aggression on provocation.

The beneficial effects of Ω-3 EPA and DHA may also be explained by their ability to reduce inflammation as opposed to the Ω-6 arachidonic acid, which has pro-inflammatory effects.[52–54] Brain structure and optimal brain function depend on a constant and sufficient supply with EPA and DHA by blood (perfusion and, in some cases, on the absence of inflammatory processes).[46] In addition, the fatty acid composition of a cell's membrane impacts on physical stability, signal transduction, ion channel behavior, and many other cell properties and functions.

GROUP MUSIC THERAPY

Definitions: Music therapy (MT) is evidence-based psychotherapy (with emphasis on credentialed music therapist–patient relationship) with individualized goals. Music medicine (MM) involves professionals other a credentialed music therapists (eg, medical personnel, music teachers, or clinicians) who prescribe music as a medicine for symptom management. MM may use prerecorded or live music, depending mainly on the direct effects of music.

Ye,[55] in a meta-analysis of 10 trials of music-based interventions in children aged ≤16 years (N = 3465), found that relative to controls, MT (but not MM) was more effective in reducing aggression and improving self-control (SMD = −1.79; 95% CI = −3.23 to −0.35). Subgroup analyses showed that greater efficacy was associated with: a frequent number of sessions (≥2 per week), age of 10 years or older, and more severe aggression at baseline. Despite the limitations of their study (small sample sizes and lack of blinding), Ye provided a cost-effective model of music groups (involving ≥2 weekly sessions with a 12-week duration) that may be generalizable to other school systems. Music-based interventions are recommended, awaiting better research, because they may have minor positive neurodevelopmental effects. Hudziak[56] found that playing a musical instrument was associated with more rapid cortical thickness maturation within areas in motor planning and coordination, visuospatial ability, and emotion and impulse regulation.

RESTRICTION OF VIOLENT VIDEO GAMES (VVG)

Based on an analysis of four meta-analyses, a task force American Psychological Association (APA) found evidence for the small but consistent effect of violent video games on increasing aggression in laboratory experiments, cross-sectional, and longitudinal studies.[57]

A major limitation of APA[57] studies was insufficient data on youth 16 years or younger and dearth of data on children younger than 10 years. A recent meta-analysis of 30 effect sizes from 21 longitudinal studies (N=15,836, mean age 13.5 years, range 8.9 to 23.1 years) examined age-dependent effects of VVG on aggression.[58] A significant and relevant positive effect of VVG on subsequent physically aggressive behavior (r = .21), with a peak of effect sizes in early adolescence. VVG increase negative outcomes (aggressive behavior, cognitions, and affect) and decrease positive outcomes (prosocial behavior, empathy, and sensitivity to aggression). These findings lead to the recommendation that parents should strictly enforce "https://www.esrb.org/" Entertainment Software Ratings Board age ratings, and manage VVG watching in youth 16 years old and younger.

INCREASE PARTICIPATION IN MARTIAL ARTS

A meta-analysis demonstrated that traditional martial arts (karate, aikido, judo, taekwondo, and kempo) reduced aggressive behavior in 507 children and adolescents (n = 12 studies, including four experimental) studies with disruptive disorders.[59] In addition, findings of 6-month nonrandomized martial arts in at-risk aggressive youth at risk[60] showed reduced aggression, improved cognition function (improved inhibition and speed of processing), and executive functions (which are highly impaired in youth with disruptive disorders). This exploratory trial supported the need for a high-quality RCT on martial arts and aggressive youth at high risk for disruptive disorders and delinquency.

PREVENTING EXPOSURE TO LEAD

Exposure to lead is a preventable cause of ADHD, disruptive disorders, aggressiveness, delinquency, and decreased 1Q according to the American Academy of Pediatrics.[61] Lead toxicity has been directly linked with externalizing behaviors in children that persist into adolescence. However, a direct association between lead exposure and externalizing disorders in adolescents could not be established, suggesting that early-life impairments may put children on a riskier developmental trajectory, possibly leading to aggressive and antisocial behavior.[62] Adolescents with higher bone lead concentrations were also found to have higher scores and aggression.[63] This study means that advocacy to prevent lead toxicity will also help prevent aggression.

UNMET NEEDS FOR PRIMARY PREVENTION

The "war on lead" spanning more than a century remains unfinished business.[67] Although there is no safe body lead level (BLL),[64] a sharp decline in the Geometric Mean BLL (GMBLL) in the US population is noteworthy. For example, the GMBLL in US children ages 1–5 y dropped from 15.2 μg/dL (95% CI: 14.3,0 16.1) in 1976–1980 to 0.83 μg/dL (95% CI: 0.78, 0.88) in 2011–2016, representing a 94.5% decrease over time.[65] This decrease in lead level has largely been achieved through federal regulations (removal of lead in gasoline and the banning of lead-based paint and lead plumbing solder for residential uses) and public health efforts.[66] Despite this impressive accomplishment, the Centers for Disease Control and Prevention (CDC) estimates indicate that nearly 385,775 children ages 1–11 y have BLLs > or = to the CDC blood lead reference value (BLRV) of 5 μg/dL. Higher GM BLLs were associated with non-Hispanic Black race/ethnicity, lower family income-to-poverty ratio, and older housing age. Sadly, at least 500,000 children or 2.5% of the population of children in the 1 to 5 year age range, above the CDC BLRV, are exposed to more lead than the other 97.5% of children of the same age. The CDC has recently updated its BLRV from 5 to 3.5 μg/dL based on the new BLL values above 97.5%.[67] Advocacy for preventing lead toxicity is still needed, especially in food insecurity and low-income areas, which are risk factors. Also, zip codes with elevated blood lead levels and high-poverty areas should be included.[68] Attention to nutrition (adequate iron, zinc, calcium) may have a protective role in lead toxicity.

Environmental Factors

Green space

Green space is a natural treatment that can improve overall well-being, decrease stress levels, and reduce symptoms of depression, anxiety, and disruptive behavior.[69] The normalized difference vegetation index (NDVI) is a scientific technique used to measure green space by comparing areas with more green vegetation to those without by calculating the ratio of visible red and near-infrared reflectance, as land surfaces with greener vegetation reflect more near-infrared and absorb more visible red wavelength. Data were analyzed from the Cincinnati Childhood Allergy and Air Pollution Study,[69] an ongoing prospective birth cohort study. At age 7 years, a 0.1-unit increase in NDVI was associated with decreased conduct scores ($\beta = -1.10$, 95% CI [-2.14, -0.06], 200 m). At age 12 years, a 0.1-unit increase in NDVI was associated with a decrease in anxiety scores ($\beta = -1.83$, 95% CI [-3.44, -0.22], 800 m), decreased depression scores ($\beta = -1.36$, 95% CI [-2.61, -0.12], 200 m), and decreased somatization scores ($\beta = -1.83$, 95% CI [-3.22, -0.44], 200 m). The study demonstrated that increased exposure to residential green space is associated with reduced youth's problematic internal and external behaviors, measured by Behavioral Assessment System for Children, Second Edition, at ages 7 and 12 years. Younan[70] found that increased exposure to green (foliage) reduces aggressive behaviors in urban-dwelling adolescents by an analysis of aggressive behaviors over the preceding 6 months of 76 monozygotic and 364 dizygotic twin pairs who had at least two assessments of aggressive behaviors at ages 9–18, by assessment with the parent-reported version of the widely used the Achenbach Child Behavior Checklist (6–18).[71]

Blue (water) space. Blue (water) space is generally defined as visible, outdoor, natural surface waters with the potential for promoting human health and well-being. Some research also includes aquariums and modified, artificially constructed spaces such as canals, dammed lakes, or urban streams/rivers. Blue spaces offer different sensory experiences, including surfing, swimming, boating, and kayaking. For example, a systemic review done by Britton[72] found that blue spaces can potentially reduce physically aggressive behaviors of adolescents in a surfing program. Other students (primarily adults and a few youths and young adults) found improvement in aggression and symptoms of PTSD, depression, and social skills, possibly by improvement in resilience and general well-being.

Exposure to secondhand smoking. Living with a smoker increases the odds of a young child showing problems with attention/behavior.

Poor Sleep and Noise Impact

A recent meta-analysis in 2021 by Van Ween[74] found up to 80% correlation between poor sleep with pediatric aggression. Environmental factors such as noise from aviation or other sources can contribute to poor sleep. The etiology of poor sleep often is multifactorial; health factors such as chronic pain, restless legs, autism, ADHD, and environmental factors can contribute to worsening of sleep. Undisturbed sleep is a prerequisite for high daytime performance, well-being, and health. Environmental noise can be a factor that causes disturbed sleep and impair sleep recuperation, and "white" noise[75] may be helpful for restorative sleep.

A summary of these studies can be found in **Table 1** using the United States Preventative Services Task Force ratings for the strength of the recommendation and level of certainty for each study.

SUMMARY

The need for CIM treatments for youth with ED, irritability/aggression is high, especially as some therapies are effective, safe, and cheap. The evidence for supplementation[32] with BSM (medium effects, $d = 0.16$ to $d = 1.1$; RR 2.97; 97.5% CI 1.50, 5.90) and Ω-3 fatty acids (low effect, $d \sim .20$)[42] is the strongest and is supported by double-blind randomized controlled trials. However, measuring levels of EPA and DHA effects were larger than when comparing EPA and DHA to placebo groups. Future studies may require dosing EPA and DHA using the Ω-3 Index of 8% to 11%.[47] Studies may also get better results when studies go for longer periods or when the pre-inflammatory status of the individual is taken into account. The use of MT, martial arts, and team sports are helpful interventions. In addition, the preventive approaches should be considered despite the small individual effect sizes, such as restricting exposure to media violence, preventing lead toxicity, decreasing sleep deprivation, and increasing exposure to green–blue spaces, as when instituted in combination may be quite impactful.

CLINICS CARE POINTS

- The DSM-5 has recently approved the use of an R code, R 45.89, for Impairing Emotional Outbursts defined as "displays of anger or distress manifested verbally and/or behaviorally that lead to significant functional impairment [4]. Not to be used concurrently with DMDD or intermittent explosive disorder (IED), the billable R code would provide an accurate descriptive label for children younger than 6 years, who cannot be diagnosed with DMDD or IED. In the presence of comorbid ADHD or disruptive disorders, the R code will improve the accuracy about reason for referral.

- Based on their narrative literature review (2019-2021), the AACAP Presidential Task Force [4] concluded that currently available interventions for emotional outbursts yield only modest effects but optimization of treatment of underlying conditions can help. These findings indicate unmet needs that can be addressed by CIM treatments for ED/irritability/aggression common to disruptive disorders.

- Broad spectrum micronutrient supplementation (BSM) is a safe (including height growth>placebo unlike stimulants) and evidence-based treatment with medium effect sizes like those of psychosocial treatment. Clinicians are encouraged to use this treatment in their practice, preferably in children who are medication naïve or after consultation with a clinician with experience in using BSM [24].

- Augmentation with Ω-3 fatty acids is also recommended, even though effect, size was low as we suspect that low effect may be explained by available studies not using the Ω-3 Index to guide the treatment.

DISCLOSURE

The authors have nothing to disclose.

REFERENCES

1. American psychiatric association. American psychiatric association: diagnostic and statistical manual of mental disorders. 5th edition. Washington, DC: American Psychiatric Association; 2022. Text revision.

2. Costello EJ, Egger H, Angold A. 10-Year research update review: the epidemiology of child and adolescent psychiatric disorders. I. Methods and public health burden. J Am Acad Child Adolesc Psychiatry 2005;44:972–86.

3. Larson K, Russ SA, Kahn RS, et al. Patterns of comorbidity, functioning, and service use for US children with ADHD, 2007. Pediatrics 2011;127:462–70.

4. Carlson GA, Singh MK, Amaya-Jackson L, et al. Narrative review: impairing emotional outbursts: what they are and what we should do about them. J Am Acad Child Adolesc Psychiatry 2022. https://doi.org/10.1016/j.jaac.2022.03.014.

5. Blader JC. Attention-deficit hyperactivity disorder and the dysregulation of emotion generation and emotional expression. Child Adolesc Psychiatr Clin N Am 2021;30(2):349–60.

6. Blader J, Pliszka S, Kafantaris V, et al. Stepped treatment for attention-deficit/hyperactivity disorder and aggressive behavior: a randomized, controlled trial of adjunctive risperidone, divalproex sodium, or placebo after stimulant medication optimization. J Am Acad Child Adolesc Psychiatry 2021;60:236–51.

7. Stevenson J. Editorial: accumulating evidence for the benefit of micronutrients for children with attention-deficit/hyperactivity disorder. J Am Acad Child Adolesc Psychiatry 2022;61(5):599–600.

8. Faraone SV, Rostain AL, Blader J, et al. Practitioner review: emotional dysregulation in attention-deficit/hyperactivity disorder - implications for clinical recognition and intervention. J Child Psychol Psychiatry 2019;60(2):133–50.

9. Shaw P, Stringaris A, Nigg J, et al. Emotion dysregulation in attention deficit hyperactivity disorder. Am J Psychiatry 2014;171:276–93.

10. Masi G, Sesso G, Pfanner C, et al. An exploratory study of emotional dysregulation dimensions in youth with attention deficit hyperactivity disorder and/or bipolar spectrum disorders. Front Psychiatry 2021;12:1–10.

11. Silverman MR, Bennett R, Feuerstahler L, et al. Measuring emotion dysregulation in children with attention deficit/hyperactivity disorder: revisiting the factor structure of the emotion regulation checklist. Behav Ther 2022;53:196–207.

12. Vachar C, Romo L, Dereure M, et al. Efficacy of cognitive behavioral therapy on aggressive behavior in children with attention deficit hyperactivity disorder and emotion dysregulation: study protocol of a randomized control trial. Trials 2022;23:124.

13. Connor DF, Doerfler LA. The many faces (and names) of mood dysregulation. Child Adolesc Psychiatr Clin N Am 2021;30:299–306.

14. Freeman AJ, Youngstrom EA, Youngstrom JK, et al. Disruptive mood dysregulation disorder in a community mental health clinic: prevalence, comorbidity and correlates. J Child Adolesc Psychopharmacol 2016;26(2):123–30.

15. Roy AK, Lopes V, Klein RG. Disruptive mood dysregulation disorder: a new diagnostic approach to chronic irritability in youth. Am J Psychiatry 2014;171:918–24.

16. Carlson GA, Pataki C. Disruptive mood dysregulation disorder among children and adolescents. Focus 2016;14(1):20–5.

17. Brotman MA, Schmajuk M, Rich BA, et al. Prevalence, clinical correlates, and longitudinal course of severe mood dysregulation in children. Biol Psychiatry 2006;60(9):991–7.

18. Copeland WE, Shanahan L, Egger H, et al. Adult diagnostic and functional outcomes of DSM-5 disruptive mood dysregulation disorder. Am J Psychiatry 2014;171:668–74.

19. Zelkowitz P, Guzder J, Paris J, et al. Borderline pathology of childhood: implications of early axis II diagnoses. Can Child Adolesc Psychiatr Rev 2004;13(3):58–61.

20. Webermann A, Brand B. (Mental illness and violent behavior: the role of dissociation Borderline Personal Disord. Emot Dysregul 2017;4:2.

21. McIntyre RS, Berk M, Brietzke E, et al. Bipolar disorders. Lancet 2020; 396(10265):1841–56.

22. Aman MG, Bukstein OG, Gadow KD, et al. What does risperidone add to parent training and stimulant for severe aggression in child attention-deficit/hyperactivity disorder? J. Amer. Acad Child Adolesc. Psychiatry 2014;53(1): 47–60.

23. Carlson GA, Klein DN. Editorial: antidepressants to the rescue in severe mood dysregulation and disruptive mood dysregulation disorder? J Am Acad Child Adolesc Psychiatry 2020;59(3):339–41.

24. Johnstone JM, Hughes A, Goldenberg JZ, et al. Multinutrients for the treatment of psychiatric symptoms in clinical samples: a systematic review and meta-analysis of randomized controlled trials. Nutrients 2020;12(11):3394.

25. Popper C. Single-micronutrient and broad-spectrum micronutrient approaches for treating mood disorders in youth and adults. Child Adolesc Psychiatr Clin N Am 2014;23(3):591–672.

26. Kaplan BJ, Rucklidge JJ. The better brain: overcome anxiety, combat depression, and reduce adhd, and stress with nutrition. Boston, MA, USA: Houghton Mifflin Harcourt; 2021.

27. Rucklidge JJ, Matthew JF, Eggleston MJF, et al. Vitamin-mineral treatment improves aggression and emotional regulation in children with ADHD: a fully blinded, randomized, placebo-controlled trial. J Child Psychol Psychiatry 2018; 59:232–46.

28. Johnstone JM, Leung B, Gracious B, et al. Rationale and design of an international randomized placebo-controlled trial of a 36-ingredient micronutrient supplement for children with ADHD and irritable mood: the Micronutrients for ADHD in Youth (MADDY) study. Contemp Clin Trials Commun 2019;16:100478.

29. Karalunas SL, Gustafsson HC, Fair D, et al. Do we need an irritable subtype of ADHD? Replication and extension of a promising temperament profile approach to ADHD subtyping. Psychol Assess 2019;31(2):236–47.

30. Tzang RF, Chang YC, Chang CH. Structural equation modeling (SEM): childhood aggression and irritable ADHD associated with parental psychiatric symptoms. Int J Environ Res Public Health 2021;18(19):10068.

31. Harding KL, Judah RD, Gant C. Outcome-based comparison of Ritalin versus food-supplement treated children with AD/HD. Altern Med Rev 2003;8(3):319–30.

32. Rucklidge J, Frampton C, Gorman B, et al. Vitamin-mineral treatment of attention-deficit hyperactivity disorder in adults: double-blind randomised placebo-controlled trial. Br J Psychiatry 2014;204:306–15.

33. Pike V, Zlotkin S. Excess micronutrient intake: defining toxic effects and upper limits in vulnerable populations. Ann NY Acad Sci 2019;1446:21–43.

34. Meiser J, Weindl D, Hiller K. Complexity of dopamine metabolism. Cell Commun Signal 2013;11(1):34.

35. Swanson JM, Kinsbourne M, Nigg J, et al. Etiologic subtypes of attention-deficit/hyperactivity disorder: brain imaging, molecular genetic and environmental factors and the dopamine hypothesis. Neuropsychol Rev 2007;17(1):39–59.

36. Johnstone JM, Hatsu I, Tost G, et al. Micronutrients for attention-deficit/hyperactivity disorder in youths: a placebo-controlled randomized clinical trial. J Am Acad Child Adolesc Psychiatry 2022;61(5):647–61.

37. Rucklidge J, Taylor M, Whitehead K. Effect of micronutrients on behavior and mood in adults with ADHD: evidence from an 8-week open label trial with natural extension. J Atten Disord 2011;15(1):79–91.
38. Catalá-López F, Hutton B, Núñez-Beletrán A, et al. The pharmacological and non-pharmacological treatment of attention deficit hyperactivity disorder in children and adolescents: a systematic review with network meta-analyses of randomised trials. PLoS One 2017;12:e0180355.
39. Correll CU, Cortese S, Croatto G, et al. Efficacy and acceptability of pharmacological, psychosocial, and brain stimulation interventions in children and adolescents with mental disorders: an umbrella review. World Psychiatry 2021;20(2):244–75.
40. Hatsu IE, Eiterman L, Stern M, et al. Household food insecurity is associated with symptoms of emotional dysregulation in children with attention deficit hyperactivity disorder: the MADDY study. Nutrients 2022;14(6):1306.
41. American pediatric association (AAP), Council on community pediatrics; committee on nutrition. Promoting food security for all children. Pediatrics 2015;136(5):e1431–8.
42. Choy O, Raine A. Omega-3 supplementation as a dietary intervention to reduce aggressive and antisocial behavior. Curr Psychiatry Rep 2018;20(5):32.
43. Gajos JM, Beaver KM. The effect of omega-3 fatty acids on aggression: a meta-analysis. Neurosci Biobehav Rev 2016;69:147–58.
44. Cooper R, Tye C, Kuntsi J, et al. The effect of omega-3 polyunsaturated fatty acid supplementation on emotional dysregulation, oppositional behaviour and conduct problems in ADHD: a systematic review and meta-analysis. J Affective Disord 2016;190:474–82.
45. von Schacky C. Omega-3 index in 2018/19. Proc Nutr Soc 2020;79(4):381–7.
46. von Schacky C. Importance of EPA and DHA Blood levels in brain structure and function. Nutrients 2021;13(4):1074.
47. von Schacky C. Omega-3 fatty acids in pregnancy—the case for a target omega-3 index. Nutrients 2020;12:898.
48. Cheng-Ho C, Ping-Tao T, Nai-Yu C, et al. Safety and tolerability of prescription omega-3 fatty acids: a systematic review and meta-analysis of randomized controlled trials. Prostaglandins Leukot Essent Fatty Acids 2018;(129):1–12.
49. Germano M, Meleleo D, Montorfano G, et al. Plasma, red blood cells phospholipids and clinical evaluation after long chain omega-3 supplementation in children with attention deficit hyperactivity disorder (ADHD). Nutr Neurosci 2007;10(1–2):1–9.
50. Königs A, Kiliaan AJ. Critical appraisal of omega-3 fatty acids in attention-deficit/hyperactivity disorder treatment. Neuropsychiatr Dis Treat 2016;12:1869–82.
51. Bloch MH, Qawasmi A. Omega-3 fatty acid supplementation for the treatment of children with attention-deficit/hyperactivity disorder symptomatology: systematic review and meta-analysis. J Am Acad Child Adolesc Psychiatry 2011;50(10):991–1000.
52. Rosell DR, Siever LJ. The neurobiology of aggression and violence. CNS Spectrums 2015;20(3):254–79.
53. Antalis CJ, Stevens LJ, Campbell M, et al. Omega-3 fatty acid status in attention deficit/hyperactivity disorder. Prostaglandins Leukot Essent Fatty Acids 2006;75(4–5):299–308.

54. Bellino S, Bozzatello P, Badino C, et al. Efficacy of polyunsaturated fatty acids (PUFAs) on impulsive behaviours and aggressiveness in psychiatric disorders. Int J Mol Sci 2021;22(2):620.

55. Ye P, Huang Z, Zhou H, et al. Music-based intervention to reduce aggressive behavior in children and adolescents: a meta-analysis. Medicine (Baltimore) 2021;100(4):e23894.

56. Hudziak JJ, Albaugh MD, Ducharme S, et al. Cortical thickness maturation and duration of music training: health-promoting activities shape brain development. J Am Acad Child Adolesc Psychiatry 2014;53(11): 1153–61.e11612.

57. American Psychological Association, Task Force on Violent Media. Technical report on the review of the violent video game literature. Washington, DC: Author. APA; 2015.

58. Burkhardt J, Wolfgang L. A meta-analysis on the longitudinal, age-dependent effects of violent video games on aggression. Media Psychology 2022;25(3): 499–512.

59. Harwood A, Lavidor M, Rassovsky Y. Reducing aggression with martial arts: a meta-analysis of child and youth studies. Aggress Violent Behav 2017;34:96–101.

60. Harwood GA, Lambez B, Feldman R, et al. The effect of martial arts training on cognitive and psychological functions in at-risk youths. Front Pediatr 2021;9. https://doi.org/10.3389/fped.2021.70704.

61. American Academy of Pediatrics (AAP) Council on Environmental health. Prevention of childhood lead toxicity. Pediatrics 2016;138(1):e201614.

62. Desrochers-Couture M, Courtemanche Y, Forget-Dubois N, et al. Association between early lead exposure and externalizing behaviors in adolescence: a developmental cascade. Environ Res 2019;178:108679.

63. Needleman HL, Riess JA, Tobin MJ, et al. Bone lead levels and delinquent behavior. JAMA 1996;275(5):363, 36enters for Disease Control and Prevention.

64. Ettinger A, Ruckart P, Dignam T. Lead poisoning prevention: the unfinished agenda. J Public Health Manag Pract 2019;25(Suppl 1):S1–2.

65. ACCLPP (Advisory Committee on Childhood Lead Poisoning Prevention). Low level lead exposure harms children: a renewed call for primary prevention. Report of the advisory committee on childhood lead poisoning prevention of the centers for disease control and prevention. Atlanta, GA: Centers for Disease Control and Prevention; 2012.

66. Egan KB, Cornwell CR, Courtney J, et al. Blood lead levels in U.S. Children ages 1-11 years, 1976-2016. Environ Health Perspect 2021;129(3):37003.

67. Dignam T, Kaufmann RB, LeStourgeon L, et al. Control of lead sources in the United States, 1970–2017: public health progress and current challenges to elim- inating lead exposure. J Public Health Manag Pract 2019;251: S13–22.

68. Ruckart PZ, Jones RL, Courtney JG, et al. Update of the blood lead reference value - United States, 2021. MMWR Morb Mortal Wkly Rep 2021;70(43):1509–12.

69. Madzia J, Ryan P, Yolton K, et al. Residential greenspace association with childhood behavioral outcomes. J Pediatr 2019;207:233–40.

70. Younan D, Tuvblad C, Li L, et al. Environmental determinants of aggression in adolescents: role of urban neighborhood greenspace. J Am Acad Child Adolesc Psychiatry 2016;55:591.

71. Achenbach T.M., Rescorla L.A., McConaughey S., et al. Achenbach System of Empirically Based Assessment 2015 Update. ASEBA; CBCL/1 1/2-5; C-TRF;

CBCL/6-18; TRF; YSR; DOF; SCICA; YASR; YABCL; BPM; TOF. In The twentieth mental measurements yearbook. 2017.

72. Britton E, Kindermann G, Domegan C, et al. Blue care: a systematic review of blue space interventions for health and wellbeing. Health Promotion Int 2020; 35(1):50–69.

73. Mahabee-Gittens EM, Vidourek RA, King KA, et al. Disparities in Neighborhood Characteristics among U.S. Children with Secondhand and Thirdhand Tobacco Smoke Exposure. Int J Environ Res Public Health 2022;19(7):4266. https://doi.org/10.3390/ijerph19074266. PMID: 35409946; PMCID: PMC8998580.

74. Van Veen M, Lancel M, Beijer E, et al. The association of sleep quality and aggression: a systematic review and meta-analysis of observational studies. Sleep Med Rev 2021;59:101500.

75. Reidy S, Smith M, Rocha S, et al. Noise as a sleep aid: a systematic review. Sleep Med Rev 2021;55:101385.

Post-Traumatic Stress Disorder/Developmental Trauma Disorder/Complex Post-Traumatic Stress Disorder and Complementary and Integrative Medicine/Functional Medicine

Deborah R. Simkin, MD, DFAACAP

KEYWORDS

- Complementary and integrative medicine (CIM) • Child • Adolescents
- Post-traumatic stress disorder (PTSD) • Abuse
- Developmental trauma disorder (DTD) • Epigenetics • Inflammation
- Research domain criteria

KEY POINTS

- Traditional therapies may also be insufficient because the underlying root of prolonged post-traumatic stress disorder (PTSD) may be related to early effects on the developing brain that sustain through adulthood.
- Even when adaptations to criteria are made to identify more children with PTSD, some children who are not identified continue to suffer.
- Developmental Trauma Disorder (based on biology rather than symptoms) may be better suited to identify PTSD in children and more in line with the Research Domain Criteria designed to develop treatment.
- CIM interventions like EMDR, EFT and imagery rescripting are more effective for PTSD when the treatment is adjusted to fit the developmental age at which the trauma occurred.
- CIM interventions like Meditation, Yoga, EFT, and EMDR, are promising due to the possible normalization of epigenetic effects, inflammatory cytokines, and cortisol that can occur with early abuse.

INTRODUCTION

Research has shown that antidepressants are ineffective for post-traumatic stress disorder (PTSD) in youth. A review by Strawn, 2014[1] did not support SSRIs as a first-line treatment for PTSD. Alpha-2 agonists, alpha-antagonists, and beta-blockers may be a better

Department of Psychiatry, Emory University School of Medicine, 8955 Highway 98 West, Suite 204, Miramar Beach, FL 32550, USA
E-mail address: Deb62288@aol.com

Child Adolesc Psychiatric Clin N Am 32 (2023) 317–365
https://doi.org/10.1016/j.chc.2022.08.011
1056-4993/23/© 2022 Elsevier Inc. All rights reserved.

fit as first-line medications. In addition, the effectiveness of antidepressants in regard to depression (a common co-morbid condition associated with PTSD) is also reduced when early childhood abuse occurs. The International Study to Predict Optimized Treatment for Depression (iSPOT-D), randomized participants to 8 weeks of treatment with escitalopram, sertraline, or venlafaxine. Patients ($n = 1008$) meeting Diagnostic and Statistical Manuel-IV (DSM-IV) criteria for Major Depressive Disorder (MDD), and 336 matched healthy controls comprised the study sample (age 18–65). A 50% or greater improvement on the 17-item Hamilton Rating Scale for Depression (HRSD17) or the 16-item Quick Inventory of Depressive Symptomatology-Self-Rated defined remission (QIDS SR16) was used to denote a positive response. Abuse, especially abuse/trauma occurring at ≤7 years of age-predicted poorer outcomes after 8 weeks of antidepressants across the three medication treatment arms. Given the efficacy of SSRIs in those who did not experience early childhood abuse, one must consider early abuse a moderator of antidepressant outcomes. Specific types of early-life trauma, mainly physical, emotional, and sexual abuse, in this age group inhibited response to antidepressant therapy for MDD.[2]

Much of the research in this article was done using DSM criteria. However, this research set the stage to allow researchers to explore whether one size fits all when it comes to treating individuals who experienced trauma early on. Some complementary and integrative medicine/functional medicine (CIM/FM) interventions will be discussed, which have played a role in attempting to normalize the dysregulation of systems that occur with early trauma. The dysregulation of systems may be a major reason why traditional psychotherapies/medications may have no therapeutic effect.

NEW APPROACHES TO THE DIAGNOSTIC CRITERIA BASED ON CHILDHOOD ABUSE
Complex Post-Traumatic Stress Disorder

Failure to identify the underlying effects of prolonged abuse may be why traditional therapies seem to have varying effects or insufficient long-term effects. Childhood traumas constitute a significant public health issue, as they occur at ominously high rates. Over 30%–40% of the general adult population has experienced some form of disrupting early life adversity.[3] The World Health Organization (WHO) International Classification of Diseases (ICD-11) has recognized that complex post-traumatic stress disorder (C-PTSD) is uniquely associated with childhood traumas. The C-PTSD diagnosis in ICD-11 includes the following symptoms: re-experiencing the traumatic event(s); avoidance of thoughts, memories, and activities that serve as reminders of the event; and persistent perceptions of heightened current threat (all found in the DSM-5 criteria for PTSD). In addition, however, C-PTSD also includes: (1) affect dysregulation; (2) negative self-concept; and (3) disturbed relationships.[4,5]

Changes to the Diagnostic and Statistical Manual of Mental Disorders, Fifth Edition
Diagnosis of Post-Traumatic Stress Disorder in Children

Some approaches to diagnosing PTSD in children have been made to more accurately denote symptoms than may be found in children under age 6 that do not appear in DSM-V. Scheeringa[6] developed an alternative algorithm for PTSD (PTSD-AA) based on behaviors rather than thoughts and feelings. PTSD-AA requires only one symptom in criterion C instead of the DSM-IV requirement of three symptoms. Developmental modifications to the wording of A2 acute reaction, B1 intrusive recollections, B2 nightmares, B3 dissociative experiences, C5 detachment or estrangement, and D2 irritability was done based on prior empirical work.[7]

However, in a study comparing DSM-IV, DSM-V, and PTSD-AA criteria, some children with substantial impairment were not diagnosed with PTSD using any of these algorithms because they lacked symptoms in the intrusion cluster or the hyperarousal cluster.[8] Therefore, impairing symptoms of abuse may not be picked up using any of these criteria in children under age 6.

Types of traumas and chronicity
In a systemic review and meta-analysis,[9] the type of trauma and the chronicity of the trauma proved to be more sensitive to uncovering PTSD. The percentage of PTSD identified using DSM-IV criteria (4.9%, 95% CI = 2.5%–8.0%) was lower than the percentage of PTSD using the PTSD-AA (19.9%, 95% CI =; 12.1%–29.0%) in pre-school children (N = 1,941). However, PTSD prevalence was higher following exposure to interpersonal trauma (32.6%) than non-interpersonal trauma (10.7%; p = .0010). In addition, the prevalence was significantly higher following repeated traumas (35.3%) than single traumas (11.3%; p = .0003).

In summary, many factors can contribute to correctly identifying children with PTSD.

Developmental trauma disorder
Developmental trauma disorder (DTD) may be a better way to identify children who are substantially suffering but do not fit any of the diagnostic criteria used to diagnose PTSD. DTD takes into account the effect of trauma during the developmental age, the effects on the developing brain, the faulty misperceptions of cues, the long-term effects of inflammation, and epigenetics.[10] Therefore, using DTD criteria may increase the ability to target vulnerable children who have gone undiagnosed by other traditional criteria.

Trauma during childhood takes a toll on the developing brain. Different symptoms are likely to occur depending on when the developmental stages were disrupted. For instance, between birth and 18 months of age, the child attaches to a caregiver who the child relies upon during periods of increasing frustration. In this way, the child learns that there is someone there to depend upon if the world seems frightening. Overwhelming feelings can and will find a way to be resolved. If the child does not have a nurturing caregiver, the child may feel intense feelings without any means to modulate them. The resulting helpless feeling can lead to excessive clinginess and anxiety, internally or externally directed aggression, and dissociation.[11–13] Chronic traumatization during early developmental stages (ages 1–4) may lead to an incorrect categorization of information. Almost all stimuli and experiences will be interpreted as potentially traumatic and responded to accordingly.[14] These misperceptions may result in an "over-developed memory for traumatic events and deficits in attention, problem-solving, semantic organization, and short-term and delayed semantic memory."[15] Somatic complaints such as headaches, stomach aches, sleep disturbances, and decreased appetite may develop as a response to intense feelings rather than verbalization of these feelings. These can intensify to include conversion symptoms or forms of dissociation such as pseudo-seizures.[12,16] Repeated experiences of rejection, betrayal and, abuse lead to children feeling bad, worthless, or not worthy of being loved—especially between ages 3 to 7 when they normally think they are the center of the world and the cause of what happens. The above events, combined with poor developmental competencies and subsequent feelings of inadequacy, can lead to self-blame and guilt.[12,13] In addition, of course, injuries and traumatic brain injuries (TBIs) can occur, which sets the stage for the long-term effects of inflammation in the brain, causing declining hippocampal volume, increasing amygdala, and interference with maturational amygdala-prefrontal coupling. Individuals reporting three or more adverse childhood events (ACEs) had significantly greater odds of reporting TBI than respondents with no ACEs.[17]

Based on these criteria, "DTD may be more helpful in identifying.

- neural substrates (neuroendocrine, neuroimaging, and EEG abnormalities);
- familiarity (evidence of the intergenerational transmission);
- epi-genetic risk factors (G x E); specific environmental risk factors (that predict developmental trauma disorder);
- biomarkers (changes in stress hormones);
- temperamental antecedents (behavioral inhibition, social avoidance);
- symptom similarity (affective, behavioral, relational, and stress response systems);
- abnormality of cognitive or emotional processing (various studies validate this);
- course of illness (chronic deterioration with episodic spikes in severity in children and persistence over the lifespan);
- high rates of co-morbidity (a wide spectrum); and lastly,
- treatment response (poor so far)".[13,18]

Therefore, DTD using biologically-based rather than symptom-based criteria, allows the application to components of the Research Domain Criteria (RDoC). The RDoC is not meant to replace current diagnostic systems. However, rather than define mental disorders by signs and symptoms which may not correlate to brain neurobiological systems, the RDoC starts with psychological/biological systems that correlate to the observed behavior/cognitive process and looks for dysregulation as the reasons for the expression of these processes. In the RDoC, these biological systems are also considered from a neurodevelopmental perspective with attention to environmental insults. This allows mental disorders to be considered as malfunctions in neural circuits or systems rather than just as neurotransmitter imbalances. The long-term goals of RDoC are to help improve diagnosis and shed light on potential new treatments for mental disorders with the hope of reversing mental disorders in some cases.[19]

Given the ineffectiveness of treatments for depression, often co-morbid with PTSD, when early abuse occurs,[2] and given the abnormal frontolimbic development in youth with a history of childhood abuse,[20] future research should focus on treatments that are capable of restoring healthy neurodevelopment using the RDoC framework. If healthy neurodevelopment can be restored, other devastating effects of early childhood trauma, such as psychosis[21] or the use of substances to cope with overwhelming feelings, leading to substance abuse, may be avoided.

STUDIES USING THE CRITERIA OF POST-TRAUMATIC STRESS DISORDER TRADITIONALLY FOUND IN DIAGNOSTIC AND STATISTICAL MANUAL OF MENTAL DISORDERS OR RELATED SCALES
N-Acetylcysteine

Early chronic/repeated stress activates a cascade of interrelated pathways. The hypothalamus–pituitary axis (HPA) dysregulates glucocorticoid signaling, which, in turn, activates the expression of pro-inflammatory cytokines and increases glutamate. Increased inflammation then decreases the expression of anti-inflammatory pathways, which leads to oxidative stress identified as increases in reactive oxygen species and decreases in glutathione. Oxidative stress plays a role in epigenetic changes. The interaction of increased inflammation and oxidized stress affects the brain leading to neuropsychiatric disorders and, peripherally, causes chronic diseases.[22] Inflammation and oxidative stress can influence hippocampal neurogenesis. N-acetylcysteine (NAC) is known to decrease oxidative stress, increase glutathione (GSH), and modulate glutamate.[23]

In an 8-week double-blind placebo-controlled trial (DBPCT)[24] NAC 2400 mg/day plus cognitive behavior therapy (CBT) was compared with placebo plus CBT for PTSD and substance use disorders (SUDs) in 35 participants (18 and over). The Clinician-Administered PTSD Scale (CAPS) total score decreased by 46% in the NAC treated group (58.8 to 32.0), compared with 25% decrease in the placebo group (58.6 to 51.5). The treatment-group difference was not statistically significant in this sample size, but the NAC within-group improvement on the CAPS total score from baseline to week 8 ($d = 1.27$, $p < .001$) and baseline to week 12 ($d = 1.48$, $p < .05$) were large. In addition, significant within-group effects on the CAPS-R (re-experiencing), CAPS-A (avoidance), and CAPS-H (hyperarousal) subscales were observed in the NAC group from baseline to Week 8 ($d = 1.01$, $d = 1.03$, and $d = 1.16$, respectively, p's $< .01$) and baseline to Week 12 ($d = 1.04$, $d = 1.34$, and $d = 1.57$, respectively, p's $< .01$). Among the placebo group, no significant within-group effects on the CAPS total were observed at Week 8 or 12. The only significant within-group effects on the CAPS-R subscale score in the placebo group were observed from baseline to Week 8 ($d = .73$, $p < .05$) and Week 12 ($d = .67$, $p < .05$). The amount of craving decreased by 81% from baseline to Week 8 with NAC (3.7 to 0.7) compared with 32% with placebo (4.1 to 2.8). As an aside, depression in the NAC and the CBT group significantly improved by week 12. In addition, NAC combined with CBT decreased cravings better than CBT alone.

Omega 3 Fatty Acids (Polyunsaturated Fatty Acids)

Recent studies have begun to delineate the importance of Omega 3 fatty acids in memory, learning, mood, and affect regulation involved in PTSD. The use of PUFAs used early after injury to prevent the development of PTSD has been studied in a DBPCT by Matsumura and colleagues.[25] Eighty-three participants (age 18 and older) received either PUFAs containing 1470 mg docosahexaenoic acid (DHA) and 147 mg eicosapentaenoic acid (EPA) per day or a placebo daily for 12 weeks within 10 days after a severe accidental injury. After 12 weeks of supplementation, participants performed script-driven imagery of their traumatic event while monitoring their heart rate (HR) and skin conductance (SC). During rest and script-driven imagery, the HR was significantly lower in the omega-3 group than in the placebo group. The two groups did not differ in the total score of CAPS (t [81] = 0.99, $p = .33$, $d = 0.22$), with their mean values (SD) for the omega-3 and placebo groups being 6.51 (7.47) and 8.43 (9.76). These findings suggest that post-trauma supplementation with a higher DHA/EPA ratio might be effective for the secondary prevention of psychophysiological symptoms of PTSD but not for the primary symptoms of PTSD. In a similar RDBPC study,[26] 110 accident-injured patients (18 and older) received 1470 mg of DHA and 147 mg of EPA or placebo for 12 weeks. There were no differences in PTSD symptoms between the 2 groups at the 3-month follow-up.

However, DHA may not be the primary contributor to the prevention of PTSD. A meta-analysis of depression found that higher EPA/DHA ratios of >60% of total EPA and DHA effectively treated depression.[27] A secondary analysis of the above RDBPC trial[28] showed that a higher level of erythrocyte EPA was associated with lower development of PTSD. Changes in EPA + DHA ($p = .023$) and EPA ($p = .001$) as well as a higher EPA: AA ratio ($p = .000$) and EPA: DHA ratio ($p = .013$) inversely correlated with PTSD severity. Change in the omega 6 arachidonic acid (AA), known to activate inflammation, was positively correlated with PTSD severity ($p = .001$). Therefore, higher ratios of EPA/DHA immediately after an injury show promise in decreasing the risk of developing PTSD.

COMPLEMENTARY AND INTEGRATIVE MEDICINE/FUNCTIONAL MEDICINE INTERVENTIONS IN OLDER CHILDREN, ADOLESCENTS, AND YOUNG ADULTS
Meditation

A RCT ($N = 173$, age = 18 and older) in a military population compared Mantram repetition versus patient-centered therapy (PCT) for 8 weeks with a 2-month follow-up. The percentage of participants who experienced clinically meaningful changes (>10-point improvements) in CAPS score did not differ significantly between the mantram group (75%) and the PCT group (61%). However, reductions in insomnia were significantly greater for the mantram group at both post-treatment assessment and 2-month follow-up. Therefore, mantram therapy may have an advantage over PCT regarding insomnia.[29]

A meta-analysis of meditation, mindfulness training, yoga, and a study that combined mindfulness and mantra meditation[30] included 19 RCTs (ages 18 & over, $N = 1173$). A random-effects model yielded a statistically significant ES in the small to medium range (ES = −.39, $p < .001$, 95% CI [−.57, −.22]). However, findings were comparable to medication management of PTSD (ES = .42), Most notably, in a review of meditation in children and adolescents, meditation was found to be effective in catastrophic circumstances when there are few resources available (discussed below).[31]

A case comparison was made[32] with a random assignment of 76 (7–17-year-olds) to Yoga or aerobic dance control (DC) plus a nonrandomized wait-list control (WLC) group. The UCLA PTSD Reaction Index[33,34] and the Strengths and Difficulties Questionnaire measured trauma-related symptoms. The intervention included an 8-week yoga intervention (YI) to reduce trauma-related symptoms and emotional and behavioral difficulties (EBDs) among children living in orphanages in Haiti. Analyses of variance revealed a significant effect (F [2,28] = 3.30; $p = 0.05$) of the YI on the trauma-related symptom scores, although this finding was not statistically significant.

Meditation may be helpful when used as an adjunct for PTSD. However, youth may more directly benefit from meditation after experiencing a catastrophe when there are insufficient services that can be provided individually or due to staff shortages. Catani and colleagues randomly assigned 31 children[8-14] who had experienced the Tsunami of Sri Lanka to six sessions of either Narrative Exposure Therapy for children (KIDNET) or meditation-relaxation (MED-RELAX). Outcome measures included severity of PTSD symptoms, level of functioning, and physical health. In both treatments, PTSD symptoms (avoidance, intrusions, and hyperarousal) and functional impairment significantly decreased at one-month post-test and remained stable over time and at a 6-month follow-up. The p-value for functional impairment was < .001. The pre-post effect size for the KIDNET group was 1.76 (CI 0.9–2.5) at the treatment end and 1.96 (CI 1.1–2.8) at 6-month follow-up. The corresponding effect sizes for MED-RELAX were 1.83 (CI 0.9–2.6) and 2.20 (CI 1.2–3.0). At 6 months of follow-up, recovery rates were 81% for the KIDNET group and 71% for the MED-RELAX group. DSM IV criteria without a time element determined the diagnosis of PTSD.[35]

Meditation with Culturally Appropriate Changes to the Diagnosis of Post-Traumatic Stress Disorder

Another example of meditation used in the face of disaster showed promising results. However, an effort was made to identify more individuals with PTSD by making culturally specific changes in the scales used to diagnose PTSD. An RCT study[36] randomly assigned 77 high school students to a 12-session mind-body group program or a WLC group in Kosovar war-traumatized high school students 2 hours per week for 6 weeks with 10 students per group. Modifications to the Harvard Trauma Questionnaire based on the culture were used to diagnose PTSD. Each session started and ended with meditation, Other Mind-Body techniques used were guided imagery, autogenic training, and biofeedback. Dancing and drawings were used to relieve stress and express feelings. Students in the immediate intervention group had significantly lower PTSD symptoms following the intervention than those in the WLC group (F = 29.8, df = 1.76; $p < .001$). The initial intervention group maintained the decreased PTSD symptom scores at the 3-month follow-up. After the WLC group received the intervention, there was a significant decrease ($p < .001$) in PTSD symptom scores compared with the pre-intervention scores.

A single-blind, randomized control design study[37] included spiritual-hypnosis assisted treatment (SHAT-meditation with guided imagery) in 30-minute groups versus wait-list. Given the absence of a widely accepted, cross-culturally valid, and applicable standardized self-report assessment of PTSD in Bali, a questionnaire was devised based on the DSM-IV TR criteria for PTSD. It included the three symptoms of re-experiencing (flashbacks), hyperarousal, and avoidance. Forty-eight children were in the treatment group and 178 in the control group (ages = 6–12 in both groups). The technique included meditation with guided imagery in a group setting for 30 minutes. Statistically significant results found that SHAT produced a 77.1% improvement rate at a 2-year follow-up, compared with 24% in the control group with significantly lower mean PTSD symptom scores.

In summary, meditation/mindfulness techniques may effectively reduce PTSD symptoms especially after catastrophic events occur but culturally specific changes in the criteria used to diagnose PTSD should be used. When an effort is made to be culturally sensitive to youth who have PTSD, they may feel the trainers are more sincerely invested in them and this may play a role in the youths' dedication to the use of the technique.

Art therapy
A randomized pilot study by Lyshak-Stelzer and colleagues[38] (ages 13–18, $N = 29$) examined the efficacy of an adjunctive trauma-focused art therapy intervention in reducing chronic child PTSD symptoms in an inpatient psychiatric facility for youth. The study compared a trauma-focused expressive art therapy protocol (TF-ART) delivered for one hour in group sessions over 16 weeks and a treatment-as-usual (TAU) control condition. Youth were randomized to either treatment condition and assessed before and after treatment using the UCLA PTSD Reaction Index, administered as an interview. There was a significant treatment-by-condition interaction[1,27] F 7.1 $p = .01$ indicating that adolescents in the TF-ART condition had a significantly greater reduction in PTSD symptom severity than those in the TAU condition.

Schouten and colleagues[39] (ages 12–60, $N = 223$, 6 controlled comparison studies) did a review of art therapy and trauma. Types of art therapy included Mandela Coloring, Trauma-Focused Mandela Coloring, group art therapy, and art therapy with psychotherapy. Mandela Coloring involves focusing on filling in geometrical shapes rather than focusing on a person's worries. Statistically significant decreases in anxiety (1.95 [0.30, 3.22]), re-experiencing (1.63 [0.07, 2.87]), and avoidance (1.25 [0.21, 2.46]) were found in 1 study using art therapy and psychotherapy. In addition, a moderate decrease in trauma symptoms severity (0.76 [0.07, 1.42]) was found in an RCT using trauma-focused Mandela coloring. In this review, art therapy combined with psychotherapy produced the most statistically significant decrease in trauma symptom severity.

In summary, art therapy may be a helpful adjunct to treating PTSD.

Eye movement desensitization and reprocessing (EMDR)
In a review by Manzoni and colleagues,[40] seven RCTs ($n = 150$, ages 8–18) met the inclusion criteria. Preliminary analyses showed that EMDR has comparable efficacy to CBT in reducing PTSD, anxiety symptoms, and depressive symptoms and was superior to waitlist/placebo conditions. Three RCTs compared CBT to EMDR in children ($N = 207$, ages 4–18). EMDR and CBT were equally effective. One study noted that EMDR is briefer than cognitive behavioral writing therapy (CBWT) in a number of

sessions (EMDR = 4.1 vs CBWT = 5.4; t [64.52] = −5.44) and length of treatment in minutes (EMDR = 140 vs CBWT = 227; t [80.17] = −5.49). Both EMDR (t = −4.51) and CBWT (t = −4.87) reduced PTSD symptoms compared with WL conditions. The authors noted that EMDR does not require a person to detail traumatic events, complete homework, or access maladaptive beliefs, which may be difficult for a child to undertake. Even though further research is needed, it seems that improvements were maintained at 3-month follow-ups. In addition, EMDR is an evidence-based therapy with a protocol in place for children, considering age and developmental modification which may also contribute to its effectiveness.

In a meta-analysis of CBT vs EMDR, Khan and colleagues[41] pooled 11 RCTs (N = 257, ages ≥10, 197 were children with mean age of 11). The variants of CBT used were imaginal exposure (IE), trauma treatment protocol (TTP), prolonged exposure (PE), trauma-focused cognitive behavioral therapy (TF-CBT), stress inoculation training with prolonged exposure (SITPE), exposure plus cognitive restructuring (E + CR), and brief eclectic psychotherapy. The EMDR was better than CBT in reducing posttraumatic symptoms [SDM (95% CI) = −0.43 (−0.73 to −0.12)]. The results were statistically significant (p = 0.006). However, the studies included in this quantitative meta-analysis had a high level of heterogeneity (I2 = 62%). To address this, a funnel plot of publication bias was done. The results did not show any asymmetry and no bias was found among the included studies mentioned. Three months later three RCTs showed EMDR = CBT (p = 0.15), 2 of which were RCTs with children. Five studies including 239 patients revealed that EMDR is better than CBT in reducing anxiety symptoms [SDM (95% CI) = −0.71 (−1.21 to −0.21)]. Of these, 2 were RCTs of children (n = 90). The result was statistically significant (p = 0.005) but there was marked heterogeneity between included studies (I2 = 70%). Of note, there was no evidence of publication bias in those included studies. This meta-analysis provides strong evidence that EMDR is better than CBT for PTSD and anxiety in children, but EMDR =CBT for PTSD after 3 months.

Rodenburg and colleagues[42] did a meta-analysis of children using EMDR. Seven RCTs were included (n = 109 for EMDR, 100 for controls, ages 4–18). and compared EMDR to CBT. The overall effect size for EMDR was d − .56 (medium), which indicates that children receiving EMDR appear to benefit from their treatment. This meta-analysis also showed that fewer sessions were associated with better treatment outcomes. Moderator analyses showed that studies using a combination of parent and child reports showed medium-to-large effect sizes (ES), whereas studies using child reports yielded small effect sizes. ES for the effect of EMDR on trauma status at the post-test was d = .56, p < .001. The combined ES for comparisons between TAU or waitlist was significantly larger (d = .66, p < .001) than ES for comparisons with CBT (d = .25, p < .05).

In summary, EMDR and CBT seem to have equal efficacy in reducing PTSD symptoms over time. However, EMDR takes fewer sessions, improves child- and parent-reported quality of life, and reduces anxiety better than CBT.

Emotional freedom technique

Recent research has begun to focus on emotional freedom techniques (EFT) for PTSD. Research in this area began after acupuncture studies showed corresponding changes on Functional MRI,[43,44] demonstrating that specific acupuncture points send deactivating signals to the amygdala, hippocampus, and other brain regions associated with fear and pain. In addition, Fang and colleagues[45] showed that acupuncture resulted in "extensive deactivation of the limbic–paralimbic–neocortical system". EFT incorporates tapping or percussion of these acupuncture points preceded by exposure therapy and cognitive reframing. A double-blinded study comparing penetration with nonpenetrating pressure on acupuncture points found equivalent clinical improvement.[46]

A meta-analysis by Church and colleagues[47] (to determine if the use of acupressure points was the sole mediator during an intervention) included 6 studies with active controls, such as diaphragmatic breathing or sham acupoints, which were used in place of tapping on the actual acupoint (N = 403 subjects). All six studies had the experimental group tap on acupoints. The studies included participants from kindergarten to age 65. Pretest vs posttest EFT treatment showed a large effect size, Cohen's d = 1.28 (95% confidence interval [CI], 0.56 to 2.00) and Hedges' g = 1.25 (95% CI, 0.54 to 1.96). The EFT groups showed moderately stronger outcomes than controls, with weighted posttreatment effect sizes of d = −0.47 (95% CI, −0.94 to 0.0) and g = −0.45 (95% CI, −0.91 to 0.0). This meta-analysis indicated that the acupressure component was an active ingredient, and outcomes were not due solely to placebo, nonspecific effects of any therapy, or non-acupressure components.

In a meta-analysis by Sebastian and Nelms[48] the effects of EFT on PTSD (seven RCTs, N = 257, ages 16 and above) were reviewed. The weighted effect size for PTSD among all seven studies was 2.96 (95% CI 1.96–3.97, p < .01). A significant treatment by-time effect was found, with a weighted Cohen's d = 2.96 (95% CI 1.96–3.97; p < 0.001) for the studies that compared EFT to usual care or a waitlist. No significant differences were found in studies comparing EFT to other evidence-based therapies such as eye movement desensitization and reprocessing (EMDR; 1 study ≥ 18) and CBT (one study). In the EFT vs EMDR in ≥ 18, the effect size was equally large (d = 0.80). No adverse events were observed and reported.

Another RCT included 13-17-year-olds (N = 16) who were assessed thirty days after receiving one session of EFT. No improvement occurred in the wait list (Impact of Events Scale total mean pre = 32 SD ± 4.82, post = 31 SD ± 3.84). Posttest scores for all experimental-group participants improved to the point where all were nonclinical on the total score, as well as the intrusive and avoidant symptom subscales, and subjective distress (IES total mean pre = 36 SD ± 4.74, post = 3 SD ± 2.60, p < .001).[49]

In summary, EFT is as effective as EMDR and CBT in adolescents and young adults. However, EFT can be effective after one session and may have an additional effect by using acupuncture points that send deactivating signals to brain regions associated with fear and pain.

Eye movement desensitization and reprocessing versus trauma-focused cognitive behavior therapy

In an RCT, participants were randomly assigned to eight sessions of trauma-focused CBT (TF- CBT) or EMDR (n = 48 youth, ages 8–18).[50] Assessments included a Clinician-Administered PTSD Scale for Children and Adolescents (CAPS-CA). TF-CBT (with parent training education and a relaxation component) and EMDR showed large reductions from pre- to post-treatment on the CAPS-CA (−20.2; 95% CI -12.2 to −28.1 and −20.9; 95% CI –32.7 to −9.1). The extension of treatment improved the effectiveness of both therapies. Therefore, EMDR seems to have equal effectiveness to TF-CBT.

Early History of Trauma and Response to Psychological and/or Medication Treatment

Maltreated and non-maltreated individuals with the same primary DSM-5 diagnoses appear to be clinically, and neurobiologically distinct which may require different treatment interventions.[51] A meta-analysis of adults, young adults and adolescents with Complex-PTSD (C-PTSD) and early onset abuse and adult-onset PTSD by Karatzias and colleagues[52] compared the use of CBT, exposure alone (EA), and EMDR. CBT, EA, and EMDR found that all interventions were superior to usual care for PTSD symptoms. However, the multivariate meta-regression found that psychological therapies for C-PTSD were less effective if early childhood trauma had occurred. Studies with predominantly childhood-onset trauma were associated with a reduction in Hedges' g of 0.35 (95% CI 0.02–0.69) compared with trials where most participants had adult-onset trauma.

Twenty-six studies were included in a meta-analysis by Nanni and colleagues.[53] No bias was found in the studies. The studies included epidemiological studies ($N = 16$) with 23,544 participants and clinical trials ($N = 10$) with 3,098 participants (mean age 14.7 and above). The association between childhood maltreatment (CM) and the outcome of treatment for depression with psychotherapy or CBT, antidepressant medication, or combined treatment was studied in 10 clinical trials (15 active treatment arms). The association between CM and psychotherapy outcome was studied in four studies. A meta-analysis of these studies revealed that maltreated individuals showed a non-significantly higher risk for poor psychotherapy outcomes (odds ratio = 1.12, 95% CI = 0.68–1.85). The association between CM and the outcome of pharmacological treatment was studied in six studies. A meta-analysis of these studies revealed that maltreated individuals showed a poorer pharmacological treatment outcome than those without a history of CM (odds ratio = 1.26, 95% CI = 1.01–1.56). The association between CM and the outcome of combined treatment (psychotherapy and antidepressant medications) was studied in five studies. A meta-analysis of these studies revealed that maltreated individuals showed poorer combined treatment outcomes than those without a history of CM (odds ratio = 1.90, 95% CI = 1.40–2.58). Overall, this meta-analysis showed that psychotherapy alone, medication alone, and psychotherapy combined with medication in adolescents, young adults and adults with a history of CM were unlikely to respond to treatment for depression. A meta-analysis of these studies showed that maltreated individuals were twice as likely as those without a history of CM to develop persistent depressive episodes (odds ratio = 2.34, 95% CI = 1.65–3.32). Another meta-analysis of these studies showed that compared with those without a history of CM, maltreated individuals were twice as likely to have an unfavorable longitudinal course of depression (odds ratio = 2.27, 95% confidence interval [CI] = 1.80–2.87). In one RCT of 107 adolescent outpatients, 13 to 18 years old, with DSM-III-R major depression were randomly assigned to CBT, systemic behavioral family therapy (SBFT), or nondirective supportive therapy (NST). CBT was more efficacious than NST in absence of sexual abuse but was not better than NST in those with a history of sexual abuse.

In an RCT, 88 PTSD subjects diagnosed according to DSM-IV criteria were randomly assigned to EMDR, fluoxetine, or pill placebo (ages ≥ 18). They received 8 weeks of treatment and a blind rater assessed subjects post-treatment and at 6-month follow-up. The primary outcome measure was the Clinician-Administered PTSD Scale, DSM-IV version, and the secondary outcome measure was the Beck Depression Inventory-II. The psychotherapy intervention was more successful than pharmacotherapy in achieving sustained reductions in PTSD and depression symptoms, but this benefit occurred primarily in adult-onset trauma survivors. At 6-month follow-up, 75.0% of adult-onset versus only 33.3% of child-onset trauma subjects receiving EMDR achieved asymptomatic end-state functioning compared with none in the fluoxetine group. For most childhood-onset trauma patients, EMDR was less effective in regard to depression and PTSD than those with adult-onset PTSD, and no one receiving pharmacotherapy treatment produced symptom remission after 6 months post-treatment.[54]

Hence, a history of early childhood abuse, especially ≤7, was the significant indicator of poorer response to the treatment of depression and PTSD when psychological therapies alone, medication alone, or the combination was used. In addition, EMDR was not as effective for the treatment of PTSD in young adults or adults with an early history of child abuse. This confirms that early childhood abuse may require specific interventions designed to address the effect of early abuse either by modifying the interventions or addressing such things as inflammation or oxidative stress often associated with early childhood abuse.

TREATMENT OF POST-TRAUMATIC STRESS DISORDER IN ADOLESCENTS, YOUNG ADULTS AND ADULTS WITH CHILDHOOD HISTORY OF TRAUMA WITH MODIFICATION OF THE INTERVENTION BASED ON THE AGE OF THE ABUSE
Eye Movement Desensitization and Reprocessing and Imagery Rescripting

An RCT[55] by Boterhoven de Haan and colleagues imagery rescripting (ImR) and EMDR as a treatment for young adults with PTSD from childhood trauma before 16 years of age documented in the Life Events Checklist for DSM-5 (N = 128, ages 18–70) were compared. Participants were eligible if they had a primary diagnosis of PTSD related to their childhood trauma, and symptoms had to be present for 3 months or more. Assessments included the Structured Clinical Interviews for DSM-IV-TR (SCID-IV) 15 or the Mini International Neuropsychiatric Interview. Emotional abuse and emotional or physical neglect were distinguished. Treatment comprised twelve 90-min sessions twice a week for 6 to 8 weeks using ImR. The treatments were modified based on the age at which the abuse occurred. In the ImRs protocol, in phase one, the patient recalls a trauma memory from their child-self perspective, identifying their thoughts, feelings, and needs. The patient is then guided to imagine a different ending, such as someone intervening by stopping the abuse and caring for the child's other needs. The therapist enters the image for the first six treatment sessions and intervenes. From session seven onward, the patient steps into the image as their adult self and intervenes (phase two). In phase three, the patient re-experiences the event from the child's perspective, with the patient as the adult intervening. The other study used the eight-phase EMDR protocol. The general assessment, preparation, and key memory components of the first trauma to be processed (phases one, two, and three), were incorporated into the first session. Phases three to eight, the active trauma processing phases, were repeated from session two onward. At session 12 or earlier, the session focused on current triggers and anticipatory anxiety related to future events. A generalized linear mixed model of repeated measures showed that observer-rated PTSD symptoms significantly decreased for both ImRs (d = 1.72) and EMDR (d = 1.73) at the 8-week post-treatment assessment and continued one year later when modifications were made based on the age of the child. ImRs and EMDR reduce the burden on both patients and therapists, as individuals are not required to relive their trauma experiences in great detail and this may be the reason for the low dropout rate. Similar results occurred with secondary outcome measures and self-reported PTSD symptoms. There were no significant differences between the two treatments on any standardized measure post-treatment and follow-up.

An 8-week RCT of EMDR vs WLC involved 36 youth ages 6-16.[56] The study used the Posttraumatic Stress Symptom Scale for Children (PTSS-C scale), to identify the severity of post-trauma symptoms (PTS) not specific to PTSD. The treatment differed from the adult-focused EMDR protocol when recalling the traumatic events, identifying negative cognitions and emotions, and primarily identifying the alternative positive cognitions. For example, if difficulties arose in identifying negative or positive emotions and expressing them verbally, face pictures expressing various emotions were shown to the child to point out the most relevant feeling. Post-treatment scores of the EMDR group were significantly lower than the WLC. However, the improvement in re-experiencing symptoms proved to be the most significant between-group difference over time. Only one EMDR session was sufficient for treating PTSD in children.

In additon, EMDR interventions seem to have flexibility and can be adapted to the type of trauma experienced.

In a case-controlled study by Tang and colleagues,[57] 83 students (ages 12–15) were randomized to either a modified EMDR intervention or TAU using psycho-education. Students selected had PTSD related to Typhoon Morakot and depression, or current moderate or high suicide risk. The EMDR was adapted because it was felt that after a catastrophic event, experiences are not processed properly. This EMDR technique sought to decrease excessive physical distress associated with flashback memories, correct distorted memories about themselves, and remove the avoidance behavior and negative cognitive thoughts associated with traumatic events. The initial sessions lasted 60 minutes and began with an explanation of the EMDR process. Sessions lasted 30-40 minutes two to three times per week for 3 months. Those in the EMDR group had to identify their most vivid flashback image, a negative belief about themselves, and bodily and emotional associations. They then had to identify a positive image of themselves to confront the negative, distorted image of themselves and rate it to the intensity of the negative image. Then the therapist did desensitization. The EMDR group showed significantly lower pre-intervention severity values of general anxiety and depression than did the TAU group. In addition, the pre-intervention severity value of disaster-related anxiety in the EMDR group was lower than that in the TAU psychoeducational group ($p = 0.05$). The severity of psychological impact on the Chinese version of Impact of Event Scale Revised (C-IES-R) in the EMDR group changed from 34.02 ($SD = 19.85$) to 18.37 ($SD = 19.60$). The severity of anxiety on the Multidimensional Anxiety Scale for Children (MASC-T) in the EMDR group changed from 69.78 ($SD = 19.54$) to 30.61 ($SD = 19.39$). The severity of depression on the Center for Epidemiologic Studies Depression Scale (CES-D) in the EMDR group changed from 25.10 ($SD = 11.50$) to 14.78 ($SD = 11.36$). The size (Cohen's d) of the EMDR effect on the C-IES-R, MASC-T, and CES-D was 0.16, 0.49, and 0.59, respectively. There were no significant changes in the TAU group on any of these scales. The results of this study support that EMDR could alleviate general anxiety and depressive symptoms and reduce disaster-related anxiety in adolescents experiencing major traumatic disasters when the EMDR is modified for traumatic disasters.

There seems to be evidence from these three studies that the outcomes improve when adaptations are used in EMDR and ImR based on the child's developmental age for which the trauma occurred or based on the extraordinary emotional distress experienced during a catastrophic condition.

PROMISING THERAPIES THAT MAY NOT REQUIRE ADAPTATIONS OF TREATMENT WITH HISTORY OF CHILDHOOD ABUSE
Neurofeedback for complex post-traumatic stress disorder

A randomized, wait-list (TAU) controlled trial of EEG neurofeedback training (NF) in patients with chronic PTSD and a history of childhood abuse was conducted by van der Kolk, 2016. Fifty-two individuals with chronic PTSD were randomized to either NF ($n = 28$) or wait-list (WL) ($n = 24$) twice weekly for 12 weeks. Clinicians completed four evaluations, at baseline (T1), after week 6 (T2), at post-treatment (T3), and one-month follow-up (T4). Assessment measures were: 1) Traumatic Events Screening Inventory (T1); 2) the Clinician-Administered PTSD Scale (CAPS; T1, T3, T4); 3) the Davidson Trauma Scale (DTS; T1-T4), and 4) the Inventory of Altered Self-Capacities (IASC; T1-T4). The most frequently endorsed events were childhood caregiver emotional abuse (78.8%), sexual abuse (69.2%), and domestic violence, 61.5%. NF training occurred two times per week for 12 weeks. The NF training protocol used a standard of inhibiting frequencies of 2–6 HZ for slow activity and 22–36 HZ for fast EEG activity. Participants had experienced an average of 9.29 ($SD = 2.90$) different traumatic events. Post-treatment, a significantly smaller proportion of NF (6/22, 27.3%) met the criteria for PTSD than the WL condition (15/22, 68.2%). Measures of tension reduction activities, affect dysregulation, and affect instability showed a significant Time × Condition interaction. The effect sizes of NF ($d = -2.33$ within, $d = -1.71$ between groups) are comparable to those reported for the most effective evidence-based treatments.[58]

A pilot RCT of Neurofeedback Training on Children with Developmental Trauma was done by Rogel and colleagues[59] ($N = 37$, ages 6–13). Baseline assessment included PTSD Reaction Index (PTSD-RI) history, trauma history, and the child's demographics. The same caregiver and the child completed a self-report NF Symptom Checklist questionnaire during and after every NF session. This pilot study showed that 24 sessions of NF significantly decreased PTSD symptoms, internalizing, externalizing, and other behavioral and emotional symptoms. In addition, NF significantly improved the executive functioning of children with severe histories of abuse and neglect who had not benefited from any previous therapy. However, treatment gains had started to revert at the 1-month follow-up assessment. The study indicated that more sessions might be needed to increase and consolidate substantial gains. However, no studies have shown that the P4-T4 protocol used in this study is the most effective. Nor have any studies shown the optimal number of sessions needed for any early traumatized population, including adults and children with PTSD. Further, comparisons to WLC are suspect for novel treatments requiring significant time/effort and caregiver investment in keeping appointments. More research is needed for NF in children.

The default-mode network (DMN) and salience network (SN) display altered connectivity in PTSD. Nicholson and colleagues[60] did a DBPCT of alpha-rhythm EEG-NF vs sham in participants with PTSD ($n = 36$, ages 21–79) over 20-weeks to observe changes in network connectivity via fMRI. PTSD severity scores significantly decreased in the experimental NFB group post-NF (DZ = 0.71) and at 3-month follow-up (DZ = 0.77) to baseline measures. The study found a shift towards normalization of DMN and SN connectivity post-NFB only in the experimental group. Improved PTSD severity and NFB performance correlated with DMN and SN connectivity changes. Critically, remission rates of PTSD were significantly higher in the NF group (61.1%) than in the sham control group (33.3%). The use of fMRI may indicate actual changes in brain connectivity correlated to decreases in PTSD symptoms. Quantitative EEGs (QEEG) using low-resolution electromagnetic tomography (LORETA) can map brain connectivity changes in the same way fMRI does at a lower cost and identify changes in these circuits during and after NF.[61] More research is needed to identify particular circuits which should be targeted when doing LORETA NF in patients with PTSD.

TREATMENT IN INDIVIDUALS WITH AN EARLY HISTORY OF CHILDHOOD ABUSE TARGETING UNDERLYING ROOT CAUSES AND THE EFFECT ON EPIGENETICS, INFLAMMATION, HYPOTHALAMIC–PITUITARY AXIS, CORTISOL, AND OXIDATIVE STRESS

Epigenetic Factors

Early traumatic experiences are associated with hyper- and hypo-methylation of specific regulatory sites in key biological stress system genes.[62] Increased methylation of essential biological stress system genes can silence a gene's activity by making the gene inaccessible for transcription, whereas demethylation may make a gene more accessible for transcription. Klengal and colleagues[63] showed an increased risk of PTSD and childhood trauma with FKBP5 single-nucleotide polymorphisms (SNPs). Binder and colleagues[64] identified 4 SNPs in the FKBP5 locus (rs9296158, rs3800373, rs1360780, and rs9470080; minimum $P = .0004$) associated with the severity of child abuse to predict the level of adult PTSD symptoms. When demethylation of the FKBP5 gene occurs, rapid induction of FKBp5 occurs which binds to the glucocorticoid receptor (GR) blocking the ability of cortisol to bind to GRs in the Hypothalamic-Pituitary-Adrenal Axis (HPA). In this scenario, negative feedback of the HPA axis cannot occur, increasing the risk of developing PTSD. In addition, increased expression of FKBP5 also leads to alterations of neuronal circuits, as reflected by structural changes in the hippocampus, and gene expression changes in the immune system, resulting in immune and metabolic disorders. The FKBP5 genotype and early trauma can predispose an individual to PTSD and depression, indicating shared diagnostic boundaries due to stress sensitivity. These effects on DNA demethylation seem to only be restricted to early experiences of trauma and not in adulthood.

On the other hand, methylation of the exon NR3C1 promoter (GR), the homolog of the exon NR3C1 promoter, decreases hippocampal GR expression and increases HPA responses to stress. In this case, increased CpG methylation of the NR3c1 promoter decreases NGFI-A binding and reduces hippocampal GR expression. There is a link between the severity of abuse and increased NR3C1 (GR) methylation in adults with a history of CM and depression.[65] Hence, childhood abuse is associated with the demethylation of high-risk SNPs of the gene FKBP5 and methylation of the gene NR3C1. These early epigenetic effects may be the reason that traditional psychotherapies and medication do not work when there is a history of childhood abuse. Research is beginning to focus on the effects of treatment in adults with genetic risk factors for PTSD and childhood trauma.

In an RCT study ($N = 22$, ages 33 and above) using mindfulness-based stress reduction (MBSR), participants had 7 weekly 2.5-hour group sessions and a 6.5-hour retreat, for a total of nine sessions over the course of 9 weeks. There was a significant time x responder group interaction for methylation in FKBP5 intron 7 bin 2 [$F^{1,19} = 7.492$, $p = 0.013$] whereby responders had an increase in methylation and non-responders had a decrease in methylation post-treatment. These preliminary findings suggest that DNA methylation signatures within FKBP5 are potential indicators of response to meditation treatment in PTSD and require validation in larger cohorts and especially in younger children.[66]

Early priming of the hypothalamic–pituitary–adrenal axis

Increased GR sensitivity in PTSD may initially upregulate the HPA axis, increasing cortisol.[67] There seems to be an increase in cortisol in children enduring multiple traumas. However, the cortisol levels seem to decline after puberty and only rise when a new emotional stressor or traumatic reminder is experienced. These changes in cortisol may be due to the "priming" of the Limbic-Hypothalamic–Pituitary–Adrenal axis (LHPA).[68,69]

Childhood trauma may also be related to a mixed state of PTSD, depression, and anxiety associated with an increased sensitivity to stress found in victims of childhood abuse. Women with a history of childhood abuse and a current major depression diagnosis showed a more than 6-fold greater ACTH response to stress than age-matched controls. Eighty-five percent of women with PTSD and childhood trauma have depression.[70] Therefore, when looking at refractory depression, one may have to be cognizant of co-occurring PTSD and the increased response to stress and childhood trauma which may play a factor in response to treatment.

The Role of Cortisol

Probiotics reduce the overactivation of the HPA axis by the vagal nerve in adults, but research on PTSD in youth is limited. Efforts to focus on interventions that may reduce cortisol using EMDR and meditation in children and adolescents is critical. Cortisol levels were reduced after acute stress in an RCT ($n = 40$, healthy university students) using PsychoNeuroEndocrinoImmunology-based meditation (PNEIMED) meditation The intervention design included 30 hours of face-to-face learning (over four consecutive days).[71] PNEIMED includes philosophical lectures and meditative and stress-control practices from the Buddhist Mahayana tradition, integrated with modern theories. The cortisol levels post-test (after the PNEIMED course) was lower than at pre-test (before the PNEIMED course), showing a significant difference of cortisol salivary concentration between the 2 measures ($F = 5.326$; $p = 0.032$). In the control group, the pre-test vs post-test did not show significant differences. A study of 40 adolescents (age 12–18) diagnosed with PTSD using the child post-traumatic stress reaction index (CPSRI) were given six sessions of EMDR.[72] Pre- and post-levels of DHEA-S and cortisol levels were drawn. Receiver operator analysis (ROC) analysis showed that the DHEA-S/cortisol ratio predicts treatment response at a medium level (AUC: 0.703, p: .030, sensitivity: 0.65, specificity: 0.86). However, a positive response was recorded when a 30% or greater improvement was seen. Usually a 50% or greater response is used to determine a positive response.

In a pilot study by West and colleagues[73] ($n = 69$ Hatha yoga decreased salivary cortisol levels. Overall, these studies suggest that EMDR, meditation, and yoga may be good alternatives when patients are unresponsive to medications and psychotherapy.

An RCT study (Church 2012) examined the effect of EFT on cortisol levels. Random assignment occurred in eighty-three nonclinical subjects to either an EFT group, a psychotherapy group receiving a supportive interview (SI), or a no-treatment (NT) group. Salivary cortisol assays were performed immediately before and 30 minutes after the intervention. Psychological distress symptoms were assessed using the symptom assessment-45. The EFT group showed statistically significant improvements in anxiety (-58.34%, $p < 0.05$), depression (-49.33%, $p < 0.002$), the overall severity of symptoms (-50.5%, $p < 0.001$), and symptom breadth (-41.93%, $p < 0.001$). The EFT group experienced a significant decrease in cortisol level (-24.39%; SE, 2.62) compared with the decrease observed in the SI (-14.25%; SE, 2.61) and NT (-14.44%; SE, 2.67) groups ($p < 0.03$). The decrease in cortisol levels in the EFT group mirrored the observed improvement in psychological distress.[74]

Oxidized Stress

As noted, PTSD can increase oxidized stress. NAC decreases oxidative stress, increases glutathione, and modulates glutamate.[23] The reduction in PTSD and craving using NAC has previously been discussed.[24] In addition, polyunsaturated fatty acids

(PUFAs) reduce components of oxidized stress found in PTSD. Increased oxidative stress markers have been reported recently in otherwise healthy early life stress/child trauma-exposed adolescents.[75] These include reduced glutathione (GSH), oxidized glutathione (GSSG), GSH/GSSG ratios, thiobarbituric acid reactive substances (TBARSs) levels, and the activity of catalase and glutathione peroxidase (GPx). All of these components are measurements of oxidized stress. More research on NAC and PUFAs and their role in reducing components of oxidized stress in PTSD are needed.

Role of inflammation

The GR lower expression and function due to epigenetic suppression may allow for exacerbated inflammatory activity. Notably, increased inflammation can then maintain and exacerbate the impaired GR function leading to sustained GR resistance into adulthood.[76] In a study of women with PTSD secondary to physical or sexual abuse during childhood, these women showed increased inflammatory and immune activity.[77] In women who had experienced early maltreatment, those diagnosed with PTSD had higher activation levels of T cells than those who did not have PTSD. More specifically, investigators found a positive correlation between T-cell activation levels and intrusive symptoms of PTSD.[78] Other investigators showed that greater concentrations of interleukin-6 (IL-6), a pro-inflammatory cytokine, were seen during the Trier Social Stress Test in adults with child maltreatment histories compared with adults without such histories.

The association between childhood trauma and adulthood inflammation is stronger for inflammatory pathways related to TNF-α; and, indeed, the GR is crucial in regulating TNF-α signaling and TNF-induced cytokine production, as well as conveying protection against TNF-related tissue damage.[79] Different types of trauma may be associated with different inflammatory cytokines. In a meta-analysis[80] of peripheral C-reactive protein, interleukin-6, and tumor necrosis factor-α in adults who had experienced childhood trauma before age 18, individual types of trauma exposure impacted differentially on the inflammatory markers. Sub-group analyses for childhood sexual abuse showed this trauma type was significantly associated with a small effect size for TNF-α ($z = 0.24$, df = 2, $P = 0.02$, 95% CI = 0.05–0.44) and a trend toward a small effect size for IL-6 ($z = 0.08$, df = 4, $P = 0.08$, 95%CI = $-$ 0.01–0.16), whereas no such results were found for CRP ($z = -$ 0.001, df = 4, $P = 0.98$, 95% CI = $-$ 0.05–0.05). Subgroup analyses for childhood physical abuse similarly showed significant associations with small effect sizes for TNF-α ($z = 0.25$, df = 2, $P = 0.01$, 95% CI = 0.05–0.45) and IL-6 ($z = 0.08$, df = 5, $P = 0.02$, 95%CI = 0.02–0.15), but not for CRP ($z = 0.007$, df = 5, $P = 0.91$, 95% CI = $-$ 0.12–0.13). Subgroup analyses for parental absence during childh was only possible for CRP, revealing a significant association with a small effect size ($z = 0.11$, df = 2, $P = 0.001$, 95% CI = 0.02–0.19) and significant heterogeneity ($P = 0.006$, I 2 = 80.4%, τ 2 = 0.004).

COMPLEMENTARY AND INTEGRATIVE MEDICINE TREATMENTS THAT TARGET INFLAMMATION

Omega 3 Fatty Acids (Polyunsaturated Fatty Acids)

Some CIM interventions reduce inflammatory responses found in PTSD. For instance, decreased hippocampal neurogenesis promoted a prolonged hippocampal period of associative fear memories associated with PTSD.[81] In addition, PUFAs may promote adult neurogenesis to facilitate the clearance of fear memories.[82] They may also maintain endocannabinoid-mediated neuronal functions[83,84] that facilitate the extinction of fear memories.[85] In addition, higher levels of PUFAs may increase greater gray matter volume in the subgenual ACC, the right hippocampus, and the right amygdala, which is involved in affect regulation.[86] In addition, fish oil can reduce sympathetic nerve activity,[87] playing a pivotal role in developing PTSD.[88]

An open-label pilot study in adults has shown the efficacy of using PUFAs in reducing symptoms of PTSD[89] and preventing the symptoms of PTSD.[90] As noted previously, increased EPA, lower AA, and a lower ratio of AA/EPA is related to a lower risk of developing PTSD.[28]

Meditation

In a review by Krapalani and colleagues,[91] meditators had increased global histone modifications (H4ac) and also had lower expression of pro-inflammatory genes, such as RIPK2 (Receptor Interacting Pro-Kinase2) and cyclooxygenase-2 (COX-2). Also, meditators had lower expression of histone deacetylase 2 (HDAC2) genes which increase the expression of pro-inflammatory genes, such as IL-12 and TNF-α. Furthermore, RIPK2 and HDAC2 genes have decreased expression in meditators, which are associated with faster cortisol-related recovery from stress. Krapalani's study supports evidence for mindfulness meditation downregulating the expression of the HDACs genes and reducing pro-inflammatory cytokines, thus, suggesting preventive and therapeutic potentials. Furthermore, individuals who practiced yoga and mindfulness meditation have reduced methylation levels conducive to decreasing PTSD and reduced pro-inflammatory markers in preliminary research. In addition, research on participants who practice tai-chi has shown a slower decline in DNA methylation in loci implicated in aging.

Emotional Freedom Techniques

In an RCT pilot study by Church and colleagues,[92] after 10 sessions of EFT compared with TAU with 6-month follow-up, PTSD symptoms declined significantly in the EFT group (53%, $P < .0001$). Participants maintained their gains on follow-up ($n = 16$). After EFT, significant differences ($P < .05$) occurred for six genes—chemokine receptor 3 (CXCR3), interleukin 18 (IL-18), interleukin 10 receptor beta, tumor necrosis factor-alpha-induced protein 6, leukocyte-endothelial cell adhesion molecule 1 (selectin L), and interferon-induced transmembrane protein 1. These target genes are generally involved in regulating cellular immunity and inflammation and are associated with stress. In another study of treatment responders using Eye Movement Desensitization and Reprocessing, significant decreases in cortisol levels occurred after session 9.[93]

Flavonoids and Probiotics

Lipopolysaccharides (LPS) produced due to dysbiosis (which occurs in the gut after chronic stress) induces the production of TNF-α and IL-6. These cytokines activate NF-kB expression, producing more inflammatory molecules leading to oxidative stress.[94,95] A study of flavonoids with anti-oxidative effects revealed that they might help reduce oxidative stress and glucocorticoid resistance.[96] In addition, individuals who scored higher on the PTSD clinician administered post-traumatic stress disorder scale (CAPS) had decreased Actinobacteria, Lentisphaerae, and Verrucomicrobia. Decreased exposure to these bacteria led to increased vulnerability for PTSD due to the decreased anti-inflammatory and immunoregulatory effects these microbes possess. Therefore, studies using flavonoids and probiotics may prove helpful in treating PTSD.[97]

Inflammation due to childhood abuse can increase the risk of medical conditions later in life. In a study of ACEs by Felitti,[98] there was a 10-year decrease in lifespan and increases in chronic diseases like diabetes, asthma, stroke, substance abuse,

Table 1
Summary of treatments for PTSD

Treatment	Level of certainty based on benefit and quality of evidence	Strength of recommendation based on Benefit and Safety	Evidence of studies in Youth/basis for recommendation	Passes SECS	Personal Recommendations Of the Reviewer
I. Meditation					
a. Meditation and yoga (Gallegos et al, 2017[30]). N=1,173, 19 RCT's, Ages ≥18	Low-more than 2 RCTs but limited quality of studies	C	1 meta-analysis	YES	• Meta-analysis had few studies, many with high bias and no estimate of the severity of PTSD in studies • Recommended as adjunct
b. Meditation/ Mindfulness (Simkin, Black et al, 2014[104]), children and adolescents	Moderate	B (During disasters Catani,2009 &Gordon,2008)	Review 2 RCT's Several comparative studies, pilots and case studies.	YES	• Two studies stand out as 1st line in disaster situations. • Catani, 2009 (35) after the Sri Lanka Tsunami & Gordon, 2008 (36) post-war in Kosovar for PTSD where emergent interventions are needed. *Catani's study* (n=31, ages 8-14, 6 sessions), recovery at 6 months was 81% for the children in the narrative exposure group (KIDNET) and 71%for those in the meditation-relaxation group (MED-RELAX)

		(ES for KIDNET=1.96 six months and MED-Relax=2.20). *Gordon's study*, after 12 sessions (n=77 high school students) there was a significant decrease (df=1.76, p <.001) in PTSD maintained at 3 months. • Benefits insomnia. • Better effect size (ES) in groups<30. • Research outcomes improve with increased amounts of time spent practicing, or participating in formal guided practice, with increased effectiveness of the techniques. • Diagnosis used to detect PTSD must be culturally sensitive, Recommend as 1st line for disasters Recommend as adjunct			
c. Spiritual-hypnosis-assisted treatment (SHAT-meditation with guided imagery) (Lesmana et al, 2009[37]), N = 48 treated, 178 controls, ages 6-12	Low	• SHAT produced a 77.1% improvement rate at a 2-year follow-up, compared to 24% in the control group.	C	1 RCT	YES

(continued on next page)

Table 1
(continued)

Treatment	Level of certainty based on benefit and quality of evidence	Strength of recommendation based on Benefit and Safety	Evidence of studies in Youth/basis for recommendation	Passes SECS	Personal Recommendations Of the Reviewer
					• Used culturally adapted diagnostic criteria for Bali Recommend
II. Yoga					
Yoga vs. aerobic dance control plus non-randomized WLC (Culver et al, 2015[32]), N = 76, ages 7-17	Low	C	1 RCT	YES	• No statistically significant results for PTSD. • Recommended as adjunct to decrease anxiety which is often co-morbid with PTSD
III. EMDR/CBT/ImR/ Exposure Therapy (ET)					
a. Comparison CBT & other psychological therapies (Gillies et al, 2013[103]), N = 758, ages 2-24, 14 RCTs	Low - more than 2 RCTs but limited quality limited quality of studies	C	Meta analysis	Yes	a. -No difference between CBT and EMDR None of therapies effects lasted >1 month. Differences in scales used to diagnose PTSD, types of trauma, methodological biases, & the small number & size of

Study	Bias	Grade	Type		Findings
					identified studies did not allow authors to determine if one modality was better than another. Poor study. Does not mean it is not recommended. Recommendation based on other studies
b. EMDR and EMDR vs CBT (Khan et al, 2018[41]), N=257, of which N=217 were children mean age 11, ages in entire study ≥10	High-very little bias in studies	A	Systemic review & Meta-analysis (11 RCT's) (4 of which were children)	YES	b. -No bias in child studies • EMDR >CBT post treatment in 11 studies (p=0.006) (4 of which were children) • 3 mos later EMDR =CBT in 2 of 4 child RCTs (p=0.15) • EMDR as effective as CBT • EMDR also effective for PTSD with anxiety in 2 of 4 child RCTs • EMDR=less sessions Recommend in children
c. Review EMDR and EMDR vs CBT	High	A	Review (8 RCTs) 3 RCTs compared CBT vs		EMDR & CBT are equally effective.

(continued on next page)

Table 1
(continued)

Treatment	Level of certainty based on benefit and quality of evidence	Strength of recommendation based on Benefit and Safety	Evidence of studies in Youth/basis for recommendation	Passes SECS	Personal Recommendations Of the Reviewer
(Manzoni et al, 2021[40]), n=150, ages 8-18			EMDR in children (N=207, ages 4-18)		EMDR is briefer than cognitive behavioral writing therapy (CBWT) in number of sessions (EMDR = 4.1 vs. CBWT = 5.4; t [64.52] = −5.44) and length of treatment in minutes (EMDR = 140 vs. CBWT = 227; t [80.17] = −5.49). Both EMDR (t = −4.51) and CBWT (t = −4.87) reduced PTSD symptoms compared to WL conditions Recommend
d. EMDR vs CBT in children (Rodenburg et al, 2009[42]), n=109 experimental group and 100 controls, ages 4-18) (42)	High	A	Meta-analysis (7 RCTs)	YES	• The overall effect size for EMDR was d − .56 (medium). • The overall effect size for EMDR was d − .56 (medium), which indicates that children receiving EMDR appear to benefit from their treatment. Parent and child ratings had

a moderate to large ES. ES for the effect of EMDR on trauma status at the post-test was d = .56, p < .001. The combined ES for comparisons between TAU or waitlist was significantly larger than (d=.66, p<.001) than ES for comparisons with CBT (d=.25, p<.05). Recommend

IV. Studies that clarified that treatments for PTSD where abuse

a. Psychological interventions for C-PTSD (Karatzias et al, 2019[52]) ages >16	Moderate for individuals without childhood trauma	B	Meta-analysis (51 RCTs) Did not indicate RCTs with individuals *16-24 years of age*	YES but not as effective with individuals with a history of childhood abuse	CBT, exposure therapy alone (EA) EMDR helps reduce symptoms of negative self-concept and disturbances in relationships found with C-PTSD in adolescents and young adults but not for affect dysregulation. • All effective as compared to treatment as usual.
	Low with history of childhood trauma	C			

(continued on next page)

Table 1
(continued)

Treatment	Level of certainty based on benefit and quality of evidence	Strength of recommendation based on Benefit and Safety	Evidence of studies in Youth/basis for recommendation	Passes SECS	Personal Recommendations Of the Reviewer
					• *However, for those with early childhood abuse, all interventions have less effect,* (Reduction in Hedges' g of 0.35 (95% CI 0.02– 0.69), • Recommend with modifications for early childhood abuse in adolescents & young adults • Recommend adolescents and young adults for those without history of childhood abuse
b. Psychotherapy or CBT alone, medication alone or combined treatment for depression in individuals with or without childhood abuse (Nanni et al, 2020[53] 26 studies, N=23,544 for epidemiological	Moderate for individuals without history of childhood abuse Low for those with a history of childhood abuse	B C	Meta-analysis-10 combined treatment clinical trials (15 active treatment arms) 2 RCTs for adolescents CBT, Family & supportive therapy 2 RCTs meds-not effective	YES for CBT in those without history of child hood abuse No for Medica-tion for depression with childhood history of child abuse	Lack of response or remission during treatment for depression (odds ratio=1.43, 95% CI=1.11–1.83) with history of Childhood abuse. A meta-analysis of these studies showed that maltreated

studies, N=3,098 for clinical trails, mean age ≥ 14.7)

individuals were twice as likely as those without a history of childhood maltreatment to develop persistent depressive episodes (odds ratio=2.34, 95% CI=1.65–3.32) and twice as likely to have an unfavorable longitudinal course of depression (odds ratio=2.27, 95% confidence interval [CI]=1.80–2.87) Recommend CBT for depression in those without history of childhood abuse. Do not recommend medication for depression

c. EMDR or fluoxetine or placebo in individuals with or without childhood abuse. (van Der Kolk et al, 2007[54]) N=85, ages ≥ 18	Low Low	RCT	C for those without childhood abuse. C for those with childhood history of abuse	EMDR more effective for those without history of childhood abuse • Medication was not effective whether or not there was childhood abuse. • EMDR less effective for those with childhood abuse

(continued on next page)

Table 1 (continued)					
Treatment	Level of certainty based on benefit and quality of evidence	Strength of recommendation based on Benefit and Safety	Evidence of studies in Youth/basis for recommendation	Passes SECS	Personal Recommendations Of the Reviewer
					At 6-month follow-up, 75.0% of adult-onset versus only 33.3% of child-onset trauma subjects receiving EMDR. • (Fluoxetine & SSRIs do not pass SECS-(Robb, 2010, Boaden, 2020)
V. EMDR with modification based on the age abuse occurred					
a. Imagery rescripting (ImR) and EMDR for young adults with childhood trauma (Boterhoven de Haan et al, 2020⁵⁵), N-128, age ≥18	Low	C	RCT	YES	For ImR and EMDR in young adults with childhood trauma, effectiveness may improve by adjusting the intervention based on the developmental age in which the abuse occurred. PTSD symptoms significantly decreased for both ImRs (d = 1.72) and EMDR (d = 1.73) at the 8-week post-treatment assessment

and continued one year later. ImR & EMDR do not have to relive the trauma and may be a reason for low drop-out rates.

					• Recommend in adolescents & young adults with a history of childhood trauma
b. EMDR with deviations from the adult protocol based on the age of the child (Ahmad et al, 2009[56]), n = 36, ages 6-16	Low	C	RCT	YES	• Deviations from the adult-focused EMDR protocol were mainly found in the: • moments of recalling the traumatic events, • identification of negative cognitions and emotions, and • mostly regarding the identification of the alternative positive cognitions. • The improvement in re-experiencing symptoms proved to be the most significant between-group difference over time. Modifications improve outcome. • Recommend
c. EMDR vs TAU depression and PTSD	Low	C	RCT		The size (Cohen's *d*) of the EMDR effect on

(continued on next page)

Table 1
(continued)

Treatment	Level of certainty based on benefit and quality of evidence	Strength of recommendation based on Benefit and Safety	Evidence of studies in Youth/basis for recommendation	Passes SECS	Personal Recommendations Of the Reviewer
with modification after a typhoon (Tang, et al 2015[74]), N = 83, ages 12-15 (57)					the Chinese version of Impact of Event Scale-Revised (C- IES-R), Multidimensional Anxiety Scale for Children (MASC-T), and Chinese version of the Center for Epidemiologic Studies Depression Scale (CES-D) was 0.16, 0.49, and 0.59, respectively. EMDR is effective after a major disaster
VI. Art Therapy					
a. Trauma Focused art therapy (TF-ART) (Lyshak-Stelzer et al, 2007[38]) ages 13-18, N=29	Low	C	Pilot RCT	YES	TF-ART significant treatment-by-condition interaction F (1,27) 7.1 p=.01 indicating that adolescents in the TF-ART condition had a significantly greater reduction in PTSD symptom severity -Recommend as adjunct in adolescents and young adults

b. Art Therapy (Schouten et al, 2015[39], ages 18-22, n=187)	Low -no RCTs	C	YES	Review 6 controlled comparative studies	Art therapy combined with psychotherapy produced the moderate decrease in trauma symptoms severity (0.76 [0.07, 1.42]) • Recommend as adjunct in young adults
V. Emotional Freedom Technique (EFT)					
a. EFT 7 RCT's, N=257 ≥ 12; (Sebastian & Nelms, 2017[48])	Moderate	B	YES	Meta-analysis (one RCT was with children, N=16, age 12-17) And one RCT > 18, N=52)	• Significant effect EFT vs TAU was 2.96 (95% CI 1.96-3.97, p< .01) RCT in adolescents 30 days after 1 session, none were symptomatic (p<.001). In RCT > 18, treatment effect sizes were large (d = 0.80) for both EMDR and EFT • Recommend for adolescents
b. EFT to determine if acupressure points were the sole mediator (3 studies, N=102, ages college students to age 65	Moderate	B	YES	Meta-analysis 3 randomized blinded studies with active controls 2 of the 3 involved college students	• Pretest vs. posttest EFT treatment showed a large effect size, Cohen's d= 1.28 (95% confidence interval [CI], 0.56 to 2.00) and Hedges' g =

(continued on next page)

Table 1
(continued)

Treatment	Level of certainty based on benefit and quality of evidence	Strength of recommendation based on Benefit and Safety	Evidence of studies in Youth/basis for recommendation	Passes SECS	Personal Recommendations Of the Reviewer
qualified) (Church et al, 2020[47])					1.25 (95% CI, 0.54 to 1.96). • Acupressure points were active component & not due to placebo in all 3 studies • Recommend
VI. Use of medication for PTSD in children and adolescents					
a. N-acetylcysteine (NAC) and CBT For PTSD and Substance Use Disorders (SUD) (Back et al, 2016[24]), n=35, ages ≥18	Low	C	DBPCT	YES	• Both groups got CBT • PTSD Scale (CAPS) total score was reduced by 46% in the NAC group and by 25% in control from baseline to Week 8 on 1200 mg BID • Cravings reduced by 81% in NAC group and 32% in control. • NAC can be used as an adjunctive to reduce PTSD symptoms in SUD and cravings.

Intervention	Evidence Level	Outcome	Study Design	Effective	Findings
a. High DHA/EPA Omega 3 fatty acids (PUFAs) given shortly after accident to determine if it would decrease physiological effects. (Matsumura et al, 2017[25]), N= 83, ages ≥18	Low Low	C=preventing physiological effects of PTSD in young adults D= preventing PTSD in young adults	DBPCT	YES for decreasing physiological effects	• Both groups improved depressive symptoms • Recommended in young adults • In patients with kidney disorders, it is not recommended. • DHA =1,470 mg and EPA= 147 mg. given 10 days post-injury. • Heart Rate and Skin Conductance improved in the Omega group. • No difference for control or omega group for CAPS. • Higher DHA/EPA does not prevent PTSD but may decrease secondary physiological effects. • Recommended for preventing physiological effects of PTSD in young adults, not PTSD
b. High DHA/EPA PUFs given after injury to determine if it would prevent PTSD	Low with high DHA and low EPA	D	RDBPC	YES but not effective	• Same formula as in the study "a" was given for 12 weeks after injury.

(continued on next page)

Table 1
(continued)

Treatment	Level of certainty based on benefit and quality of evidence	Strength of recommendation based on Benefit and Safety	Evidence of studies in Youth/basis for recommendation	Passes SECS	Personal Recommendations Of the Reviewer
(Matsuoka, et al 2015[26]), N= 110, ages ≥18					• No difference between 2 groups for preventing PTSD in young adults • Higher DHA/EPA does not work for preventing • Not recommended for preventing PTSD
c. Re-analysis of study b. (Matsuoka et al, 2016 [28]), N=110, ages ≥18	Low	C for higher EPA/DHA	RDBCT	YES	• Re-analysis of study b. • Higher erythrocyte EPA associated with lower development of PTSD • Higher EPA: DHA (p=.013) and EPA/AA inversely correlated with PTSD severity. • Increase AA (p=.001) correlated with PTSD severity. • Recommend a 2/1 ratio for EPAs to DHA at 1200 mg to 2000 mg as total dose in young adults to prevent PTSD

vii. Neurofeedback

a. Neurofeedback for chronic PTSD (van der kolk et al, 2016[58]), ages ≥18	Low	C for adults and young adults	RCT	NO -expensive	NF 2 x weekly for 12 weeks. In those with history of childhood abuse and chronic PTSD, ES of NF (d = -2.33 within, d = - 1.71 between groups) are comparable to those reported for the most effective evidence-based treatments • Recommended in young adults
b. Neurofeedback with children unresponsive to previous therapies (Rogel et al, 2020[59]), N=37, ages 6-13	Low	—	RCT	No -too expensive	24 sessions NF significantly improved the executive functioning of children with severe histories of abuse and neglect who had not benefited from any previous therapy. However, treatment gains reverted at the 1-month FU assessment. Protocol used by van der Kolk for this study may not be suitable to children. • This protocol is not recommended for children

(continued on next page)

Table 1
(continued)

Treatment	Level of certainty based on benefit and quality of evidence	Strength of recommendation based on Benefit and Safety	Evidence of studies in Youth/basis for recommendation	Passes SECS	Personal Recommendations Of the Reviewer
c. NF for PTSD using fMRI (Nicholson et al, 2020[60], N=36, ages ≥21)	Low	C	RCT	No expensive	• Remission rates were significantly higher than sham with normalization of Default Mode Network and Salience Network connectivity post NF-fMRI and 3-month f/u in adults & some young adults. • fMRI does help to show improvements in connectivity. • To date, no DBPCT or meta- analysis has been done using LORETA NF -can correlate to connectivity found in fMRI, but is less expensive to do. • QEEG is very helpful in looking at pre-and post-treatment effects with all interventions for PTSD. • More research has to be done on children.

VIII. Addressing Childhood PTSD, inflammatory markers, and epigenetic alterations

a. Childhood trauma, adult inflammation: meta-analysis of CRP, iL-6 and TNF-α. (Baumeister et al, 2016[80]), ages $\geq$20.9, N=16, 870=CPR, 3751=IL-6, 881=TNF-α	Low	C-needs replication	Meta analysis for inflamma-tory cytokines associated with childhood trauma,	YES	• Childhood physical and sexual abuse associated with TNF-α, modestly with IL-6. • Parental absence associated with CRP. • Recommend following inflammatory cytokines and markers and correlating to treatment success
b. Epigenetic effects of mind-body therapies in individuals with a history of childhood abuse (Kripalani et al, 2021[91]), N=646, ages mid50's	Low-no studies in children	C Needs Replication No RCTs	Review	YES	• Yoga, Tai Chi, & meditation decreased inflammatory cytokines and decreased cortisol. Recommend more research particularly in children to determine if epigenetic effects can be reversed
c. Mindfulness-Based Stress Reduction - Methylation of FKBP5 and SLC6A4 in	Low No research in children	C Needs Replication No RCTs	Review	YES	• Individuals with PTSD & childhood trauma who were responders to MSBR had

(continued on next page)

Table 1
(continued)

Treatment	Level of certainty based on benefit and quality of evidence	Strength of recommendation based on Benefit and Safety	Evidence of studies in Youth/basis for recommendation	Passes SECS	Personal Recommendations Of the Reviewer
Relation to Treatment (Bishop et al, 2018[66]), n=22, adults with PTSD					methylation of FKBp5 and non-responders had a de-methylation. • Research needed in children. Recommend more research
d. DBPCT-Measuring effect of NAC on oxidized stress in individuals with PTSD (Atkura et al, 2007[23])	Low	C Needs replication	DBPCT	YES	• NAC (1200 mg/BID) decreases oxidized stress. • Promising biological effect. • Recommend more research
e. Meditation effect cortisol levels (Bottaccioli et al, 2019[71],) university students, n=40	Low	C needs replication	RCT	YES	• Meditation decreased cortisol after acute stress in young adults. • Promising biological effect. • Recommend more research
f. EFT (Church et al, 2012[74]) Measuring EFT salivary cortisol levels in 83 adult veterans.	Low-no studies in children	C needs replication	RCT	YES	• 10 sessions of EFT decreased cortisol. • Promising biological effect. • Recommend more research especially in children with high cortisol

g. Effect of EFT on epigenetics involving inflammatory genes (Church et al, 2018[92]), n=16, veterans	Low-needs replication and no studies in children	C Needs replication and higher N	RCT pilot study	• 10 sessions of EFT decreased the expression of pro-inflammatory genes and increased the expression of anti-inflammatory genes. • Promising biological effect. • Recommend more research especially in children
h. Hatha yoga reduced cortisol levels (West et al, 2004[73]), n=69, college students	Low more studies needed for young adults and children	C needs replication	Pilot study	• Yoga decreases cortisol in young adults Recommend more research (Passes SECS) verall statement on addressing childhood PTSD, inflammation and epigenetic effects • More studies need to address the effectiveness of treatment for PTSD and corresponding decrease in inflammatory

(continued on next page)

Table 1 (*continued*)

Treatment	Level of certainty based on benefit and quality of evidence	Strength of recommendation based on Benefit and Safety	Evidence of studies in Youth/basis for recommendation	Passes SECS	Personal Recommendations Of the Reviewer
					markers, cortisol, and epigenetic changes that occurred due to early childhood abuse. • Those studies may give insight as to why traditional psychotherapies do not work in children with childhood abuse. • Although some of these studies do not involve youth, they are mentioned due to their importance for future research on children and adolescents.

Strength of Recommendations based on benefit and safety

A=Recommend Strongly. There is a high certainty that the net benefit is substantial *and safe.*

B=Recommend. There is a high certainty that the net benefit is moderate or there is moderate certainty that the net benefit is moderate to substantial *and safe.*

C=Neutral (offer or provide this service for selected patients depending on individual circumstances, based on professional judgment and patient preferences).
There is at least moderate certainty that the net benefit is small

D=Discourage. There is moderate or high certainty that the service has no net benefit or that the harms outweigh the benefits

I = Insufficient (if the service is offered, patients should understand the uncertainty about the balance of benefits and harms) Current evidence is insufficient to assess the balance of benefits and harms of the service. Evidence is lacking, of poor quality, or conflicting, and the balance of benefits cannot be determined.)

Level of certainty regarding quality:

HIGH Level of Evidence with robust positive data meta-analyses or meta-reviews involving 2 or more RCTs of excellent, robust quality. The available evidence usually includes consistent results from well-designed, well-conducted RCTs in representative child, adolescent or young adult (18-24 years old) populations, assessing the effects on mental health outcomes.

MODERATE Level of Evidence with robust positive data involving 2 or more RCTs of excellent, robust quality. The available evidence usually includes consistent results from well- designed, well-conducted RCTs in representative child, adolescent or young adult (18-24 years old) populations, assessing the effects on mental health outcomes.

LOW Level of evidence with less than 2 RCTs with good or average quality. The available evidence is insufficient to assess the effects on mental health outcomes.

SECS Criteria:

A guide to clinical decisions is that Interventions that are Safe, Easy, Cheap, *and* Sensible (SECS) require less evidence to justify individual trials than those that are Risky, Unrealistic, Difficult, *or* Expensive (RUDE). Because some of the treatments do not have much solid, compelling evidence but would be reasonable to try with a lower bar of evidence, this criterion is also taken into account. Being risky, unrealistic, difficult *OR* expensive (RUDE) disqualifies from SECS. The bolded conjunctions are essential in applying this guide.

cancer, obesity, heart disease, and cancer and a corresponding increase in inflammatory markers like CRP. The link between childhood abuse and CRP is crucial because individuals with a history of childhood trauma show an average CRP increase related to risk factors for future heart attack, stroke, and the development of diabetes.[99] A dysregulated stress system could disinhibit inflammatory processes, promoting biological aging, inflammatory-related or immunosuppressed medical conditions, and compromised overall health.[100]

Meditation and EFT, and to a lesser degree, PUFAs, flavonoids, and probiotics may be helpful in decreasing inflammation associated with PTSD.

A summary of these studies can be found in **Table 1** using the United States Preventative Services Task Force ratings for the strength of the recommendation and level of certainty for each study. (See **Table 1**).

SUMMARY

No studies have shown efficacy for antidepressants in children and adolescents with PTSD as first-line treatment.[1,54,101,102] The last American Academy of Child and Adolescent Psychiatry Practice Parameters for PTSD was done in 2010. At that time, trauma-focused-cognitive behavior therapy (TF-CBT) was recommended as the first-line treatment for PTSD. However, recent studies have shown equal efficacy for TF- CBT vs EMDR,[50] EFT vs CBT,[48] CBT vs EMDR,[40–42] and ImR versus EMDR.[55] Research on PTSD treatments for children, adolescents, and young adults differ in response based on the age the abuse occurred,[13,14] the type of criteria used to diagnose,[7,8] the type of abuse, and the chronicity of the abuse.[9] So, one must keep in mind that when comparing studies, all of these components may not have allowed the comparison of different therapy outcomes in a meta-analysis to be properly analyzed. Only one meta-analysis by Gillies listed in **Table 1** attempted to compare CBT to all psychological therapies. CBT was as effective as EMDR but there were so many compounding difficulties in making comparisons like those mentioned above, that the huge undertaking that was required to do this study gave no substantial evidence for using any of the interventions.[103]

Complementary and Integrative/Functional Medicine interventions that are effective for children adolescents, and young adults with PTSD, include EMDR, EFT, and ImR and are considered first-line in those age groups. In addition, art therapy,[39] meditation,[29,30] yoga,[32] and NAC[24] as recommended as adjunctive treatments. However, under catastrophic conditions where there are few resources, meditation[35–37] seems to have significant effects when used as a first-line treatment. The same is true for EMDR with adaptations.[57] Also, PUFAs, given soon after an injury, with a higher EPA/DHA ratio may prevent PTSD soon after an injury.[28] Finally, more research is needed on flavonoids, photobiomodulation, and probiotics.

Research has helped to clarify that although all of the first-line interventions above are effective, some research has indicated that some interventions may not be as effective when chronic abuse occurs when the individual is ≤ 7. Research that led investigators to this conclusion began when a study involving psychotherapy or CBT, medication, or a combined approach was used for depression in adolescents, young adults, and adults with a history of childhood abuse. These interventions were seldom effective in individuals with early childhood abuse.[53] Furthermore, even when new diagnostic criteria are developed to distinguish young adult-onset PTSD from adolescents, young adults, and adults with PTSD and childhood abuse (eg, ICD-11, Complex-PTSD), even proven therapies like EMDR and CBT and EA had poor results in those with a history of childhood abuse[52] and EMDR was less effective in individuals with early childhood abuse.[54]

When researchers began to make adaptations to treatment based on the age the child experienced the abuse, EMDR and ImR in RCTs[55] showed more efficacy in those ≥18. EMDR adaptations also proved effective in individuals from 6 to 16 years of age[56] and in those 12 to 15 years of age.[57] The same was true for TF-CBT.[6]

In regard to adaptations to criteria used to identify PTSD, care and attention should be given to diagnosing and treating individuals from culturally different backgrounds. Meditation had greater success when the criteria for diagnosis were adjusted appropriately for the culture.[36,37] Although well-meaning, even when adaptations to criteria (eg, PTSD-AA) were made to identify more children with PTSD,[9] children who still suffer significantly from the trauma may not be diagnosed.[8] The diagnostic criteria for developmental trauma disorder (DTD) may be beneficial in this regard. DTD[11–16] has attempted to define the developmental effects of trauma based on the age the trauma occurred, the effects on the developing brain, the faulty misperceptions of cues, and long-term effects of inflammation, and epigenetics. All of these components may reduce the effectiveness of treatments. For instance, the effect of trauma on the de-methylation or re-methylation of genes at an early age may be a primary reason why some treatments are ineffective.[62–66] DTD (based on biology) is more suited for the RDoC than a DSM diagnosis (based on symptoms).

Some CIM/FM interventions may address the effects of environmental insults left behind secondary to early abuse. Reversal of epigenetic effects of trauma has been studied. EFT[92] decreased the expression of inflammatory genes, and meditation re-methylated the FKBP5 gene associated with early abuse.[66] In addition, inflammation can be addressed by CIM/FM interventions. Yoga, Tai Chi, and meditation decreased inflammatory cytokines and decreased cortisol.[91] Cortisol levels have also been reduced with meditation,[71] yoga,[73] EMDR,[72] and EFT.[74] fMRI analysis showed that probiotic treatments with specific Lactobacillus and Bifidobacterium species could dampen brain responses to negative emotional stimuli in the amygdala and the frontal and temporal cortices in Inflammatory Bowel Disease patients,[104] which could be relevant for PTSD patients. Oxidized stress was reduced,[23] and PTSD symptoms improved in a DBPCT with the use of NAC.[24] Oxidized stress can decrease neurogenesis in the hippocampus.[105] Maintaining higher EPA than DHA, decreasing AA, and lowering the AA/EPA were found to prevent PTSD when given shortly after an injury.[28] PUFAs may promote adult neurogenesis to facilitate the clearance of fear memories.[82] They may also maintain endocannabinoid-mediated neuronal functions[83,84] that facilitate the extinction of fear memories.[85] In addition, higher levels of PUFAs may increase greater gray matter volume in the subgenual ACC, the right hippocampus, and the right amygdala, which is involved in affect regulation.[86] In addition, fish oil can reduce sympathetic nerve activity,[87] playing a pivotal role in developing PTSD.[88] Although not typically considered as a CIM/FM intervention, propranolol given 90 minutes before Script Driven Traumatic Imagery showed pre-to post-treatment effect sizes of 2.74 vs 0.55 for placebo. Propranolol is thought to alter the amount of emotional fear associated with the reconsolidation of activated memories.[106]

All of these interventions are pertinent when one considers how abuse may affect the brain during time sensitive periods of vulnerability. Periods around age 3–5 have been associated with hippocampus development, and may therefore be particularly sensitive for vulnerability for ACE and trauma fostering later dissociation and PTSD. Other windows of vulnerability affecting hippocampal development have been defined for ages 11–13. Windows affecting amygdala development (age 10–11) and the prefrontal cortex (ages 14–16) have been identified.[107,108]

Some new therapies are promising. For example, NF[58] significantly improved PTSD symptoms in young adults and adults with a history of childhood abuse. Nicholson and colleagues[60] correlated fMRI NF to track changes in neurological pathways with improvement in PTSD symptoms in patients who had not previously responded to traditional therapies. The latter is an example of how circuits may be monitored after treatment interventions and applied to the RDoC where circuits are suggested as a unit of analysis. Another promising approach may include photobiomodulation[109,110] which uses red and near-infrared light. The primary targets of photon absorption involve cytochrome c oxidase in mitochondria, and calcium ion channels. Secondary and tertiary effects include increases in nitric oxide, a decrease of ROS in damaged cells, an increase in ATP, and activation of transcription factors, all leading reduced inflammation. It has improved memory, mood and cognitive functions and improved the microbiome.

Studies by Felitti and colleagues[98] have shown a 10-year decrease in lifespan and increases in chronic diseases like diabetes, asthma, stroke, substance abuse, cancer, obesity, heart disease, cancer, and a corresponding increase in inflammatory markers like CRP in childhood with ACEs. The number of traumatic events increased the risk. Therefore, every clinician must also address the mediators that perpetuate inflammation leading to other chronic conditions and neuroinflammation in the brain, hence decreasing the effectiveness of treatment and the worsening symptoms of PTSD.

Complementary and Integrative interventions may fit into the one treatment-one disorder approach traditionally used in medicine. However, Functional Medicine requires looking at how all systems are affected by such things as inflammation. This requires monitoring all the systems affected by inflammation, including neuroinflammation, insulin resistance leading to diabetes, thyroid functioning influenced by inflammation stress, and the disruption of sex hormones and increase in cortisol, etc. all of which can affect psychiatric disorders. It looks at antecedents (like family history and genetics), triggers (like early abuse), and mediators that perpetuate inflammation (like lifestyle). Some examples of mediators may include diet, nutritional deficiencies, antibiotics, toxins in the environment, mycotoxins, sleep, poor management of stress, artificial sweeteners, conflictual relationships, and proton pump inhibitors that cause dysbiosis and inflammation (**Figure 1**).[94,95,111,112] These interventions compose the

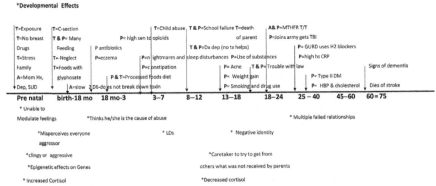

Fig. 1. Trajectory of events and effects from childhood abuse on Functional Medicine timeline. A, antecedents; P, perpetuators; T, Triggers. Some CIM/FM Approaches = Fix gut, improve vitamin deficiencies, improve sleep, organic and non-GMO foods, NAC or other researched interventions, EFT, EMDR, meditation for decreasing inflammatory cytokines, increase exercise, tx SUD, exercise to decrease inflammation, work on relationships, CBT, reverse osmosis filter, Organic Mediterranean diet, detect unresolved loss, identify LDs, tx MTHFR, Treat mold or other infections, Quercetin for hs CRP, give 2/1 ratio EPA/DHA, probiotics & prebiotics, Bright light tx, use free apps to detect toxins in household products (EWG healthy living) etc.

essence of Functional Medicine which in the long run seeks to produce a healthy emotional, spiritual, and mental state in the individual. Functional Medicine seeks to find the reason as to why the disease state transpired and to reverse the disease state, if possible.

In summary, the effectiveness of any treatment for PTSD may differ based on mitigating factors that were not considered when making the diagnosis or doing the treatment. Nevertheless, CIM/FM interventions may be of great use in treating refractory PTSD.

DISCLOSURE

None.

REFERENCES

1. Strawn JR, Keeshin' BR, DelBello MP, et al. Psychopharmacologic Treatment of post-traumatic stress disorder in children and adolescents: a review. J Clin Psychiatry 2010;71(7):932–41.
2. Williams LM, Debattista C, Duchemin A, et al. Childhood trauma predicts antidepressant response in adults with major depression: data from the randomized international study to predict optimized treatment for depression. Transl Psychiatry 2016;6:e799.
3. Edwards VJ, Holden GW, Felitti VJ, et al. Relationship between multiple forms of childhood maltreatment and adult mental health in community respondents: results from the adverse childhood experiences study. Am J Psychiatry 2003;160: 1453–60.
4. Herman JL. Complex PTSD: a syndrome in survivors of prolonged and repeated trauma. J Trauma Stress 1992;5(3):377–91. Available at: http://traumadissociation.com/complexptsd.
5. Cloitre M, Stolbach BC, Herman JL, et al. A developmental approach to complex PTSD: childhood and adult cumulative trauma as predictors of symptom complexity. J Trauma Stress 2009;22(5):399–408.
6. Scheeringa MS, Weems CF, Cohen JA, et al. Trauma-focused cognitive-behavioral therapy for post-traumatic stress disorder in three through six year-old children: a randomized clinical trial. J Child Psychol Psychiatry 2011; 52(8):853–60.
7. Scheeringa MS, Zeanah CH, Myers L, et al. New findings on alternative criteria for PTSD in pre-school children. J Am Acad Child Adolesc Psychiatry 2003; 42(5):561–70.
8. Gigengack MR, van Meijel EP, Alisic E, et al. Comparing three diagnostic algorithms of post-traumatic stress in young children exposed to accidental trauma: an exploratory study. Child Adolesc Psychiatry Ment Health 2015;9:14.
9. Woolgar F, Garfield H, Dalgleish T, et al. Systematic review and meta-analysis: prevalence of posttraumatic stress disorder in trauma-exposed preschool-aged children. J Am Acad Child Adolesc Psychiatry 2021. https://doi.org/10.1016/j.jaac.2021.05.026. S0890-8567(21)00423-8.
10. De Young AC, Landolt MA. PTSD in children below the age of 6 years. Curr Psychiatry Rep 2018;20(11):97.
11. Bailey HN, Moran G, Pederson DR. Childhood maltreatment, complex trauma symptoms, and unresolved attachment in an at-risk sample of adolescent mothers. Attach Hum Dev 2007;9(2):139–61. https://doi.org/10.1080/14616730701349721.

12. Cook A, Spinazzola J, Ford J, et al. Complex trauma in children and adolescents. Psychiatr Ann 2005;35:390–8.
13. van der Kolk BA. Developmental Trauma Disorder: toward a rational diagnosis for children with complex trauma histories. Psychiatr Ann 2005;35(5):401–8.
14. van der Kolk BA, Courtois CA. Editorial comments: complex developmental trauma. J Trauma Stress 2005;18(5):385–8. https://doi.org/10.1002/jts.20046.
15. Ford JD, Courtois CA, Steele K, et al. Treatment of complex post-traumatic self-dysregulation. J Trauma Stress 2005;18:437–47.
16. Ford JD, Cloitre M. Best practices in psychotherapy for children and adolescents. In: Courtois CA, Ford JD, editors. Treating complex traumatic stress disorders: An evidence-based guide. Guilford Press; 2009. p. 59–81.
17. Guinn AS, Ports KA, Ford DC, et al. Associations between adverse childhood experiences and acquired brain injury, including traumatic brain injuries, among adults: 2014 BRFSS North Carolina. INJ Prev 2019;25(6):514–20.
18. Bremness A, Polzin W. Commentary: developmental trauma disorder: a missed opportunity in DSM V. J Can Acad Child Adolesc Psychiatry 2014;23(2):142–5.
19. Ross CA, Margolis RL. Research domain criteria: strengths, weaknesses, and potential alternatives for future psychiatric research. Mol Neuropsychiatry 2019;5(4):218–36.
20. Herringa RJ. Trauma, PTSD, and the developing brain. Curr Psychiatry Rep 2017;19(10):69.
21. Croft J, Heron J, Teufel C, et al. Association of trauma type, age of exposure, and frequency in childhood and adolescence with psychotic experiences in early adulthood. JAMA Psychiatry 2019;76(1):79–86, published correction appears in JAMA Psychiatry. 2019 Jan 1;76(1):102] [published correction appears in JAMA Psychiatry. 2020 Feb 1;77(2):218.
22. Karanikas E, Daskalakis NP, Agorastos A. Oxidative dysregulation in early life stress and posttraumatic stress disorder: a comprehensive review. Brain Sci 2021;11(6):723.
23. Atkuri K, Mantovani JJ, Herzenberg LA, et al. N-acetylcysteine - a safe antidote for cysteine/glutathione deficiency. Curr Opin Pharmacol 2007;7(40):355–9.
24. Back SE, McCauley JL, Korte KJ, et al. A double-blind randomized controlled pilot trial of N-Acetylcysteine in veterans with PTSD and substance use disorders. J Clin Psychiatry 2016;77(11):e1439–46.
25. Matsumura K, Noguchi H, Nishi D, et al. Effects of omega-3 polyunsaturated fatty acids on psychophysiological symptoms of post-traumatic stress disorder in accident survivors: a randomized, double-blind, placebo-controlled trial. J Affect Disord 2017;224:27–31.
26. Matsuoka Y, Nishi D, Hamazaki K, et al. Docosahexaenoic acid for selective prevention of post-traumatic stress disorder among severely injured patients: a randomized, placebo-controlled trial. J Clin Psychiatry 2015;76(8):e1015–22.
27. Liao Y, Xie B, Zhang H, et al. Efficacy of omega-3 PUFAs in depression: a meta-analysis. Transl Psychiatry 2019;9(1):190 [Erratum in: Transl Psychiatry. 2021 Sep 7;11(1):465. PMID: 31383846; PMCID: PMC6683166].
28. Matsuoka YJ, Hamazaki K, Nishi D, et al. Change in blood levels of eicosapentaenoic acid and post-traumatic stress symptom: a secondary analysis of data from a placebo-controlled trial of omega3 supplements. J Affect Disord 2016; 205:289–91.
29. Bormann JE, Thorp SR, Smith E, et al. Individual treatment of posttraumatic stress disorder using mantram repetition: a randomized clinical trial. Am J Psychiatry 2018;175(10):979–88.

30. Gallegos AM, Crean HF, Pigeon WR, et al. Meditation and yoga for post-traumatic stress disorder: a meta-analytic review of randomized controlled trials. Clin Psychol Rev 2017;58:115–24.

31. Simkin DR, Black NB. Meditation and mindfulness in clinical practice. Child Adolesc Psychiatr Clin N Am 2014;23(3):487–534.

32. Culver KA, Whetten K, Boyd DL, et al. Yoga to reduce trauma-related distress and emotional and behavioral difficulties among children living in orphanages in Haiti: a pilot study. J Altern Complement Med 2015;21(9):539–45.

33. Steinberg AM, Brymer M, Decker K, et al. The UCLA PTSD reaction index. Curr Psychiatry Rep 2004;6:96–100.

34. Steinberg AM, Brymer MJ, Kim S, et al. Psychometric properties of the UCLA PTSD reaction index: part 1. J Trauma Stress 2013;26:1–9.

35. Catani C, Kohiladevy M, et al. Treating children traumatized by war and tsunami: a comparison between exposure therapy and meditation-relaxation in North-East Sri Lanka. BMC Psychiatry 2009;9:22.

36. Gordon JS, Staples JK, Blyta A, et al. Treatment of posttraumatic stress disorder in postwar Kosovar adolescents using mind-body skills groups: a randomized controlled trial. J Clin Psychiatry 2008;69(9):1469–76.

37. Lesmana CBJ, Suryani LK, Jensen GD, et al. A spiritual-hypnosis assisted treatment of children with PTSD after the 2002 Bali terrorist attack. Am J Clin Hypn 2009;52(1):23–34.

38. Lyshak-Stelzer F, Singer P, John P St, et al. Art therapy for adolescents with post-traumatic stress disorder symptoms: a pilot study, art therapy. J Am Art Ther Assoc 2007;24(4):163–9.

39. Schouten KA, de Niet GJ, Knipscheer JW, et al. The effectiveness of art therapy in the treatment of traumatized adults: a systematic review on art therapy and trauma. Trauma Violence Abuse 2015;16(2):220–8.

40. Manzoni M, Fernandez I, Bertella S, et al. Eye movement desensitization and reprocessing: the state of the art of efficacy in children and adolescent with post traumatic stress disorder. J Affect Disord 2021;282:340–7.

41. Khan AM, Dar S, Ahmed R, et al. Cognitive behavioral therapy versus eye movement desensitization and reprocessing in patients with post-traumatic stress disorder: systematic review and meta-analysis of randomized clinical trials. Cureus 2018;10(9):e3250.

42. Rodenburg R, Benjamin A, de Roos C, et al. Efficacy of EMDR in children: a meta-analysis. Clin Psychol Rev 2009;29(7):599–606. ISSN 0272-7358.

43. Hui KK, Liu J, Makris N, et al. Acupuncture modulates the limbic system and subcortical gray structures of the human brain: evidence from fMRI studies in normal subjects. Hum Brain Mapp 2000;9(1):13–25, 31.

44. Hui KK, Liu J, Marina O, et al. The integrated response of the human cerebro-cerebellar and limbic systems to acupuncture stimulation at ST 36 as evidenced by fMRI. Neuroimage 2005;27(3):479–96.

45. Fang J, Jin Z, Wang Y, et al. The salient characteristics of the central effects of acupuncture needling: limbic–paralimbic– neocortical network modulation. Hum Brain Mapp 2009;30(4):1196–206.

46. Takakura N, Yajima H. Analgesic effect of acupuncture needle penetration: a double-blind crossover study. Open Med 2009;3(2):54–61.

47. Church D, Stapleton P, Kip K, et al. Corrigendum to: is tapping on acupuncture points an active ingredient in emotional freedom techniques: a systematic review and meta-analysis of comparative studies. J Nerv Ment Dis 2020;208(8):

632–5 [Erratum for: J Nerv Ment Dis. 2018 Oct;206(10):783-793. PMID: 32740561].

48. Sebastian B, Nelms J. The effectiveness of emotional freedom techniques in the treatment of post traumatic stress disorder: a meta-analysis, explore: The J Sci Healing, https://doi.org/10.1016/j.explore.2016.10.001

49. Church D, Piña O, Reategui C, et al. Single-session reduction of the intensity of traumatic memories in abused adolescents after EFT: a randomized controlled pilot study. Traumatology 2012;18(3):73–9.

50. Diehle J, Opmeer BC, Boer F, et al. Eur Trauma-focused cognitive behavioral therapy or eye movement desensitization and reprocessing: what works in children with posttraumatic stress symptoms? A randomized controlled trial. Child Adolesc Psychiatry 2015;24(2):227–36.

51. Teicher MH, Gordon JB, Nemeroff CB. Recognizing the importance of childhood maltreatment as a critical factor in psychiatric diagnoses, treatment, research, prevention, and education. Mol Psychiatry 2022;27(3):1331–8.

52. Karatzias T, Murphy P, Cloitre M, et al. Psychological interventions for ICD-11 complex PTSD symptoms: systematic review and meta-analysis. Psychol Med 2019;49(11):1761–75.

53. Nanni V, Uher R, Danese A. Childhood maltreatment predicts unfavorable course of illness and treatment outcome in depression: a meta-analysis. Am J Psychiatry 2012;169(2):141–51.

54. van der Kolk B, Spinazzola J, Blaustein M, et al. A randomized clinical trial of eye movement desensitization and reprocessing (EMDR), fluoxetine, and pill placebo in the treatment of post-traumatic stress disorder: treatment effects and long-term maintenance. J Clin Psychiatry 2007;68(1):37–46.

55. Boterhoven de Haan K, Lee C, Fassbinder E, et al. Imagery rescripting and eye movement desensitization and reprocessing as treatment for adults with post-traumatic stress disorder from childhood trauma: a randomized clinical trial. Br J Psychiatry 2020;1–7. https://doi.org/10.1192/bjp.2020.158.

56. Ahmad A, Larsson B, Sundelin-Wahlsten V. EMDR treatment for children with PTSD: results of a randomized controlled trial. Nord J Psychiatry 2007;61(5): 349–54.

57. Tang TC, Yang P, Yen CF, et al. Eye movement desensitization and reprocessing for treating psychological disturbances in Taiwanese adolescents who experienced Typhoon Morakot. Kaohsiung J Med Sci 2015;31(7):363–9.

58. van der Kolk BA, Hodgdon H, Gapen M, et al. A randomized controlled study of neurofeedback for chronic PTSD. PLoS One 2016;11(12):e0166752. https://doi.org/10.1371/journal.pone.0166752 pmid:2799243. Available at:.

59. Rogel A, Loomis AM, Hamlin E, et al. The impact of neurofeedback training on children with developmental trauma: a randomized controlled study. Psychol Trauma 2020;12(8):918–29.

60. Nicholson AA, Ros T, Densmore M, et al. A randomized, controlled trial of alpha-rhythm EEG neurofeedback in post-traumatic stress disorder: a preliminary investigation showing evidence of decreased PTSD symptoms and restored default mode and salience network connectivity using fMRI. Neuroimage Clin 2020;28:102490.

61. Simkin DR, Thatcher RW, Lubar J. Quantitative EEG and neurofeedback in children and adolescents: anxiety disorders, depressive disorders, comorbid addiction and attention-deficit/hyperactivity disorder, and brain injury. Child Adolesc Psychiatr Clin N Am 2014;23(3):427–64 [Erratum in: Child Adolesc Psychiatr Clin N Am. 2015 Jan;24(1):197. PMID: 24975621].

62. McGowan PO, Sasaki A, D'Alessio AC, et al. Epigenetic regulation of the gluco-corticoid receptor in human brain associates with childhood abuse. Nat Neurosci 2009;12(3):342–8.

63. Klengel T, Mehta D, Anacker C, et al. Allele-specific FKBP5 DNA demethylation mediates gene-childhood trauma interactions. Nat Neurosci 2013;16:33–41, 51.

64. Binder EB, Bradley RG, LIU W, et al. Association of FKBP5 polymorphisms and childhood abuse with risk of posttraumatic stress disorder symptoms in adults. JAMA 2008;299(11):1292–305.

65. Perroud N, Paoloni-Giacobino A, Prada P, et al. Increased methylation of gluco-corticoid receptor gene (NR3C1) in adults with a history of childhood maltreat-ment: a link with the severity and type of trauma. Translational Psychiatry 2011; 1:e59.

66. Bishop JR, Lee AM, Mills LJ, et al. Methylation of FKBP5 and SLC6A4 in relation to treatment response to mindfulness-based stress reduction for posttraumatic stress disorder. Front Psychiatry 2018;9:418 [Erratum in: Front Psychiatry. 2021; 12:642245. PMID: 30279666; PMCID: PMC6153325].

67. Szeszko PR, Lehrner A, Yehuda R, et al. Glucocorticoids and hippocampal structure and function in PTSD. Clin Psychopharmacol 2018;26(3):142–57, 2010 30:217–219. Harv Rev Psychiatry. May/Jun.

68. Heim C, Newport DJ, Mletzko T, et al. The link between childhood trauma and depression: insights from HPA axis studies in humans. Psychoneuroendocrinol-ogy 2008;33(6):693–710.

69. Yehuda R. Advances in understanding neuroendocrine alterations in PTSD and their therapeutic implications. Ann NY Acad Sci 2006;1071:137–66.

70. Heim C, Newport J, Heit S, et al. Pituitary-adrenal and autonomic responses to stress in women after sexual and physical abuse in childhood. JAMA 2000; 284(5):592–7.

71. Bottaccioli AG, Bottaccioli F, Carosella A, et al. Psychoneuroendocrinoimmunol-ogy-based meditation (PNEIMED) training reduces salivary cortisol under basal and stressful conditions in healthy university students: results of a randomized controlled study. Explore (NY) 2019. https://doi.org/10.1016/j.explore.2019.10. 006. pii: S1550-8307(19)30548-8.

72. Usta MB, Gumus YY, Say GN, et al. Basal blood DHEA-S/cortisol levels predicts EMDR treatment response in adolescents with PTSD. Nord J Psychiatry 2018; 72(3):164–72.

73. West J, Otte C, Geher K, et al. Effects of Hatha yoga and African dance on perceived stress, affect, and salivary cortisol. Ann Behav Med 2004;28(2): 114–8.

74. Church D, Yount G, Brooks AJ. The effect of emotional freedom techniques on stress biochemistry: a randomized controlled trial. J Nerv Ment Dis 2012; 200(10):891–6.

75. do Prado CH, Grassi-Oliveira R, Wieck A, et al. The impact of childhood maltreatment on redox state: relationship with oxidative damage and antioxidant defenses in adolescents with no psychiatric disorder. Neurosci Lett 2016;617: 173–7.

76. Pace TWW, Hu F, Miller AH. Cytokine-effects on glucocorticoid receptor func-tion: relevance to glucocorticoid resistance and the pathophysiology and treat-ment of major depression. Brain Behav Immun 2007;21:9–19.

77. Carpenter LL, Gawuga CE, Tyrka AR, et al. Association between Plasma IL-6 response to acute stress and early-life adversity in healthy adults. Neuropsycho-pharmacology 2010;35:2617–23.

78. Lemieux A, Coe CL, Carnes M. Symptom severity predicts degree of T cell activation in adult women following childhood maltreatment. Brain Behav Immun 2008;22(6):994–1003.

79. Van Bogaert T, De Bosscher K, Libert C. Crosstalk between TNF and glucocorticoid receptor signaling pathways. Cytokine Growth Factor Rev 2010;21:275–86.

80. Baumeister D, Akhtar R, Ciufolini S. Childhood trauma and adulthood inflammation: a meta-analysis of peripheral C-reactive protein, interleukin-6 and tumor necrosis factor-α. Mol Psychiatry 2016;21:642–9.

81. Kitamura T, Saitoh Y, Takashima N, et al. Adult neurogenesis modulates the hippocampus dependent period of associative fear memory. Cell 2009;139:814–27.

82. Matsuoka Y. Clearance of fear memory from the hippocampus through neurogenesis by omega-3 fatty acids: a novel preventive strategy for posttraumatic stress disorder? Biopsychosocial Med 2011;5:3.

83. Lafourcade M, Larrieu T, Mato S, et al. Nutritional omega-3 deficiency abolishes endocannabinoid-mediated neuronal functions. Nat Neurosci 2011;14(3):345–50.

84. Yamada D, Takeo J, Koppensteiner P, et al. Modulation of fear memory by dietary polyunsaturated fatty acids via cannabinoid receptors. Neuropsychopharmacology 2014;39:1852–60.

85. Marsicano G, Wotjak C, Azad S, et al. The endogenous cannabinoid system controls extinction of aversive memories. Nature 2002;418:530–4.

86. Conklin SM, Gianaros PJ, Brown SM, et al. Long-chain omega-3 fatty acid intake is associated positively with corticolimbic gray matter volume in healthy adults. Neurosci Lett 2007;421(3):209–12.

87. Ginty AT, Conklin SM. Preliminary evidence that acute long-chain omega-3 supplementation reduces cardiovascular reactivity to mental stress: a randomized and placebo-controlled trial. Biol Psychol 2012;89(1):269–72, 4.

88. Alquraan L, Alzoubi KH, Hammad H, et al. Omega-3 fatty acids prevent posttraumatic stress disorder-induced memory impairment. Biomolecules 2019;9(3):100.

89. Matsuoka Y, Nishi D, Yonemoto N, et al. Omega-3 fatty acids for secondary prevention of post-traumatic stress disorder after accidental injury: an open-label pilot study. J Clin Psychopharmacol 2010;30(2):217–9.

90. Nishi D, Koido Y, Nakaya N, et al. Fish oil for attenuating post-traumatic stress symptoms among rescue workers after the great east Japan earthquake: a randomized controlled tr1al. Psychother Psychosom 2012;81:315–7.

91. Kripalani S, Pradhan B, Gilrain KL. The potential positive epigenetic effects of various mind-body therapies (MBTs): a narrative review. J Complement Integr Med 2021. https://doi.org/10.1515/jcim-2021-0039.

92. Church D, Yount G, Fox L, et al. Epigenetic effects of PTSD remediation in veterans using EFT (emotional freedom techniques). Am J Health Promot 2018;32(1):112.

93. Gerardi M, Rothbaum B, Astin MC, et al. Cortisol response following exposure treatment for PTSD in rape victims. J Aggress Maltreat Trauma 2010;19(4):349–56. J Aggress Maltreat Trauma. Author manuscript; available in PMC 2011 Jun 1. Published in final edited form as:.

94. Simkin DR, Arnold LE. The roles of inflammation, oxidative stress and the gut-brain axis in treatment refractory depression in youth: complementary and integrative medicine interventions. OBM Integr Complement Med 2020;5(4):25.

95. Simkin DR. Microbiome and mental health, specifically as it relates to adolescents. Curr Psychiatry Rep 2019;21(9):93.
96. Ruijters EJ, Haenen GR, Willemsen M, et al. Food-derived bioactives can protect the anti-inflammatory activity of cortisol with antioxidant-dependent and -independent mechanisms. Int J Mol Sci 2016;17(2):239.
97. Hemmings SMJ, Malan-Muller S, van den Heuvel € Leigh L, et al. The microbiome in post-traumatic stress disorder and trauma-exposed controls: an exploratory study. Psychosom Med 2017;79(8):936–46.
98. Felitti VJ, Anda RF, Nordenberg D, et al. Relationship of childhood abuse and household dysfunction to many of the leading causes of death in adults: the Adverse Childhood Experiences (ACE) Study. Am J Prev Med 1998;14(4):245–58.
99. Ridker PM. Cardiology Patient Page. C-reactive protein: a simple test to help predict risk of heart attack and stroke. Circulation 2003;108:e81–5.
100. Rohleder N, Karl A. Role of endocrine and inflammatory alterations in comorbid somatic diseases of post-traumatic stress disorder. Minerva Endocrinol 2006; 31:273–88.
101. Robb AS, Cueva JE, Sporn J, et al. Sertraline treatment of children and adolescents with post-traumatic stress disorder: a double-blind, placebo-controlled trial. J Child Adolesc Psychopharmacol 2010;20(6):463–71.
102. Boaden K, Tomlinson A, Cortese S, et al. Antidepressants in children and adolescents: meta-review of efficacy, tolerability and suicidality in acute treatment. Front Psychiatry 2020;11:717.
103. Gillies D, Taylor F, Gray C, et al. Psychological therapies for the treatment of post-traumatic stress disorder in children and adolescents (Review). Evid Based Child Health 2013;8(3):1004–116.
104. Pinto-Sanchez MI, Hall GB, Ghajar K, et al. Probiotic Bifidobacterium longum NCC3001 reduces depression scores and alters brain activity: a pilot study in patients with irritable bowel syndrome. Gastroenterology 2017;153:448–59.
105. Huang TT, Zou Y, Corniola R. Oxidative stress and adult neurogenesis–effects of radiation and superoxide dismutase deficiency. Semin Cell Dev Biol 2012;23(7): 738–44.
106. Brunet A, Saumier D, Liu A, et al. Reduction of PTSD symptoms with pre-reactivation propranolol therapy: a randomized controlled trial. Am J Psychiatry 2018;175(5):427–33.
107. Andersen SL, Teicher MH. Stress, sensitive periods and maturational events in adolescent depression. Trends Neurosci 2008;31:183–91.
108. Pechtel P, Lyons-Ruth K, Anderson CM, et al. Sensitive periods of amygdala development: the role of maltreatment in preadolescence. Neuroimage 2014;97:236–44.
109. Hamblin MR. Mechanisms and applications of the anti-inflammatory effects of photobiomodulation. AIMS Biophys 2017;4(3):337–61. Epub 2017 May 19. PMID: 28748217; PMCID: PMC5523874.
110. Salehpour F, Mahmoudi J, Kamari F, et al. Brain photobiomodulation therapy: a narrative review. Mol Neurobiol 2018;55(8):6601–36.
111. Danese A, Moffitt TE, Harrington H, et al. Adverse childhood experiences and adult risk factors for age-related disease: depression, inflammation, and clustering of metabolic risk markers. Arch Pediatr Adolesc Med 2009;163(12):1135–43.
112. Danese A, Lewis SJ. Psychoneuroimmunology of Early-Life Stress: the Hidden Wounds of Childhood Trauma? Neuropsychopharmacology 2017;42(1):99–114.

Mood Disorders in Youth
Complementary and Integrative Medicine

Kirti Saxena, MD[a,b,*], Sherin Kurian, MD[a,b], Reena Kumar, DO[c],
L. Eugene Arnold, MD, MEd[d], Deborah R. Simkin, MD, DFAACAP[e]

KEYWORDS

- Mood disorders • Depression • Bipolar disorder • Omega-3 fatty acids
- Complementary and integrative medicine • Vitamins • Children and Adolescents

KEY POINTS

- Several randomized control trials for complementary and integrative medicine appear promising.
- Biological mechanisms involved in mood disorders include inflammation, oxidative stress, and mitochondrial dysfunction.
- Beneficial effects on mood have been associated with omega-3 essential polyunsaturated fatty acids; Vitamins, Probiotics and others.
- Physical exercise may have a mild-to-moderate effect on mood in nonmedicated adolescents with MDD and Yoga as monotherapy or adjunctive therapy shows positive effects, particularly for depression.
- School-based interventions may reduce the risk of depressive symptoms in students with mild-to-moderate depression.

INTRODUCTION

Global estimates from the World Health Organization indicate that roughly 10% to 20% of adolescents experience mental illness.[1]

Indeed, recurrent major depression and bipolar disorder (BD) are lifelong illnesses that often become clinically apparent in late teens or early 20s.[2] Long-term prognosis of mood disorder in youth is poor,[2] and there is particular concern about the safety of psychotropic medication in the youth.[3,4] Despite advances in the development of antidepressants, the prevalence of mood disorders, especially treatment-resistant, is

[a] Department of Child and Adolescent Psychiatry, Texas Children's Hospital, 8080 North Stadium Drive, Houston, TX 77054, USA; [b] Department of Psychiatry, Baylor College of Medicine, 1 Moursund Street, Houston, TX 77030, USA; [c] Andrew Weil Center for Integrative Medicine, University of Arizona, 655 N Alvernon Way, Suite 120, Tuscon, AZ 85711, USA; [d] Department of Psychiatry and Behavioral Health, The Ohio State University College of Medicine, 395E McCampbell Hall, 1581 Dodd Drive, Columbus, OH 43210, USA; [e] Department of Psychiatry, Emory University School of Medicine, 8955 Highway 98 West, Suite 204, Miramar Beach, FL 32550, USA
* Corresponding author.
E-mail address: kxsaxen1@texaschildrens.org

Child Adolesc Psychiatric Clin N Am 32 (2023) 367–394
https://doi.org/10.1016/j.chc.2022.08.012
1056-4993/23/© 2022 Elsevier Inc. All rights reserved.

increasing globally.[5] Approximately one-third of individuals with major depressive disorder (MDD) do not respond to 2 or more antidepressant trials.[6,7] Nevertheless, in those patients, various forms of medical treatment are often continued for substantial duration. Given the concerns about the adverse effects and effectiveness of psychotropics in symptom resolution, parents may seek other treatment options, such as complementary and integrative treatments/functional medicine (CIM/FM).

Articles in this volume of *Child and Adolescent Psychiatric Clinics of North America*, will review the available evidence on a broad range of CIM/FM treatments to provide an overview of the current options for treating psychiatric disorders in youth. This one focuses on mood disorders. We begin with the mechanisms involving nutrition and inflammation, describing how several CIM/FM interventions can evoke an anti-inflammatory response, including polyunsaturated fatty acids (PUFAs), probiotics, vitamins, folic acid, and L-methyl folate, N-acetylcysteine (NAC), melatonin, bright-light therapy (BLT), meditation, exercise, etc. Although these supplements and lifestyle skills are relatively well-known, they may be infrequently used. We then review other less-known CIM treatments for youth, such as saffron, school-based therapies, and transcranial photobiomodulation.

BIOLOGICAL MECHANISMS INVOLVED IN MOOD DISORDERS
Inflammation and Mood Disorders

There is robust association between inflammation or immune activation and mood disorders.[7,8] Elevated circulating levels of proinflammatory markers, such as tumor necrosis factor-alpha (TNFα), interleukin (IL)-6, and C-reactive protein (CRP), have been consistently reported in individuals with MDD and BD.[9–11] A systematic review corroborated that proinflammatory cytokines are increased, while anti-inflammatory cytokines are reduced in individuals with BD, mainly during manic and depressive episodes, compared with healthy controls. These peripheral changes attenuate during euthymia, indicating that inflammation may be associated with acute mood episodes of BD.[12] Several dietary components can evoke an anti-inflammatory response, including PUFAs, flavonoids, vitamins, and minerals.[13]

Although inflammatory markers play a role in childhood depression, in a meta-analysis by Kim and colleagues,[14] 3 studies evaluating depression and early adversity revealed inflammation was more significantly related to adversity than depression.

Current drugs approved to treat mood disorders also display some anti-inflammatory properties. For instance, antidepressants decrease peripheral levels of IL-4, IL-6, and IL-10 in MDD subjects. IL-1ß decrease was significantly associated with serotonin reuptake inhibitors (SSRI) whereas no significant difference was observed for other cytokines, such as IL-2, TNF-α, and IFN-γ. Accordingly, antidepressants may improve depressive symptoms but lower the levels of only some proinflammatory cytokines.[15] Lithium also has anti-inflammatory properties, decreasing proinflammatory cytokines IL-2, IL-6, and IFN-γ however increasing anti-inflammatory cytokines IL-4 and IL-10 in human whole-blood cell culture.[16]

Inflammation linked to refractory depression in children and adolescents has been reviewed by Simkin and Arnold[17] and Simkin.[18] Dysbiosis (changes in the normal flora of the gut) releases lipopolysaccharides from gram-negative bacteria, which activates the inflammatory process leading to the production of IL-6 and TNF-α. The gut wall breaks down ("leaky gut") due to the shortage of short-chain fatty acids (SCFA), like butyrate and acetate, which are normally produced by healthy gut bacteria. SCFA ordinarily helps to maintain gut integrity. In addition, these inflammatory cytokines signal the vagal nerve. This results in 3 important effects on the brain that may decrease the effectiveness of treatment. First, it causes an upregulation of the hypothalamus–pituitary–adrenal (HPA) axis by inflammatory molecules blocking the glucocorticoid receptors and, therefore, preventing negative feedback from damping down the release of the adrenocorticotropic hormone. The result is a greater sensitivity to stress and an increase in the perception of pain. Second, indoleamine 2,3-dioxygenase (IDO) is activated by inflammatory cytokines so that tryptophan (which normally converts to serotonin) is redirected to produce quinolinic acid (a glutamate receptor agonist). Third, microglia, which normally act as scavengers to fight infection and clean up damaged neurons, are activated to release proinflammatory cytokines and attack neurons. The symptoms associated with the activation of microglia is called sickness behavior (lethargy, anhedonia, somnolence, weight loss, decreased concentration, and anxiety).

Role of the Folate and Methylation Cycles in Depression

Dysbiosis can lead to poor absorption of vitamins necessary for the folate and methylation cycles. Vitamin B12 must be available to combine with the active form of vitamin B9 (folate), called L-methylfolate, and homocysteine to produce S-adenosyl-L-methionine (SAMe) needed for the production of neurotransmitters and maintenance of DNA methylation. If there is a B12 deficiency, then homocysteine levels will increase and SAMe levels will decrease (**Fig. 1**) with a corresponding decrease in the production of monoamine neurotransmitters.[17] In fact, in a study by Esnafoglu, and colleagues,[19] there was an increase in the severity of depression when vitamin B12 was low and homocysteine high in children with depression. High homocysteine levels were also correlated to depression in children in a study by Paduchova and colleagues.[20]

The conversion of vitamin B9 to L-methylfolate is influenced by the methylenetetrahydrofolate reductase (MTHFR) gene. With the alleles T/C, B9 is converted to L-methylfolate 65% of the time, and with alleles T/T, L-methylfolate is produced 35% of the time that it would have been with alleles CC. MTHFR polymorphism may enhance the environmental risks of low folate intake associated with gut inflammation or

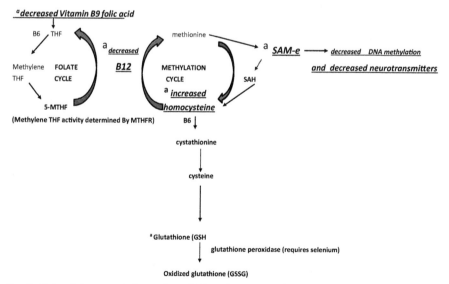

Fig. 1. Role of decreased absorption of B9 and B12 secondary to dysbiosis in the gut. [a]Low B12 and increased homocysteine cysteine in children with depression (Paduchova, 2021) (Esnafoglu, 2020) (Courtesy of Simkin and Arnold, 2020.)

traumatic stress in childhood. In fact, in children with a history of childhood trauma, the MTHFR T/T genotype carriers developed a more severe form of depression.[21,22]

Oxidative Stress

Multiple studies have confirmed the association between oxidative stress and mood disorders. In both MDD and BD, oxidative stress markers are increased.[23,24] Katrenčíková investigated markers of oxidative stress, including urinary 8-isoprostane (8-isoP-U) and lipoperoxides (LP), advanced oxidation protein products (AOPP), and nitrotyrosine (NT), and markers of antioxidant defense, such as the Trolox equivalent antioxidant capacity of serum (TEAC), Cu/Zn superoxide dismutase (SOD), glutathione peroxidase (GPx), and catalase (CAT) enzyme activities.[25] The children's depression inventory (CDI) severity correlated significantly positively with NT and negatively with TEAC, SOD, and GPx. NT correlated positively with the baseline omega-6/omega-3 ($\Omega6/\Omega3$) FA ratio and negatively with SOD.

Role of oxidative stress in mitochondrial dysfunction

Mitochondrial dysfunction directly reflects energy metabolism, as measured by the production of ATP. Hippocampal neurogenesis (ie, formation of new neurons in this brain area) and neuroplasticity (ie, adaptive capacity of the brain in the face of environmental changes) can be impaired by the deficiency in energy metabolism, and these two phenomena are implicated in mood disorders.[26,27] One role of mitochondria is to neutralize reactive oxygen species (ROS) produced during oxidative stress. However, when the mitochondria are overwhelmed with ROS, this results in damage to the mitochondrial electron transport chain, which has been associated with depression and BD.[17,18]

Role of oxidative stress and the folate and methylation cycles

During oxidative stress, homocysteine is shifted to glutathione. Glutathione is used to reduce ROS, like H_2O_2 to H_2O. This occurs with the help of glutathione peroxidase. However, the shift of homocysteine to glutathione will leave less homocysteine to combine with L-methhylfolate and B12 to produce SAM-E.[17] Thus, fewer neurotransmitters will be formed and less maintenance of DNA methylation will occur (**Fig. 2**).

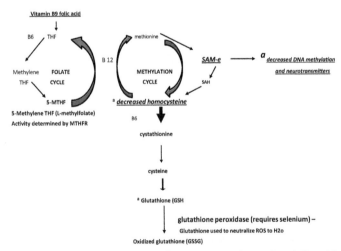

Fig. 2. Role of oxidative stress caused by inflammation in depression. [a]Glutathione is sacrificed to decrease oxidative stress, less homocysteine is available to produce neurotransmitters and less DNA is methylate (Courtesy of Simkin and Arnold, 2020.)

Role of Brain-Derived Neurotrophic Factor

Decreased brain-derived neurotrophic factor (BDNF), which is an important mediator of neurogenesis and neuroplasticity, is associated with mood disorders.[28–30] Most studies on neurotrophins in BD have focused on BDNF. A meta-analysis revealed reduced BDNF levels during manic and depressive episodes but not euthymia.[29] Prior studies have found no significant difference in BDNF in euthymic BD youth,[31] and in youth with BD in various mood states versus healthy controls (HC).[32,33] One study reported a decrease in BDNF expression (mRNA in lymphocyte, protein in platelets) in unmedicated BD versus HC youth.[34] In a more recent study, both the CDI and $\Omega6/\Omega3$ ratio correlated positively with thromboxane (TXB) and negatively with BDNF at baseline.[20] This was probably due to the omega-6 arachidonic acid (AA) producing TXB, which is proinflammatory.

COMPLEMENTARY AND INTEGRATIVE MEDICINE/FUNCTIONAL MEDICINE TREATMENTS
Essential Polyunsaturated Fatty Acids

Research reveals beneficial effects on mood with $\Omega3$ fatty acids with little evidence of adverse side effects or deleterious drug interactions.[35,36] Indeed, $\Omega3$ might function as either a primary or adjunctive treatment with a more favorable risk–benefit ratio for children with BP-not otherwise specified than currently available drugs.[35] Specifically, evidence has implicated dietary deficiency in essential long-chain omega-3 (LCn-3) fatty acids, including eicosapentaenoic acid (EPA) and docosahexaenoic acid (DHA), in the pathophysiology and etiology of MDD. This is supported by converging evidence from cross-national and cross-sectional epidemiologic surveys, case-control LCn-3 fatty acid biostatus studies, prospective observational and LCn-3 fatty acid intervention studies, rodent neurodevelopmental studies, and recent neuroimaging findings. Additionally, accumulating evidence suggests that LCn-3 fatty acid deficiency may increase the risk for suicide and cardiovascular disease, two primary causes of excess premature mortality in individuals with MDD.[37]

Omega-3 ($\Omega3$, n-3) and omega 6 ($\Omega6$, n-6) PUFAs are necessary for neuronal membrane structure, fluidity, and function, providing a nest for receptors and facilitating electrical transmission. They are also the substrate for the production of prostaglandins and other eicosanoids. They are called essential fatty acids because mammalian metabolism cannot synthesize them, so they must be ingested. The main $\Omega3$ acids are eicosapentaenoic (EPA, 20-carbon) and docosahexaenoic (DHA, 22-C), which can be derived from alpha-linolenic (ALA, 18-C) by intact desaturation and elongation metabolism. The main $\Omega6$ acids are gamma-linolenic (GLA, 18-C) and arachidonic (AA, 20-C), which can be derived from linoleic (18-C) by intact metabolism.

Owen and colleagues[38] posited possible pathways for linking $\Omega3$ depletion to depression: (1) Ratios of docosahexaenoic acid (DHA) to other fatty acids affect membrane fluidity and the functioning of enzymes, ion channels, and receptor binding; (2) $\Omega3$ concentrations impact neuroplasticity and cell survival; (3) $\Omega3$ concentrations affect gene expression; and (4) $\Omega3$ availability affects production of proinflammatory and anti-inflammatory eicosanoids (prostaglandins, thromboxanes, and cytokines); inflammatory eicosanoids are elevated in depressed individuals. High-resolution structural magnetic resonance imaging shows people with higher intake levels of $\Omega3$ have greater gray matter volume in the anterior cingulate cortex (ACC), the right hippocampus, and the right amygdala. Notably, these are brain areas involved in emotional arousal and emotion regulation and are smaller in people with mood disorders.[39]

Ω3 may improve symptoms of many psychiatric disorders in youth including mood disorders,[36,37,40,41] autism,[42] attention-deficit/hyperactivity disorder (ADHD),[43,44] and psychosis.[45]

The omega-3 and therapy studies (OATS) were a pair of 2 × 2 pilot RCTs of Ω3 fatty acids and psychoeducational psychotherapy (PEP) for youth 7 to 14 year old with mood disorders. Additionally, all study participants were given a daily multivitamin. Twelve weeks' Ω3 1.6 g/d with an EPA:DHA ratio of 7:1 increased the blood levels of EPA (proportion of total measured lipids) sevenfold and DHA by almost half. The increase in EPA blood levels mediated Ω3 improvement in global function in the unexpected direction of greater improvement with smaller EPA increase, suggesting that the optimal dose may have been exceeded for smaller children.[46] In the same study, Ω3supplementation was associated with decreased impairment in executive function.[47]

The OATS depression study included 72 youth (7–14 year old) with diagnoses of major depression, dysthymia, or depression not-otherwise-specified randomized to Ω3 versus placebo and individual family psychoeducational psychotherapy (IF-PEP) versus active monitoring (AM) using a 2 × 2 design. Although the main analysis was not significant, maternal history of depression and psychosocial stress moderated treatment response such that youth whose mothers had a history of depression or who had low levels of family psychosocial stress responded significantly better to both omega 3 and psychotherapy treatments (compared with placebo) than those with no maternal depression or high levels of family stress. With high psychosocial stress or no maternal depression, all four treatment assignments, including placebo, showed a significant improvement (P = .01–.001) whereas with maternal depression or low psychosocial stress only the three active treatments (Ω3, PEP, and the combination) did.[48]

Another 23 youth (7–14 years) with BP-NOS (not otherwise specified) or cyclothymia (CYC) constituted the OATS bipolar sample, with similar randomization to 4 treatments: Ω3 + PEP: n = 5; Ω3 + AM: n = 5; placebo + PEP: n = 7; placebo + AM: n = 6. Intent-to-treat analyses indicated a significant improvement in Kiddie SADS depression rating scale (KDRS) for combined treatment relative to placebo and AM (P = .01). Across groups, manic symptoms improved over time without significant treatment effects. IF-PEP and Ω3 are well tolerated and associated with improved depressive symptoms among youth with BP-NOS and CYC.[49]

In a pilot, randomized, double-blind controlled study 38 youth (11–17 years) were randomized 1:1 to Ω3 FA (N = 19) or Ω6 FA (N = 19), alongside their standard antidepressant therapy. Seventeen in the Ω3 group and 18 in the Ω6 group completed the 12-week study. Both treatment groups were stratified into 2 subgroups: Ω3 group—depressive disorder (DD);(N = 10/17) and mixed anxiety depressive disorder (MADD) (N = 7/17) and Ω6 group (DD—N = 10/18 and MADD—N = 8/18). Only those in the Ω3 group had a significantly decreased CDI (P = .034). Moreover, in the Ω3 groups, the DD subgroup had a significantly greater improvement in depressive symptoms (P = .0001) than the MADD subgroup (P = .271). For the treatment of depression in children, an Ω3 fatty acid-rich fish oil emulsion was noted to be an effective adjuvant supplement.[50]

In a pilot randomized, double-blind, controlled trial,[51] youth (N = 24; age = 5–12) with bipolar spectrum disorders (BSD) were randomized to 1 of 3 treatment arms: inositol plus placebo, Ω3 fatty acids plus placebo, and the combined active treatment of Ω3fatty acids plus inositol. Youth randomized to the Ω3 fatty acids plus inositol arm had the largest decrease in scores for the Young mania rating scale (YMRS), children's depression rating scale (CDRS), and the brief psychiatric rating scale (P < .05).

Therefore, the combination of Ω3 fatty acids plus inositol decreased manic and depressive symptoms in prepubertal children with mild-to-moderate BSD.

In 28 children (ages 6–12 years) with major depression,[52] 70% of those receiving Ω3 at a 2:1 ratio of EPA:DHA (380–400 mg EPA; 180–200 mg DHA) but none receiving placebo enjoyed greater than 50% reduction in depressive symptoms.

In an RCT by Katrenčíková,[53] 60 patients aged 7 to 18 years with DD and MADD, were supplemented with either emulsions of Ω3-enriched fish oil (Om3 group) or with emulsions of Ω6-rich sunflower oil (Om6 group) during the 12-week intervention period, in addition to their standard treatment with selective serotonin reuptake inhibitors (SSRIs). The emulsion of fish oil consisted of 2.4 g of total Ω3 FA (1.0 g of EPA and 0.75 g of DHA, ratio EPA:DHA = 1.33:1), and the emulsion of sunflower oil contained 2.467 g of Ω6linoleic acid. Supplementations with Ω3 FA, in contrast to Ω6 FA, reduced the severity of depression, as assessed by the children's depressive inventory (CDI) scores of 6.3 (22%) and 6.5 (24%), respectively. The Ω6/ Ω3 ratio decreased from 24.2/1 to 7.6/1 after 6 weeks of Ω3 FA supplementation and to 9.9/1 after 12 weeks (69% and 60% decreases, respectively). EPA correlated negatively and the ratio of Ω6/ Ω3 FA positively with the severity of depression (CDI score). The study found a significant positive correlation of the CDI with nitrotyrosine (NT), a marker of protein damage, and a negative correlation with TEAC, Cu/Zn SOD, and GPx, all of which are used to fight the formation of free radicals formed during oxidative stress. NT correlated positively with the baseline Ω6/ Ω3 FA ratio and negatively with SOD. Supplementation with Ω3FA, but not with Ω6 FA, decreased 8-isoprostane in urine (8-IsoP-U), a marker of increased oxidative stress, advanced oxidation protein products (AOPP), and NT, another marker of protein damage; and increased TEAC and SOD activity. Omega-3 FA supplementation reduces oxidative stress in patients with DD.

A systemic review suggested the appropriate ratio of EPA/DHA for MDD is 2/1 and the total dose of EPA and DHA is 1000 to 2000 mg/d for at least 12 to 16 weeks in children and adolescents.[54] In the International Society for Nutritional Psychiatry Research Practice Guidelines for Omega-3 Fatty Acids in the Treatment of Major Depressive Disorder in pregnant women, children, and the elderly, and for prevention in high-risk populations, the following recommendations were based on a review of the literature by an expert panel. In the therapeutic settings with respect to formulation and dosage, both pure EPA or an EPA/DHA combination of a ratio higher than 2 (EPA/DHA >2) are considered effective, and the recommended dosages should be 1 to 2 g of net EPA daily, from either pure EPA or an EPA/DHA (>2:1) formula. However, they recognized that personalizing the clinical application of n-3 PUFAs in subgroups of MDD with a low Ω3 index or high levels of inflammatory markers might be regarded as areas that deserve future research.[55]

Probiotics

A meta-analysis showed that probiotics significantly decreased the depression scale score ($P = .005$) in the subjects (ages 20 and above). Probiotics had an effect on both the healthy population ($P = .03$) and patients with MDD ($P = .03$). Probiotics had an effect on the population aged under 60 ($P = .005$) whereas it had no significant effect on people aged over 65 ($P = .22$). Overall, probiotics were associated with a significant reduction in depression, underscoring the need for additional research on this potential preventive strategy for depression.[56]

Vitamin C

Vitamin C (ascorbic acid) has become of interest in adjuvant therapy settings for depressive symptoms because psychological abnormalities are among the characteristics of vitamin C deficiency.[57] There is also preliminary evidence that the administration of vitamin C may be able to reduce the severity of MDD in children.[58]

Depressed youth younger than 18 years taking fluoxetine (10–20 mg/d) for 6 months (N = 24) had a greater depression decrease with adjunctive vitamin C (1000 mg/d) than with adjunctive placebo measured by both the CDRS ($P < .0001$) and CDI ($P < .0001$).[57] This synergistic antidepressant effect of vitamin C and fluoxetine suggests that this vitamin could be helpful in improving conventional pharmacotherapy for pediatric MDD and potentially reduce side effects.

Vitamin D

Vitamin D is known to transcriptionally activate tryptophan hydroxylase 2, which forms serotonin from tryptophan,[59] modulates the HPA axis, and regulates catecholamine production through vitamin D receptors.[60] Vitamin D was negatively correlated with the CDI in 2 studies on children and adolescents.[19,20] Vitamin D 3 deficiency has been linked to increasing levels of proinflammatory cytokines and insulin resistance.[61] In a study of 940 adolescent girls, vitamin D_3 was given as a dose of 50,000 IU/week for 9 weeks. Depression score was evaluated using the Beck depression inventory-II (BDI-II). Comparison among the four categories of depression scores (normal, mild, moderate, and severe) revealed no significant differences in demographic and anthropometric parameters at baseline. After 9 weeks of vitamin D supplementation, there was a significant reduction in mild, moderate, and severe depression scores.[62] An open trial, included 16 youth with BSDs exhibiting manic symptoms and 19 controls. Individuals with BSD took 2000 IU of vitamin D3 daily for 8 weeks.[63] Neuroimaging data were acquired in both groups at baseline, and for the BSD group at the end of 8 weeks of vitamin D3. Baseline ACC γ-aminobutyric acid (GABA)/creatine (Cr) was lower in BSD than in controls (F [1,31] = 8.91, $P = .007$). Following 8 weeks of vitamin D3BSD patients showed a significant decrease in YMRS scores (t = −3.66, $P = .002$, df = 15) and the CDRS scores (t = −2.93, $P = .01$, df = 15); and a significant increase in ACC GABA (t = 3.18, $P = .007$, df = 14). In a study of vitamin D in adults with depression, the depressive symptoms did not improve until after the levels were above 42 ng/mL.[64] The original range considered to be within normal limits (30–100 ng/mL) was set to prevent rickets. Given the above information, levels from 30 to 42 ng/mL should be considered subclinical and levels between 50 to 80 ng/mL should be targeted. Vitamin D should be taken with a fatty meal to promote absorption.[17]

Folic Acid and L-Methyl-Folate

Nutritional supplements are a feasible intervention for primary prevention because they are likely to be acceptable and intuitively would seem to have a greater chance of being effective at a preventative stage, rather than later when clinical mood disturbances have occurred.

Folate is a water-soluble B vitamin, also known as B9, and is found in leafy vegetables like spinach. Folic acid is the oxidized synthetic compound used in food fortification and dietary supplements. Although similar in structure, the body absorbs folic acid more easily than folate.[65]

Relative folate deficiency is known to be associated with several neuropsychiatric disorders including mood disorders, and there are a few mechanisms by which folate deficiency might produce neurobiological changes relevant to the development of mood disorders.[66]

Low plasma and red blood cell folate have long been associated with clinical depressive disorders. A meta-analysis showed a significant relationship between low folate status and risk of depression[67] and treatment with folic acid has been shown to improve the therapeutic effect of fluoxetine in depressed individuals.[68,69]

Moreover, long-term treatment of poststroke survivors with folic acid, B6, and B12 was associated with a reduction in the hazard of major depression.[70]

In a randomized, placebo-controlled, parallel-group, double-blind study of youth ($N = 112$; age 14–24) with a high familial risk of mood disorders, participants were randomized to folic acid (2.5 mg daily) or an identical placebo for 36 months. Although posthoc analyses suggest folic acid delayed the time to onset of mood disorder, results did not suggest folic acid reduced the incidence of a mood disorder in comparison to those on placebo.[65]

MTHFR mutations should be considered when treatment for refractory depression occurs. Ten adolescents with a single mutation among the 2-methylene tetrahydrofolate reductase (*MTHFR*) gene variants (50% *A1298 AC*; 30% *C677 CT*) all had treatment-resistant depression. When prescribed adjunctive L-methylfolate (LM), 8 (80%) demonstrated improvement in depression, anxiety, and irritability.[71]

Broad Spectrum Micronutrients

The equivocal results with some single nutrients underscore the complexity of brain nutrition, in which many nutrients are involved. Broad-spectrum micronutrients, with all known vitamins and essential minerals, "cover the bases," operating through numerous mechanisms. In the brain, broad-spectrum micronutrients appear to have effects in (1) treating a variety of psychiatric symptoms, (2) enhancing a diverse range of normal brain functions, and (3) appearing to increase the potency of most central nervous system (CNS)-active drugs.[72]

Broad spectrum mineral–vitamin combinations have been evaluated in youth for treating aggressive behavior and conduct problems[73–77] and mood disorders[78,79] In youth with ADHD, improvements in sleep, anxiety, and irritability were noted.[80,81] Broad-spectrum interventions have also been examined in nonclinical populations for improving mood, anxiety, and stress,[82,83] also cognition in youth.[84]

N-Acetylcysteine

Approximately 11% of adolescents experience depression[85] and chronic use of cannabis is associated with depression.[86] This is particularly problematic because approximately 25% of high school seniors report past 30-day cannabis use and 6% use cannabis almost daily.[87] Further, adolescents are at a greater risk for developing cannabis use disorder (CUD) than adults.[88]

NAC, an over-the-counter medication thought to regulate glutamate transmission and reduce oxidative stress, has some promising findings in both enhancing the efficacy of abstinence-based cannabis treatment programs[89] and reducing depressive symptoms.[90]

A secondary analysis in an 8-week randomized controlled trial of NAC for cannabis cessation (1200 mg twice/day) was done in 74 youth with a DSM-IV-TR *Cannabis Dependence* diagnosis, ages 13 to 21 years.[91] Of those with depressive symptoms measured as a score of 14 or above on the BDI-II, NAC was negatively associated with positive urine cannabinoid tests during treatment and the difference between NAC and placebo was stronger for adolescents who had greater severity of baseline depressive symptoms ($b = -0.09$, SE $= 0.04$, $P = .034$). More studies are required with larger samples in order to confirm whether NAC would be more beneficial in reducing cannabis use in those with depression.

Physical Activity

Exercise can increase peroxisome proliferation activated receptor gamma (PPAR-γ), coactivator 1α (PGC1α) gene expression, which reduces synthesis and release of proinflammatory cytokines and decreases glutamatergic neurotoxicity, thereby reducing inflammatory cytokines associated with depression.[92] The Depressed Adolescents Treated with Exercise (DATE) study studied the effects of a standardized aerobic exercise protocol to treat nonmedicated adolescents who met DSM-IV-TR criteria for MDD. Thirty adolescents aged 12 to 18 years were randomized to either vigorous exercise (EXER) (>12 kg/kcal/wk [KKW]) or a control stretching activity (<4 KKW) for 12 weeks. By week 12, the exercise group had a 100% response rate (86% remission) whereas the stretch group response rate was 67% (50% remission) ($P = .02$).[93]

The intensity of the exercise may matter. Sixty-one healthy young adults (72% female) (aged 18–30 year old) were assigned to 6 weeks of high-intensity interval training (HIIT), moderate continuous training (MCT), or no exercise (CON). Changes in depression (BDI -II), anxiety (Beck Anxiety Inventory), and perceived stress (Perceived Stress Scale) along with proinflammatory cytokines, TNF-α, IL-6, IL-1β, and CRP were measured. Depression increased for CON. In contrast, MCT decreased depression and proinflammatory cytokine TNF-α levels. HIIT did decrease depressive symptoms, but it also increased perceived stress, TNF-α, and IL-6 relative to MCT. Taken together, the results suggest that moderate-intensity exercise may be optimal for the promotion of mental health by decreasing TNF-α and depression.[94]

Herbs

Adaptogens are herbs used in Ayurvedic and Chinese medicine. They reduce oxidative stress by reducing the levels of nitrous oxide and by helping to normalize an upregulated HPA axis by unblocking the glucocorticoid receptor so that the normal homeostatic feedback process can occur.[95] In an RCT, *Acanthopanax senticosus* (Siberian Ginseng) plus lithium was compared with fluoxetine plus lithium in 76 adolescents aged 12 to 17 with bipolar depression. Remission rates (51.4% vs 48.7%) and response rates (67.6% vs 71.8%) were comparable. No significant differences between adolescents with BD treated with lithium plus adjunctive *A senticosus* or Li plus adjunctive fluoxetine were seen. Three of the adolescents on fluoxetine experienced a manic switch, compared with none in the *A senticosus* group.[96]

Bright Light Therapy

BLT has been examined in youth with a delayed sleep-phase disorder, in which disruptions in circadian rhythm led to a regular pattern of late bedtimes and late morning awakening times, with changes in diurnal hormonal and body temperature cycles, slow alerting upon awakening, decreased energy patterns, and often depressive moods.[97] Meta-analytic evidence has proven that BLT leads to a significant reduction of depressive symptoms in seasonal affective disorder[98,99] and nonseasonal depression.[100]

Sixty-two depressed adolescents (13–18 years) were randomly assigned to BLT alone for 2 weeks or a combination of BLT and wake therapy (WT; COMB). After one night of WT, adolescents in the COMB-group had longer sleep durations, earlier sleep onset, less awakening during the night, and an improved sleep efficiency.[101,102]

Twenty-eight youth (ages 7–17) with a seasonal affective disorder were randomized to receive active treatment (1 hour of BLT plus 2 hours of dawn simulation) or placebo (1 hour of clear goggles plus 5 minutes of low-intensity dawn simulation) for 1 week. During light therapy, scores from The Structured Interview Guide for the Hamilton Depression Rating Scale, Seasonal Affective Disorders parent version, significantly decreased from baseline in comparison with placebo. 80% of children and 78% of parents stated the child "felt best," during the light therapy phase.[103]

Melatonin

Melatonin is a natural hormone that regulates sleep. In a randomized, double-blind, placebo-controlled trial in youth with BD (N = 48; age = 11–17 years), in comparison to the placebo, melatonin decreased olanzapine-induced metabolic side effects by significantly inhibiting the rise in cholesterol and systolic blood pressure.[104] Also, coadministration of melatonin with olanzapine and lithium carbonate in adolescents with BD may reduce the weight gain associated with these drugs to marginal significance.[105]

Saffron (Crocus sativus L.)

Saffron, a spice derived from the stigmas of the C sativus flower, has several pharmacologic actions including anti-inflammatory, anticancer, antioxidant, antiplatelet, and neuroprotective properties.[106] As an antidepressant agent, saffron has been shown through several RCTs to be more effective than placebo[107,108] and of equivalent efficacy to the antidepressants, including fluoxetine,[109–111] imipramine,[112] and citalopram[113] for the treatment of mild-to-moderate depression.

In an 8-week, randomized, double-blind, placebo-controlled study in 80 youth aged 12 to 16, saffron was associated with greater self-reported improvements in overall internalizing symptoms (P = .049), separation anxiety (P = .003), social phobia (P = .023), and depression (P = .016).[106]

Current evidence suggests beneficial effects of saffron on parameters of mental health and treatment of CNS disorders in individuals with and without depression. However, RCTs of the effects of saffron for treatment of depression and anxiety have not been systematically evaluated and the results are controversial.[114]

Transcranial Photobiomodulation

Current treatments for MDD have significant limitations in efficacy and side effect burden. FDA-approved devices for MDD are burdensome (due to repeated in-office procedures) and are most suitable for severely ill patients. There is a critical need for device-based treatments in MDD that are efficacious, well-tolerated, and easy to use. Neuromodulation strategies can be an option for individuals who do not respond to or tolerate antidepressant medications, which include FDA-approved electroconvulsive therapy (ECT), transcranial magnetic stimulation (rTMS), and vagus nerve stimulation (VNS). Other neuromodulation options, such as transcranial direct current stimulation (tDCS), magnetic seizure therapy (MST), and deep brain stimulation (DBS), remain experimental.

Transcranial photobiomodulation (t-PBM) is a novel form of neuromodulation, based on nonretinal exposure to light at specific wavelengths. t-PBM with near-infrared (NIR) has yielded promising early results for the treatment of neuropsychiatric disorders.[115] The t-PBM method penetrates the cerebral cortex, stimulating the mitochondrial respiratory chain, and significantly increases cerebral blood flow. Animal and human studies, using a variety of t-PBM settings and experimental models, suggest that t-PBM may have significant efficacy and good tolerability in MDD.

In a pilot study of 10 adults with MDD and anxiety disorders, four 4-min treatments in random order were performed: NIR to the left forehead at F3, to the right forehead at F4, and placebo treatments (light off) at the same site. At 2 weeks post-treatment, 6 of 10 patients had a remission (a score ≤ 10) on the Hamilton depression rating scale (HAM-D), and 7 of 10 achieved this on the Hamilton anxiety rating scale (HAM-A). Patients experienced highly significant reductions in both HAM-D and HAM-A scores following treatment, with the greatest reductions occurring at 2 weeks. Mean rCBF across hemispheres increased from 0.011 units in the off condition to 0.043 units in the on condition, for a difference of 0.032 (95% CI: −0.016, 0.080) units, though this result did not reach statistical significance.[116] These data support the need for large confirmatory studies for t-PBM as a possible novel, safe, and easy-to-administer antidepressant treatment.[117]

Meditation

In a study of 58 individuals (age 19–50 year old) with major depression diagnosed with DSM-5 criteria, participants were randomly assigned to yoga and meditation or a control group for 12 weeks. There was a significant decrease compared with controls [difference between means, (95% CI)] in BDI-II score [−5.83 (−7.27, −4.39), $P < 0.001$] and significant increase in BDNF (ng/mL) [5.48 (3.50, 7.46), $P < 0.001$] after yoga meditation lifestyle intervention (YMLI). Among the mind–body communicative biomarkers, there was a significant increase in circulating dehydroepiandrosterone (DHEAS—an indication of reduced inflammation) and sirtuin 1 (used in the repair of DNA) and a significant decrease in circulating cortisol and IL-6 (a proinflammatory cytokine) after YMLI compared baseline level and control group. A total of 12 weeks YMLI showed improvement in cellular health biomarkers that included a significant decrease in 8 Oxo-2′- deoxyguanosine (8OH2dG-a marker of DNA damage); a significant increase in TAC and a decrease in ROS (markers of oxidative stress); and a significant increase in telomerase activity compared with that of control group (all $P < 0.05$). However, change in telomere length was not significant in both groups. Also, the control group showed significantly increased ROS and IL-6 levels compared with baseline ($P < .001$). As noted earlier, an overactive HPA and increased cortisol is associated with depression. In this study, increased cortisol was associated with reductions in BDNF and an increase in depression severity.[118]

Intervention in Schools

Coordinating individual and family interventions to enhance the school environment has been argued as a potentially important direction for universal depression interventions. Merry and colleagues'[119] review suggests that both psychological and educational preventative interventions in childhood and adolescence show positive reductions in symptoms of depression immediately following intervention and at follow-up 6- to 12-month post completion of intervention.

Youth ($N = 2027$; mean ages 12.3–14.5 years) from grades 7 to 9 of 24 schools participated in an RCT study where 12 schools were randomized to a universal preventative intervention (including a student social relationship/emotional health curriculum, and parent/caregiver parenting education) and 12 were randomized as control schools. Although there was no overall intervention effect on depressive symptoms, students with moderate depressive symptoms who received the intervention and whose parents attended parent education events had a significantly reduced risk of depressive symptoms at follow-up.[120]

In a double-blind, randomized, controlled study, Spanish adolescents ($N = 867$, grade 8–10) were randomized into an incremental theory intervention ($n = 456$) or an educational control intervention ($n = 411$). Adolescents with high depression scores decreased by almost 18% in those that received the intervention but increased by 37% in the control group. In the 9th grade, the effects of the intervention were in the opposite direction.[121] This requires further study to check for age/grade

Table 1
Evidence Based CIM Treatments in Youth

Treatment	Level of certainty by USPSTF Definitions	Strength of Recommendation Based on Benefit and Safety	Evidence Base in Youth	Results/Personal Recommendations of Reviewers
I. Depression and bipolar disorder (BD)				
12-weeks of omega-3 (Ω3) daily, eicosapentaenoic acid, EPA),randomized to psychoeducational psychotherapy(PEP) vs active monitoring (AM) (Fristad et al, 2015[49] Fristad et al, 2019[48] Arnold et al, 2017[46] Vesco et al, 2018[47]) Age 7–14; N = 95: 72 depression, 23 bipolar not-otherwise specified (BD-NOS) or cyclothymic (CYC)	Low	C	2 × 2 pilots	Significant improvement with Ω3 in overweight/obese subgroup, Ω3 decreased impairment in executive functioning. PEP significantly better than placebo with maternal depression (p = 0.020) and without stress. PEP + Ω3 decreased depression significantly more than placebo + AM, P = .01. Recommend for mild depression or as adjunct Passes SECS
Bright light therapy (BLT) vs BLT and wake therapy (WT);(COMB) (Kirschbaum et al, 2018[101]) Age 13–18; N = 62: depression	Low	C	Randomized control trial	COMB-group had longer sleep durations, earlier sleep onset, fewer wakes during night, improved sleep efficiency. Recommend for mild depression or as adjunct Passes SECS
Weekly cannabis cessation counseling and abstinence-based contingency management (CM). In	Low	C	Randomized, double-blind, placebo-controlled trial	In secondary analyses adolescents with baseline depressive symptoms had significantly fewer positive urine

(continued on next page)

Table 1
(continued)

Treatment	Level of certainty by USPSTF Definitions	Strength of Recommendation Based on Benefit and Safety	Evidence Base in Youth	Results/Personal Recommendations of Reviewers
addition, participants randomized to N-acetylcysteine (NAC) or placebo. Active treatment=8 weeks (Tomko et al, 2018[91]) Age 12–21 years; N = 74: Depression in cannabis dependence				cannabinoid tests than those without depressive symptoms Recommend the intervention as adjunct Passes SECS
Randomization to 12 weeks of an Ω3 fatty acid-rich fish oil emulsion or Ω6 FA-rich sunflower oil emulsion (Trebatická et al, 2017[50]) Age 11–17; N = 35: depressive disorder (DD) and mixed anxiety depressive disorder (MADD)	Low	C	Randomized, double-blind controlled, pilot study	Depression significantly decreased in the Ω3 group. Among the Ω3 subgroups, the DD subgroup had significant improvement in depression compared to the MADD subgroup Recommend for mild depression or as adjunct Passes SECS
Fluoxetine plus vitamin C vs. fluoxetine plus placebo for 6 months (Amr et al, 2013[57]) Age < 18; N = 24: major depressive disorder (MDD) = 12, control = 12	Low	C	Randomized, Double Blind parallel-group placebo-controlled pilot study	Fluoxetine and vitamin C significantly decreased depression compared to fluoxetine plus placebo Recommend for vitamin C for mild depression as adjunct Passes SECS
Randomized to either vigorous exercise (EXER) or a control stretching activity for 12 weeks	Low	C	Pilot, randomized controlled trial	By week 12, 86% in the exercise group achieved remission, whereas the 50% stretch group achieved 50% remission

Description			Study design	Outcome
(Hughes et al, 2013[??]) Age 12–18, N = 30: nonmedicated adolescents that met DSM-IV-TR criteria for MDD				
Randomized to 6 weeks of high-intensity interval training (HIIT), moderate continuous training (MCT), or no exercise (CON) (Paolucci et al, 2018[94]) Age 18–30 years, N = 60	Low	C	Randomized	Depression decreased in both MCT and HIT groups from Beck Depression Inventory scores. MCT had additional advantages over HIT, as it further decreased inflammatory marker TNF-α, and may thus bean optimal intensity for promotion of mental health. Recommend the intervention as adjunct Passes SECS
Randomized to Ω3 fatty acids or placebo For 16 weeks. (Nemets et al, 2006[52]) Age 6–12 years; N = 28: MDD	Low	C, not risky	Randomized controlled, double-blind pilot study	Depression significantly decreased with Ω3 Recommend based on individual preferences and clinical judgment as adjunct Passes SECS
12 weeks of olanzapine, lithium carbonate, and melatonin vs olanzapine, lithium carbonate, and placebo (Mostafavi et al, 2017[104]). Age 11–17 years; N = 48: BD	Low	C, not risky	Randomized, double-blind, placebo-controlled trial	Coadministration of melatonin with olanzapine and lithium carbonate in adolescents with BD could reduce the weight gain to near significance Recommend melatonin based on clinical judgment as adjunct Passes SECS
Inositol plus placebo; Ω3 fatty acids plus placebo; Ω3 fatty acids plus inositol (Wozniak et al, 2015[51]) Age 5–12 years; N = 24: BDI or II or BD-NOS	Low	C, not risky	Randomized, double-blind, controlled clinical trial: pilot study	Ω3 fatty acids plus inositol reduced symptoms of mania and depression in prepubertal children with mild to moderate BD Recommend based on individual preferences and clinical judgment as adjunct Passes SECS

(continued on next page)

Table 1
(continued)

Treatment	Level of certainty by USPSTF Definitions	Strength of Recommendation Based on Benefit and Safety	Evidence Base in Youth	Results/Personal Recommendations of Reviewers
Randomized to folic acid or placebo for 36 months (Sharpley et al, 2014[65]) Age 14–24 years; N = 112: youth with increased familial risk of mood disorder	Low	I	Randomized, placebo-controlled, parallel group, double blind study	No evidence that folic acid reduced incidence of mood disorder Insufficient evidence to recommend
L-methyl folate supplementation for those with MTHFR mutation (Dartoisetal et al, 2019[71]) Adolescents with treatment-resistant depression; N = 10: depression	Low	C	Case series	Eight out of 10 adolescents with treatment-resistant depression and MTHFR mutation had improvement in depression, anxiety and irritability with L-methyl folate supplementation Recommend based on individual preferences and clinical judgment as adjunct Passes SECS
Randomized to Ω3 FA fish oil + SSRI or Ω6 FA sunflower oil for 12 weeks + SSRI (Katrenčiková et al, 2020[25]) Age 7–18 years; N = 60: DD and MADD	Low	C, not risky	Randomized, controlled trial	Supplementation of omega 3s, in contrast to omega 6s, reduced these verity of depression(as noted by CDI scores). Omega 3 supplementation is found to reduce markers of oxidative stress inpatients with depressive disorders. Recommend for mild depression or as adjunct Passes SECS
Vitamin D 350,000 IU/week for 9 weeks (Bahrami et al, 2018[62])	Low	C	Clinical trial, without placebo control	After 9 weeks of weekly vitamin D3 supplementation, there was a significant reduction in

Adolescent girls; N = 940: depression				depression score(as noted by BDI rating). Recommend vitamin D3 based on clinical judgment as adjunct Passes SECS
8 weeks of daily vitamin D3 in patients with manic symptoms (N = 16) vs controls (N = 19) (Sikoglu, et al, 2015[63]): youth with bipolar spectrum disorders	Low	C	Open trial	Baseline GABA was lower among youth with bipolar disorders vs controls(neuroimaging data). GABA levels increased in the ACC on follow-up imaging after 8weeks of supplementation. Significant reduction of mania and depressive symptoms noted on YMRS and CDRS rating scales respectively. Recommend vitamin D3 based on clinical judgment as adjunct Passes SECS
Randomized to 8 weeks of saffron vs placebo (Lopresti et al, 2018[106]) Age 12–16 years; N = 80: youth with depression and anxiety symptom	Low	C, Low risk	Randomized, double-blind, placebo-controlled trial	Saffron was associated with greater self-reported improvements in overall internalizing symptoms, separation anxiety, social phobia, and depression. Recommend saffron based on individual preference and clinical judgment Passes SECS
Randomized to 12 weeks of yoga and meditation lifestyle intervention (YMLI) vs control (Tolahunase et al, 2018[118]) (Simkin and Arnold et al, 2020[17]) Age 19–50 years; N = 58: DSM-5d × MDD	Low	C, Low risk	Randomized controlled trial	Intervention group (yoga/meditation) had decreased depression scores (BDI-II rating). Decreases in inflammatory biomarkers, improved BDNF were also noted. Recommend the intervention as adjunct Passes SECS

(continued on next page)

Table 1
(continued)

Treatment	Level of certainty by USPSTF Definitions	Strength of Recommendation Based on Benefit and Safety	Evidence Base in Youth	Results/Personal Recommendations of Reviewers
II. Bipolar Depression				
Randomized to —adaptogen (Eleutherococcus senticosus) plus lithium vs. fluoxetine plus lithium (Weng et al, 2007[96]) Ages 12-17; N=76	Low	C, Risk of manic switch	Randomized, double-blind, placebo-controlled trial	Remission and response rates comparable for adaptogen vs fluoxetine. Adolescents (N = 3) on fluoxetine experience damanic switch. Insufficient data to recommend Does not pass SECS due to risk of mania
III. Pediatric Seasonal Affective Disorder				
Randomization to active BLT or placebo for 1 week; treatment phase followed by a second dark-glasses phase (1–2 weeks) (Swedo et al, 1997[103]) Age 7–17 years; N = 28	Low	C	Double-blind, placebo-controlled, crossover	Depression significantly decreased from baseline during BLT. No differences between placebo and control phases. Recommend for mild depression as adjunct Passes SECS
IV. School Intervention Studies 12 schools randomized to a universal preventative intervention; 12 schools randomized as controls (Buttigieg et al, 2015[120]) Age 12.3–14.5 years; N= 2027: 24 schools	Low	C	Randomized, controlled trial	No overall intervention effect on depressive symptoms. Intervention students with moderate symptoms whose Parents attended parent education events had a significantly reduced risk of depressive symptoms at follow-up. Recommend the intervention as adjunct Passes SECS

| Incremental theory (N = 456) vs educational control (N = 411) Over 12 months (Calvete et al, 2019[121]) 8th–10th graders | Low | C | Double-blind, randomized, controlled | In adolescents, depression decreased with intervention; in controls, depression increased by 37%. Recommend the intervention as adjunct Passes SECS |

Strength of Recommendations based on benefit and safety:

A=Recommend Strongly. There is a high certainty that the net benefit is substantial and safe.

B=Recommend. There is a high certainty that the net benefit is moderate or there is moderate certainty that the net benefit is moderate to substantial and safe.

C=Neutral (offer or provide this service for selected patients depending on individual circumstances, based on professional judgment and patient preferences). There is at least moderate certainty that the net benefit is small.

D=Discourage. There is moderate or high certainty that the service has no net benefit or that the harms outweigh the benefits

I = Insufficient (if the service is offered, patients should understand the uncertainty about the balance of benefits and harms) Current evidence is insufficient to assess the balance of benefits and harms of the service. Evidence is lacking, of poor quality, or conflicting, and the balance of benefits cannot be determined.)

Level of certainty regarding quality:

HIGH Level of Evidence with robust positive data meta-analyses or meta-reviews involving 2 or more RCTs of excellent, robust quality. The available evidence usually includes consistent results from well-designed, well-conducted RCTs in representative child, adolescent or young adult (18-24 years old) populations, assessing the effects on mental health outcomes.

MODERATE Level of Evidence with robust positive data involving 2 or more RCTs of excellent, robust quality. The available evidence usually includes consistent results from well-designed, well-conducted RCTs in representative child, adolescent or young adult (18-24 years old) populations, assessing the effects on mental health outcomes.

LOW Level of evidence with less than 2 RCTs with good or average quality. The available evidence is insufficient to assess the effects on mental health outcomes.

SECS Criteria:

A guide to clinical decisions is that Interventions that are Safe, Easy, Cheap, and Sensible (SECS) require less evidence to justify individual trials than those that are Risky, Unrealistic, Difficult, or Expensive (RUDE). Because some of the treatments do not have much solid, compelling evidence but would be reasonable to try with a lower bar of evidence, this criterion is also taken into account. Being risky, unrealistic, difficult or expensive (RUDE) disqualifies from SECS. The bolded conjunctions are essential in applying this guide.

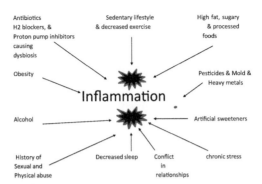

Fig. 3. Contributions to inflammation and dysbiosis. (Courtesy of Simkin and Arnold, 2020.)

developmental moderation of effect before it could be recommended as a stand alone treatment.

A summary of these studies can be found in **Table 1** using the United States Preventative Services Task Force ratings for the strength of the recommendation and level of certainty for each study.

SUMMARY

The most common treatments for depression and BD are medication and psychotherapy, but each has limited efficacy (see **Table 1** for a concise compilation of the studies). Given concerns about treatment-induced suicidal ideation and behavior in children and adolescents, other treatment options, such as complementary and alternative treatments warrant exploration. Current evidence supports trying inflammation reduction, adjunctive Ω3 PUFAs, vitamins/minerals, probiotics, NAC, physical exercise, adjunctive melatonin, yoga/meditation, BLT, FDA-approved neuromodulation, and L-methyl folate for those with MTHFR genetic deficiency. Ultimately, lifestyle changes for the child and the family may decrease the risk of developing depression or may reveal components of refractory depression that may need to be addressed (**Fig. 3**). Looking at inflammation in all systems in order to allow the patient to be balanced from a mental, emotional, and spiritual state is the art of functional medicine.

CLINICS CARE POINTS

- Clinical pearls would include clinical assessment of the patient, educating the patient and family in regard to which treatment would be indicated for their improvement.

DISCLOSURE

Drs K. Saxena, S. Kurian, R. Kumar, and D.R. Simkin have no disclosures. Dr L.E. Arnold has received research funding from Supernus Pharmaceuticals, Roche/Genentech Pharmaceuticals, Otsuka Pharmaceuticals, Axial, and Young Living Essential Oils and National Institute of Health (USA, R01 MH 100144), has consulted with Pfizer Pharmaceuticals and CHADD, and been on advisory boards for Otsuka and Roche/Genentech.

REFERENCES

1. Adolescent mental health. 2019. Available at: https://www.who.int/news-room/fact-sheets/detail/adolescent-mental-health.
2. Angst J. Course and prognosis of mood disorders. New Oxford textbook of psychiatry 2000;1:721–4.
3. Ramchandani P. A question of balance. Nature 2004;430(6998):401–2. https://doi.org/10.1038/430401a.
4. Morrison AP, Hutton P, Shiers D, et al. Antipsychotics: is it time to introduce patient choice? Br J Psychiatry 2012;201:83–4. https://doi.org/10.1192/bjp.bp.112.112110.
5. Jorm AF, Patten SB, Brugha TS, et al. Has increased provision of treatment reduced the prevalence of common mental disorders? Review of the evidence from four countries. World Psychiatry 2017;16(1):90–9. https://doi.org/10.1002/wps.20388.
6. Souery D, Papakostas GI, Trivedi MH. Treatment-resistant depression. J Clin Psychiatry 2006;67(Suppl 6):16–22.
7. Colpo GD, Leboyer M, Dantzer R, et al. Immune-based strategies for mood disorders: facts and challenges. Expert Rev Neurother 2018;18(2):139–52.
8. Fries GR, Walss-Bass C, Bauer ME, et al. Revisiting inflammation in bipolar disorder. Pharmacol Biochem Behav 2019;177:12–9. https://doi.org/10.1016/j.pbb.2018.12.006.
9. Howren MB, Lamkin DM, Suls J. Associations of depression with C-reactive protein, IL-1, and IL-6: a meta-analysis. Psychosom Med 2009;71(2):171–86.
10. Strawbridge R, Arnone D, Danese A, et al. Inflammation and clinical response to treatment in depression: a meta-analysis. Eur Neuropsychopharmacol 2015;25(10):1532–43. https://doi.org/10.1016/j.euroneuro.2015.06.007.
11. Dowlati Y, Herrmann N, Swardfager W, et al. A meta-analysis of cytokines in major depression. Biol Psychiatry 2010;67(5):446–57. https://doi.org/10.1016/j.biopsych.2009.09.033.
12. Sayana P, Colpo GD, Simões LR, et al. A systematic review of evidence for the role of inflammatory biomarkers in bipolar patients. J Psychiatr Res 2017;92:160–82. https://doi.org/10.1016/j.jpsychires.2017.03.018.
13. Phillips CM, Shivappa N, Hébert JR, et al. Dietary inflammatory index and mental health: a cross-sectional analysis of the relationship with depressive symptoms, anxiety and well-being in adults. Clin Nutr 2018;37(5):1485–91. https://doi.org/10.1016/j.clnu.2017.08.029.
14. Kim JW, Szigethy EM, Melhem NM, et al. Inflammatory markers and the pathogenesis of pediatric depression and suicide: a systematic review of the literature. J Clin Psychiatry 2014;75(11):1242–53. https://doi.org/10.4088/JCP.13r08898.
15. Więdłocha M, Marcinowicz P, Krupa R, et al. Effect of antidepressant treatment on peripheral inflammation markers - a meta-analysis. Prog Neuropsychopharmacol Biol Psychiatry 2018;80(Pt C):217–26. https://doi.org/10.1016/j.pnpbp.2017.04.026.
16. Rapaport MH, Manji HK. The effects of lithium on ex vivo cytokine production. Biol Psychiatry 2001;50(3):217–24.
17. Simkin DR, Arnold LE. The roles of inflammation, oxidative stress and the gut-brain Axis in treatment refractory depression in youth: complementary and integrative medicine interventions. 2020.

18. Simkin DR. Microbiome and mental health, Specifically as it Relates to adolescents. Curr Psychiatry Rep 2019;21(9):93. https://doi.org/10.1007/s11920-019-1075-3.

19. Esnafoglu E, Ozturan DD. The relationship of severity of depression with homocysteine, folate, vitamin B12, and vitamin D levels in children and adolescents. Child Adolesc Ment Health 2020;25(4):249–55.

20. Paduchová Z, Katrenčíková B, Vaváková M, et al. The effect of omega-3 fatty acids on thromboxane, brain-derived neurotrophic factor, homocysteine, and vitamin D in depressive children and adolescents: randomized controlled trial. Nutrients 2021;13(4):1095. https://doi.org/10.3390/nu13041095.

21. Lok A, Bockting C, Koeter M, et al. Interaction between the MTHFR C677T polymorphism and traumatic childhood events predicts depression. Transl Psychiatry 2013;3:e288. https://doi.org/10.1038/tp.2013.60.

22. Wu YL, Ding XX, Sun YH, et al. Association between MTHFR C677T polymorphism and depression: an updated meta-analysis of 26 studies. Prog Neuropsychopharmacol Biol Psychiatry 2013;46:78–85. https://doi.org/10.1016/j.pnpbp.2013.06.015.

23. Black CN, Bot M, Scheffer PG, et al. Is depression associated with increased oxidative stress? A systematic review and meta-analysis. Psychoneuroendocrinology 2015;51:164–75.

24. Andreazza AC, Kauer-Sant'anna M, Frey BN, et al. Oxidative stress markers in bipolar disorder: a meta-analysis. J Affect Disord 2008;111(2–3):135–44.

25. Katrenčíková B, Vaváková M, Paduchová Z, et al. Oxidative stress markers and antioxidant enzymes in children and adolescents with depressive disorder and impact of omega-3 fatty acids in randomised clinical trial. Antioxidants (Basel) 2021;10(8):1256.

26. Allen J, Romay-Tallon R, Brymer KJ, et al. Mitochondria and mood: mitochondrial dysfunction as a Key player in the Manifestation of depression. Front Neurosci 2018;12:386.

27. Bansal Y, Kuhad A. Mitochondrial dysfunction in depression. Curr Neuropharmacol 2016;14(6):610–8.

28. Teixeira AL, Colpo GD, Fries GR, et al. Biomarkers for bipolar disorder: current status and challenges ahead. Expert Rev Neurother 2019;19(1):67–81.

29. Rowland T, Perry BI, Upthegrove R, et al. Neurotrophins, cytokines, oxidative stress mediators and mood state in bipolar disorder: systematic review and meta-analyses. Br J Psychiatry 2018;213(3):514–25.

30. Bocchio-Chiavetto L, Bagnardi V, Zanardini R, et al. Serum and plasma BDNF levels in major depression: a replication study and meta-analyses. World J Biol Psychiatry 2010;11(6):763–73.

31. Cevher Binici N, Inal Emiroğlu FN, Resmi H, Ellidokuz H. Serum brain-derived neurotrophic factor levels among euthymic adolescents with bipolar disorder Type I. Noro Psikiyatr Ars 2016;53(3):267–71.

32. Hatch JK, Scola G, Olowoyeye O, et al. Inflammatory markers and brain-derived neurotrophic factor as potential Bridges linking bipolar disorder and cardiovascular risk among adolescents. J Clin Psychiatry 2017;78(3):e286–93.

33. Karthikeyan S, Dimick MK, Fiksenbaum L, et al. Inflammatory markers, brain-derived neurotrophic factor, and the symptomatic course of adolescent bipolar disorder: a prospective repeated-measures study. Brain Behav Immun 2022;100:278–86.

34. Pandey GN, Rizavi HS, Dwivedi Y, et al. Brain-derived neurotrophic factor gene expression in pediatric bipolar disorder: effects of treatment and clinical response. J Am Acad Child Adolesc Psychiatry 2008;47(9):1077–85.

35. Young C, Martin A. Omega-3 fatty acids in mood disorders: an overview. Braz J Psychiatry 2003;25(3):184–7.

36. Sarris J, Mischoulon D, Schweitzer I. Omega-3 for bipolar disorder: meta-analyses of use in mania and bipolar depression. J Clin Psychiatry 2012; 73(1):81–6.

37. McNamara RK. Role of omega-3 fatty acids in the etiology, treatment, and prevention of depression: current status and future directions. J Nutr Intermed Metab 2016;5:96–106.

38. Owen C, Rees AM, Parker G. The role of fatty acids in the development and treatment of mood disorders. Curr Opin Psychiatry 2008;21(1):19–24.

39. Conklin SM, Gianaros PJ, Brown SM, et al. Long-chain omega-3 fatty acid intake is associated positively with corticolimbic gray matter volume in healthy adults. Neurosci Lett 2007;421(3):209–12.

40. Wozniak J, Biederman J, Mick E, et al. Omega-3 fatty acid monotherapy for pediatric bipolar disorder: a prospective open-label trial. Eur Neuropsychopharmacol 2007;17(6–7):440–7.

41. Clayton EH, Hanstock TL, Hirneth SJ, et al. Reduced mania and depression in juvenile bipolar disorder associated with long-chain omega-3 polyunsaturated fatty acid supplementation. Eur J Clin Nutr 2009;63(8):1037–40.

42. Amminger GP, Berger GE, Schäfer MR, et al. Omega-3 fatty acids supplementation in children with autism: a double-blind randomized, placebo-controlled pilot study. Biol Psychiatry 2007;61(4):551–3.

43. Sinn N, Bryan J. Effect of supplementation with polyunsaturated fatty acids and micronutrients on learning and behavior problems associated with child ADHD. J Dev Behav Pediatr 2007;28(2):82–91. https://doi.org/10.1097/01.DBP. 0000267558.88457.a5.

44. Sorgi PJ, Hallowell EM, Hutchins HL, et al. Effects of an open-label pilot study with high-dose EPA/DHA concentrates on plasma phospholipids and behavior in children with attention deficit hyperactivity disorder. Nutr J 2007;6:16. https://doi.org/10.1186/1475-2891-6-16.

45. Amminger GP, Schäfer MR, Papageorgiou K, et al. Long-chain omega-3 fatty acids for indicated prevention of psychotic disorders: a randomized, placebo-controlled trial. Arch Gen Psychiatry 2010;67(2):146–54.

46. Arnold LE, Young AS, Belury MA, et al. Omega-3 fatty acid plasma levels before and after supplementation: Correlations with mood and clinical Outcomes in the omega-3 and therapy studies. J Child Adolesc Psychopharmacol 2017;27(3): 223–33.

47. Vesco AT, Young AS, Arnold LE, et al. Omega-3 supplementation associated with improved parent-rated executive function in youth with mood disorders: secondary analyses of the omega 3 and therapy (OATS) trials. J Child Psychol Psychiatry 2018;59(6):628–36.

48. Fristad MA, Vesco AT, Young AS, et al. Pilot randomized controlled trial of omega-3 and individual-family psychoeducational psychotherapy for children and adolescents with depression. J Clin Child Adolesc Psychol 2019; 48(sup1):S105–18.

49. Fristad MA, Young AS, Vesco AT, et al. A randomized controlled trial of individual family psychoeducational psychotherapy and omega-3 fatty acids in youth with

Subsyndromal bipolar disorder. J Child Adolesc Psychopharmacol 2015;25(10): 764–74.

50. Trebatická J, Hradečná Z, Böhmer F, et al. Emulsified omega-3 fatty-acids modulate the symptoms of depressive disorder in children and adolescents: a pilot study. Child Adolesc Psychiatry Ment Health 2017;11:30. https://doi.org/ 10.1186/s13034-017-0167-2.

51. Wozniak J, Faraone SV, Chan J, et al. A randomized clinical trial of high eicosa-pentaenoic acid omega-3 fatty acids and inositol as monotherapy and in com-bination in the treatment of pediatric bipolar spectrum disorders: a pilot study [published correction appears in J Clin Psychiatry 2016 Sep;77(9):e1153. https://doi.org/10.4088/JCP.14m09267. J Clin Psychiatry. 2015;76(11): 1548-1555.

52. Nemets H, Nemets B, Apter A, et al. Omega-3 treatment of childhood depres-sion: a controlled, double-blind pilot study. Am J Psychiatry 2006;163(6): 1098–100. https://doi.org/10.1176/ajp.2006.163.6.1098.

53. Katrenčíková B, Vaváková M, Waczulíková I, et al. Lipid Profile, Lipoprotein Sub-fractions, and fluidity of membranes in children and adolescents with depres-sive disorder: effect of omega-3 fatty acids in a double-blind randomized controlled study. Biomolecules 2020;10(10):1427.

54. Chang JP, Su KP. Nutritional Neuroscience as Mainstream of Psychiatry: the ev-idence- based treatment Guidelines for using omega-3 fatty acids as a new treatment for psychiatric disorders in children and adolescents. Clin Psycho-pharmacol Neurosci 2020;18(4):469–83. https://doi.org/10.9758/cpn.2020.18. 4.469.

55. Guu TW, Mischoulon D, Sarris J, et al. International Society for nutritional Psychi-atry research practice Guidelines for omega-3 fatty acids in the treatment of ma-jor depressive disorder. Psychother Psychosom 2019;88(5):263–73.

56. Huang R, Wang K, Hu J. Effect of probiotics on depression: a systematic review and meta-analysis of randomized controlled trials. Nutrients 2016;8(8):483. https://doi.org/10.3390/nu8080483. PMID: 27509521; PMCID: PMC4997396.

57. Amr M, El-Mogy A, Shams T, et al. Efficacy of vitamin C as an adjunct to fluox-etine therapy in pediatric major depressive disorder: a randomized, double-blind, placebo-controlled pilot study. Nutr J 2013;12:31. https://doi.org/10. 1186/1475-2891-12-31. PMID: 23510529; PMCID: PMC3599706.

58. Cocchi P, Silenzi M, Calabri G, et al. Antidepressant effect of vitamin C. Pediat-rics 1980;65(4):862–3.

59. Spedding S. Vitamin D and depression: a systematic review and meta-analysis comparing studies with and without biological flaws. Nutrients 2014;6(4): 1501–18.

60. Cernackova A, Durackova Z, Trebaticka J, et al. Neuroinflammation and depres-sive disorder: the role of the hypothalamus. J Clin Neurosci 2020;75:5–10.

61. Milaneschi Y, Hoogendijk W, Lips P, et al. The association between low vitamin D and depressive disorders. Mol Psychiatry 2014;19(4):444–51.

62. Bahrami A, Mazloum SR, Maghsoudi S, et al. High dose vitamin D supplemen-tation is associated with a reduction in depression score among adolescent girls: a Nine-week follow-up study. J Diet Suppl 2018;15(2):173–82.

63. Sikoglu EM, Navarro AA, Starr D, et al. Vitamin D3 supplemental treatment for mania in youth with bipolar spectrum disorders. J Child Adolesc Psychophar-macol 2015;25(5):415–24. https://doi.org/10.1089/cap.2014.0110.

64. Jaddou HY, Batieha AM, Khader YS, et al. Depression is associated with low levels of 25-hydroxyvitamin D among Jordanian adults: results from a national

population survey. Eur Arch Psychiatry Clin Neurosci 2012;262(4):321–7. https://doi.org/10.1007/s00406-011-0265-8.

65. Sharpley AL, Hockney R, McPeake L, et al. Folic acid supplementation for prevention of mood disorders in young people at familial risk: a randomised, double blind, placebo controlled trial. J Affect Disord 2014;167:306–11. https://doi.org/10.1016/j.jad.2014.06.011.

66. Mattson MP, Shea TB. Folate and homocysteine metabolism in neural plasticity and neurodegenerative disorders. Trends Neurosci 2003;26(3):137–46. https://doi.org/10.1016/S0166-2236(03)00032-8.

67. Gilbody S, Lightfoot T, Sheldon T. Is low folate a risk factor for depression? A meta-analysis and exploration of heterogeneity. J Epidemiol Community Health 2007;61(7):631–7. https://doi.org/10.1136/jech.2006.050385. PMID: 17568057; PMCID: PMC2465760.

68. Coppen A, Bailey J. Enhancement of the antidepressant action of fluoxetine by folic acid: a randomised, placebo controlled trial. J Affect Disord 2000;60(2):121–30. https://doi.org/10.1016/s0165-0327(00)00153-1.

69. Venkatasubramanian R, Kumar CN, Pandey RS. A randomized double-blind comparison of fluoxetine augmentation by high and low dosage folic acid in patients with depressive episodes. J Affect Disord 2013;150(2):644–8. https://doi.org/10.1016/j.jad.2013.02.029.

70. Almeida OP, Marsh K, Alfonso H, et al. B-vitamins reduce the long-term risk of depression after stroke: the VITATOPS-DEP trial. Ann Neurol 2010;68(4):503–10. https://doi.org/10.1002/ana.22189.

71. Dartois LL, Stutzman DL, Morrow M. L-Methylfolate augmentation to antidepressants for adolescents with treatment-resistant depression: a case series. J Child Adolesc Psychopharmacol 2019;29(5):386–91.

72. Popper CW, Kaplan BJ, Rucklidge JJ. Single and broad-spectrum micronutrient treatment in psychiatric practice. Complement Integr treatments Psychiatr Pract 2017;75–101.

73. Gesch CB, Hammond SM, Hampson SE, et al. Influence of supplementary vitamins, minerals and essential fatty acids on the antisocial behaviour of young adult prisoners. Randomised, placebo-controlled trial. Br J Psychiatry 2002;181:22–8. https://doi.org/10.1192/bjp.181.1.22.

74. Schoenthaler SJ, Bier ID. The effect of vitamin-mineral supplementation on juvenile delinquency among American schoolchildren: a randomized, double-blind placebo-controlled trial. J Altern Complement Med 2000;6(1):7–17. https://doi.org/10.1089/acm.2000.6.7.

75. Schoenlhaler SJ, Amos S, Doraz W, et al. The effect of randomized vitamin-mineral supplementation on violent and non-violent antisocial behavior among incarcerated juveniles. J Nutr Environ Med 1997;7(4):343–52.

76. Tammam JD, Steinsaltz D, Bester DW, et al. A randomised double-blind placebo-controlled trial investigating the behavioural effects of vitamin, mineral and n-3 fatty acid supplementation in typically developing adolescent schoolchildren. Br J Nutr 2016;115(2):361–73. https://doi.org/10.1017/S0007114515004390.

77. Zaalberg A, Nijman H, Bulten E, et al. Effects of nutritional supplements on aggression, rule-breaking, and psychopathology among young adult prisoners. Aggress Behav 2010;36(2):117–26.

78. Rucklidge JJ, Gately D, Kaplan BJ. Database analysis of children and adolescents with bipolar disorder consuming a micronutrient formula. BMC Psychiatry 2010;10:74. https://doi.org/10.1186/1471-244X-10-74.

79. Frazier EA, Fristad MA, Arnold LE. Multinutrient supplement as treatment: literature review and case report of a 12-year-old boy with bipolar disorder. J Child Adolesc Psychopharmacol 2009;19(4):453–60.

80. Gordon HA, Rucklidge JJ, Blampied NM, et al. Clinically significant symptom reduction in children with attention-deficit/hyperactivity disorder treated with micronutrients: an open-label Reversal Design study. J Child Adolesc Psychopharmacol 2015;25(10):783–98.

81. Kaplan BJ, Fisher JE, Crawford SG, et al. Improved mood and behavior during treatment with a mineral-vitamin supplement: an open-label case series of children. J Child Adolesc Psychopharmacol 2004;14(1):115–22. https://doi.org/10.1089/104454604773840553.

82. Long SJ, Benton D. Effects of vitamin and mineral supplementation on stress, mild psychiatric symptoms, and mood in nonclinical samples: a meta-analysis. Psychosom Med 2013;75(2):144–53. https://doi.org/10.1097/PSY.0b013e31827d5fbd.

83. Rucklidge JJ, Kaplan BJ. Broad-spectrum micronutrient formulas for the treatment of psychiatric symptoms: a systematic review. Expert Rev Neurother 2013;13(1):49–73. https://doi.org/10.1586/ern.12.143.

84. Eilander A, Gera T, Sachdev HS, et al. Multiple micronutrient supplementation for improving cognitive performance in children: systematic review of randomized controlled trials. Am J Clin Nutr 2010;91(1):115–30.

85. Avenevoli S, Swendsen J, He JP, et al. Major depression in the national comorbidity survey-adolescent supplement: prevalence, correlates, and treatment. J Am Acad Child Adolesc Psychiatry 2015;54(1):37–44, e2.

86. Volkow ND, Baler RD, Compton WM, et al. Adverse health effects of marijuana use. N Engl J Med 2014;370(23):2219–27.

87. Johnston LD, Miech RA, O'Malley PM, et al. Monitoring the Future national survey results on drug use 1975-2018: Overview, key findings on adolescent drug use. Ann Arbor: Institute for Social Research, University of Michigan; 2019.

88. Chen CY, O'Brien MS, Anthony JC. Who becomes cannabis dependent soon after onset of use? Epidemiological evidence from the United States: 2000-2001. Drug Alcohol Depend 2005;79(1):11–22.

89. Gray KM, Carpenter MJ, Baker NL, et al. A double-blind randomized controlled trial of N-acetylcysteine in cannabis-dependent adolescents. Am J Psychiatry 2012;169(8):805–12 [published correction appears in Am J Psychiatry. 2012;169(8):869].

90. Fernandes BS, Dean OM, Dodd S, et al. N-Acetylcysteine in depressive symptoms and functionality: a systematic review and meta-analysis. J Clin Psychiatry 2016;77(4):e457–66.

91. Tomko RL, Gilmore AK, Gray KM. The role of depressive symptoms in treatment of adolescent cannabis use disorder with N-Acetylcysteine. Addict Behav 2018; 85:26–30. https://doi.org/10.1016/j.addbeh.2018.05.014 [published correction appears in Addict Behav. 2019 Feb;89:263].

92. Ignácio ZM, da Silva RS, Plissari ME, et al. Physical exercise and Neuroinflammation in major depressive disorder. Mol Neurobiol 2019;56(12):8323–35.

93. Hughes CW, Barnes S, Barnes C, et al. Depressed Adolescents Treated with Exercise (DATE): a pilot randomized controlled trial to test feasibility and establish preliminary effect sizes. Ment Health Phys Act 2013;6(2). https://doi.org/10.1016/j.mhpa.2013.06.006.

94. Paolucci EM, Loukov D, Bowdish DME, et al. Exercise reduces depression and inflammation but intensity matters. Biol Psychol 2018;133:79–84.

95. Panossian AG. Adaptogens in mental and behavioral disorders. Psychiatr Clin North Am 2013;36(1):49–64. https://doi.org/10.1016/j.psc.2012.12.005.

96. Weng S, Tang J, Wang G, et al. Comparison of the addition of Siberian Ginseng (Acanthopanax senticosus) versus fluoxetine to lithium for the treatment of bipolar disorder in adolescents: a randomized, double-blind trial. Curr Ther Res Clin Exp 2007;68(4):280–90.

97. Okawa M. Delayed sleep phase syndrome and depression. Sleep Med 2011; 12(7):621–2. https://doi.org/10.1016/j.sleep.2011.03.014.

98. Golden RN, Gaynes BN, Ekstrom RD, et al. The efficacy of light therapy in the treatment of mood disorders: a review and meta-analysis of the evidence. Am J Psychiatry 2005;162(4):656–62.

99. Mårtensson B, Pettersson A, Berglund L, et al. Bright white light therapy in depression: a critical review of the evidence. J Affect Disord 2015;182:1–7. https://doi.org/10.1016/j.jad.2015.04.013.

100. Al-Karawi D, Jubair L. Bright light therapy for nonseasonal depression: meta-analysis of clinical trials. J Affect Disord 2016;198:64–71. https://doi.org/10.1016/j.jad.2016.03.016.

101. Kirschbaum I, Straub J, Gest S, et al. Short-term effects of wake- and bright light therapy on sleep in depressed youth. Chronobiol Int 2018;35(1):101–10.

102. Gest S, Holtmann M, Bogen S, et al. Chronotherapeutic treatments for depression in youth. Eur Child Adolesc Psychiatry 2016;25(2):151–61.

103. Swedo SE, Allen AJ, Glod CA, et al. A controlled trial of light therapy for the treatment of pediatric seasonal affective disorder. J Am Acad Child Adolesc Psychiatry 1997;36(6):816–21. https://doi.org/10.1097/00004583-199706000-0001976.

104. Mostafavi A, Solhi M, Mohammadi MR, et al. Melatonin decreases olanzapine induced metabolic side-effects in adolescents with bipolar disorder: a randomized double-blind placebo-controlled trial. Acta Med Iran 2014;52(10):734–9.

105. Mostafavi SA, Solhi M, Mohammadi MR, et al. Melatonin for reducing weight gain following administration of Atypical Antipsychotic olanzapine for adolescents with bipolar disorder: a randomized, double-blind, placebo-controlled trial. J Child Adolesc Psychopharmacol 2017;27(5):440–4. https://doi.org/10.1089/cap.2016.0046.

106. Lopresti AL, Drummond PD, Inarejos-García AM, et al. affron®, a standardised extract from saffron (Crocus sativus L.) for the treatment of youth anxiety and depressive symptoms: a randomised, double-blind, placebo-controlled study. J Affect Disord 2018;232:349–57. https://doi.org/10.1016/j.jad.2018.02.070.

107. Akhondzadeh S, Tahmacebi-Pour N, Noorbala AA, et al. Crocus sativus L. in the treatment of mild to moderate depression: a double-blind, randomized and placebo-controlled trial. Phytother Res 2005;19(2):148–51.

108. Moshiri E, Basti AA, Noorbala AA, et al. Crocus sativus L. (petal) in the treatment of mild-to-moderate depression: a double-blind, randomized and placebo-controlled trial. Phytomedicine 2006;13(9–10):607–11. https://doi.org/10.1016/j.phymed.2006.08.006.

109. Noorbala AA, Akhondzadeh S, Tahmacebi-Pour N, et al. Hydro-alcoholic extract of Crocus sativus L. versus fluoxetine in the treatment of mild to moderate depression: a double-blind, randomized pilot trial. J Ethnopharmacol 2005; 97(2):281–4. https://doi.org/10.1016/j.jep.2004.11.004.

110. Akhondzadeh Basti A, Moshiri E, Noorbala AA, et al. Comparison of petal of Crocus sativus L. and fluoxetine in the treatment of depressed outpatients: a

pilot double-blind randomized trial. Prog Neuropsychopharmacol Biol Psychiatry 2007;31(2):439–42.

111. Shahmansouri N, Farokhnia M, Abbasi SH, et al. A randomized, double-blind, clinical trial comparing the efficacy and safety of Crocus sativus L. with fluoxetine for improving mild to moderate depression in post percutaneous coronary intervention patients. J Affect Disord 2014;155:216–22. https://doi.org/10.1016/j.jad.2013.11.003.

112. Akhondzadeh S, Fallah-Pour H, Afkham K, et al. Comparison of Crocus sativus L. and imipramine in the treatment of mild to moderate depression: a pilot double-blind randomized trial [ISRCTN45683816]. BMC Complement Altern Med 2004;4(12). https://doi.org/10.1186/1472-6882-4-12. PMID: 15341662; PMCID: PMC517724.

113. Ghajar A, Neishabouri SM, Velayati N, et al. Crocus sativus L. versus citalopram in the treatment of major depressive disorder with anxious Distress: a double-blind, controlled clinical trial. Pharmacopsychiatry 2017;50(4):152–60. https://doi.org/10.1055/s-0042-116159.

114. Ghaderi A, Asbaghi O, Reiner Ž, et al. The effects of saffron (Crocus sativus L.) on mental health parameters and C-reactive protein: a meta-analysis of randomized clinical trials. Complement Ther Med 2020;48:102250.

115. Hamblin MR. Shining light on the head: photobiomodulation for brain disorders. BBA Clin 2016;6:113–24.

116. Schiffer F, Johnston AL, Ravichandran C, et al. Psychological benefits 2 and 4 weeks after a single treatment with near infrared light to the forehead: a pilot study of 10 patients with major depression and anxiety. Behav Brain Funct 2009; 5:46.

117. Askalsky P, Iosifescu DV. Transcranial photobiomodulation for the Management of depression: current Perspectives. Neuropsychiatr Dis Treat 2019;15:3255–72.

118. Tolahunase MR, Sagar R, Faiq M, et al. Yoga- and meditation-based lifestyle intervention increases neuroplasticity and reduces severity of major depressive disorder: a randomized controlled trial. Restor Neurol Neurosci 2018;36(3): 423–42. https://doi.org/10.3233/RNN-170810.

119. Merry SN, Hetrick SE, Cox GR, et al. Psychological and educational interventions for preventing depression in children and adolescents. Cochrane Database Syst Rev 2011;12:CD003380. https://doi.org/10.1002/14651858. CD003380.pub3. PMID: 22161377.

120. Buttigieg JP, Shortt AL, Slaviero TM, et al. A longitudinal evaluation of the Resilient Families randomized trial to prevent early adolescent depressive symptoms. J Adolesc 2015;44:204–13. https://doi.org/10.1016/j.adolescence.2015. 07.014. PMID: 26298674.

121. Calvete E, Fernández-Gonzalez L, Orue I, et al. The effect of an intervention Teaching adolescents that people can change on depressive symptoms, cognitive Schemas, and Hypothalamic-Pituitary-Adrenal Axis hormones. J Abnorm Child Psychol 2019;47(9):1533–46.

Complementary and Integrative Approaches to Prevention and Treatment of Child and Adolescent Obesity

Swapna N. Deshpande, MD[a],*, Deborah R. Simkin, MD[b]

KEYWORDS

- Child • Adolescent • Prevention • Treatment • Obesity
- Intensive lifestyle intervention • Microbiome • Inflammation

KEY POINTS

- The prevalence of child and adolescent obesity increased to approximately 20% between 2011 and 2012.
- In children and adolescents, obesity is characterized by activation of inflammatory markers and alteration of gut permeability. Successful interventions can reduce inflammation and reverse this process.
- Studies have demonstrated that intensive lifestyle interventions, motivational interviewing (MI)-based nutritional coaching for families, physical activity, and cognitive behavioral therapy could reduce obesity in this age group.
- Studies using mindfulness in obese children and their families may help reduce weight gain.
- Probiotics in obese children with non-alcoholic fatty liver disease and insulin resistance have shown remarkable results.
- Synbiotics as adjuncts using diet and exercise programs have made a substantial difference.
- Including parents in the intervention, especially younger children, is vital in making a long-lasting impact.

INTRODUCTION

Obesity in children is based on body mass index (BMI) and is defined as BMI at or above the sex-specific 95th percentile on the US Center for Disease Control and Prevention (CDC) BMI for age growth charts.[1] Child and adolescent obesity is a significant global challenge, with numbers consistently increasing in the last few decades since

[a] Department of Psychiatry, Oklahoma State University, 5310 E 31st St, Tulsa, OK 74135, USA;
[b] Department of Psychiatry, Emory University School of Medicine, 4641 Gulfstarr Dr., Suite 106, Destin, FL 32541, USA
* Corresponding author.
E-mail address: Swapna.deshpande@okstate.edu

Child Adolesc Psychiatric Clin N Am 32 (2023) 395–419
https://doi.org/10.1016/j.chc.2022.08.013
1056-4993/23/© 2022 Elsevier Inc. All rights reserved.

childpsych.theclinics.com

1980.[2] Prevalence of child and adolescent obesity in the United States increased from approximately 10%–11% in 1988–1994 to approximately 20% in 2011–2012.[1] Rising obesity is likely associated with consuming more calories and decreasing physical activity.[3] Much of the increase in prevalence in developed countries is related to modifiable risk factors. The risk factors that have significant impacts are high-calorie diets available at a lower cost and sedentary lifestyles.[3] Child and adolescent obesity are not only associated with physical health risks but also with psycho-social comorbidities and lower cognitive, school, and later life achievement.[4]

Obesity during adolescence increases the risk of cardiovascular and metabolic diseases in adulthood. In addition, higher BMI during adolescence is strongly associated with a higher risk of several malignancies, such as breast cancer, leukemia, Hodgkins's disease, and colorectal cancer.[5]

According to a 1998 World Health Organization definition, a lifestyle intervention aims to modify an individual's way of living and improve their physical and psychological health by changing patterns of behavior that are harmful to health.[4] Intensive lifestyle changes, including reduced calorie intake, decreased sedentary behavior, and increased physical activity, are cornerstones for preventing and treating child and adolescent obesity. However, a significant contributor to obesity is the low inflammatory state caused by lifestyle conditions that trigger or sustain a change in the normal microbiome called dysbiosis. Interventions to prevent obesity can be classified using the Mrazek and Haggerty categories of universal, selective, and indicated interventions as outlined in the report by the Institute of Medicine. Preventive interventions can be directed towards whole populations (universal), high-risk children (selective), or those with signs and symptoms of obesity (indicated).

This article reviews specific risk factors and corresponding non-pharmacological interventions that are evidence-based to address child and adolescent obesity.

THE GUT'S ROLE IN OBESITY CAUSED BY DYSBIOSIS

The influence of dysbiosis (an imbalance in the types of organisms in a person's normal microbiome) is complex but must be explained to understand the substantial role that lifestyle choices play in the increased risk for obesity.

Bifidobacterium and Lactobacillus maintain gut integrity by producing short-chain fatty acids (SCFA) like butyrate and acetate. Dysbiosis, caused by a decrease in healthy bacteria and an increase in gram-negative bacteria, decreases the production of SCFAs and the breakdown of the gut junction proteins, like occludin.

Gram-negative bacteria predominate and release lipopolysaccharides (LPS). LPS initiates an inflammatory response binding to the toll-like receptor 4 (TLR4), causing the differentiation of T cells and the production of inflammatory cytokines, interleukin-6 (IL-6), and tumor necrosis factor (TNF)-alpha. In turn, transcription of more inflammatory molecules by tumor necrosis kappa beta is produced. This inflammatory process decreases insulin sensitivity, decreases leptin signaling, and increases adipose mass.[6–9]

Dysbiosis and the decrease in SCFA contribute to other factors that lead to obesity. Typically, SCFA is produced from non-digestible starches. SCFA-mediated activation, particularly by acetate, of G-protein coupled receptor 43 (GPR43) suppresses insulin signaling in adipocytes, inhibiting fat accumulation in adipose tissue and promoting the metabolism of unincorporated lipids and glucose in other tissues. During dysbiosis, these protective factors against obesity are lost. In addition, the production of serotonin and γ-aminobutyric acid (GABA) by healthy microbes decreases. Serotonin and GABA play a major role in the central control of appetite.[10,11]

Vagal nerve stimulation is also involved in appetite signaling. Normally, SCFA binds to enteroendocrine cells in the gut, releasing anorectic (hunger-suppressing) hormones. Examples of these hormones include glucagonlike peptide-1 (GLP-1, produced by colonic L-cells), peptide YY (PYY, produced by ileal and colonic cells), and cholecystokinin (CCK). These hormones stimulate the vagal nerve, which acts on the hypothalamus to promote satiety and reduce food intake. SCFAs are believed to mediate these processes via GPR41[10] on the enteroendocrine cells.[12] Therefore, dysbiosis can decrease the production of SCFA, which, in turn, would decrease the release of anorectic hormones. In addition, SCFAs typically inhibit the release of ghrelin. Without this suppression, ghrelin is released, and appetite increases.

Dysbiosis, caused by high fat, processed sugary foods, stimulates the vagal nerve and increases the risk of depression via the vagal nerve when is LPS released.[6] However, this change in the diet also decreases leptin signaling, which has been associated with increasing the risk for depression and obesity. One study found that adolescents who were depressed had a 70% increased risk of being obese and obese adolescents had a 40% increased risk of being depressed.[13]

High-fat diets have been associated with dysbiosis leading to a decrease in Bacteroidetes and an increase in Firmicutes. In a study of obese children, strains classified as Firmicutes (*Clostridium* and *Lactobacillus*) predominated in the stool microbiota of obese children, whereas those of Bacteroidetes (Prevotella and Bacteroides) were in the minority ($p < 0.001$). The concentration of SCFAs in the stool of obese children was lower in comparison to the stool of normal-weight children ($P = 0.04$).[14]

Lastly, primary bile salts are deposited in the gut and changed to secondary bile salts by bacteria. These secondary bile salts act at GPR TGR5 (G protein-coupled bile acid receptor 1, GPBAR-1) receptor on L-cells, which activates GLP 1 to reduce insulin resistance. However, the presence of *Clostridium* prevents the production of secondary bile salts and, hence, insulin resistance increases. In addition, *Clostridium*, in the presence of these bile salt and a high-fat diet, increases Branched Chain Amino Acids, which also increases insulin resistance.[15]

Taken together, dysbiosis is by far one of the significant contributions to developing obesity.

UNIVERSAL INTERVENTIONS TO REDUCE THE RISK OF OBESITY
Inflammation and Obesity

One of the most apparent universal interventions would be addressing all factors that lead to dysbiosis and obesity. One of the factors that lead to an increased risk for obesity is environmental toxins. New data reinforce previous evidence of a link between prenatal exposure to bisphenol A (BPA) and childhood obesity and suggest associations of prenatal exposure to PFAS and phthalates with child adiposity. Evidence is increasing that exposure to polyfluoroalkyl substances (PFAS) and phthalates in adulthood might be associated with gestational diabetes, impaired glucose tolerance, and obesity and that these chemicals, as well as bisphenols, could be linked to type 2 diabetes.[16] Early-life exposure to chemicals that are common contaminants associated with food production (pesticides; imidacloprid, chlorpyrifos, and glyphosate) and processing (acrylamide), in addition to chemicals ubiquitously found in our household goods (brominated flame retardants) and drinking water (heavy metals), contribute to the development of metabolic syndrome (MetS) and obesity.[17]

Interestingly, glyphosate is sprayed on wheat and other food products and is readily found in water systems. *Escherichia coli*, *Salmonella enteritidis*, *Salmonella typhimurium*, *S galliarum*, and the *Clostridia* species have shown marked resistance to glyphosate. Knowing the role of glyphosate in dysbiosis, one can easily see why glyphosate is associated with obesity.[18] It would be prudent to avoid environmental contaminants found in food by only using organic and non-genetically modified foods (GMO) foods. Avoidance of contaminants in the water system can be best addressed with reverse osmosis water filter systems. Research-based free apps that identify household products that contain contaminants would also be wise to use.

Improving sleep would help decrease the risk of developing obesity. Decreased sleep increases obesity by decreasing glucose tolerance, insulin sensitivity, and leptin and by increasing inflammation and increasing ghrelin.[19] Insufficient sleep is associated with obesity risk, with observational studies suggesting potentially stronger associations in pediatric populations than in adults.[20–22]

Eliminating artificial sweeteners is essential. Non-caloric artificial sweeteners (NAS) are among the most widely used food additives worldwide. NAS consumption can lead to glucose intolerance through alterations in the intestinal microbiota. These alterations include increased abundance of Bacteroides species and decreased abundance of *Lactobacillus reuteri*. *L reuteri* is known to help with gut integrity.[23]

As noted, a Western diet high in high fats and processed sugary foods increases the risk of obesity by several complex interactions previously described. High fat, processed sugary foods increase dysbiosis, decreases leptin signaling, increases hunger, and increases insulin resistance.[7,9] The recommended amount of sugar a person should eat daily by the American Heart Association is 5–8 g. Most Americans eat approximately 41 g per day. Previous studies have revealed that a Mediterranean diet could positively affect gut microbial communities.[24] The CORDIOPREV study has shown that consumption of a Mediterranean diet or a low-fat diet might partially restore the gut microbiome dysbiosis in obese patients with metabolic syndrome.[25]

Stress is another risk factor for obesity. The hypothalamus–pituitary–adrenal axis (HPA) activity associated with stress affects the gut microbiota composition.[6] Thus, early exposure to stress leads to decreased diversity in gut microbiota and might have long-term effects on its composition. Moreover, chronic stress in adulthood affects the composition of the intestinal microbiota, with a decrease in Bacteroides and *Clostridium* species, and also leads to increased inflammation, which is indicative of immune activation. Furthermore, chronic stress alters the integrity of the intestinal barrier, increasing circulating concentrations of immunomodulatory bacterial cell wall components such as LPS.[26]

Early-life exposure to antibiotics or foods containing glyphosate can change the microbiome. Changes in the microbiome are important throughout life, but particularly early on when the microbiome is more fragile in the first 3 years. Microbes are necessary for the development of the HPA.[27] In addition, colonization must occur to ensure the normal development of the stress signaling pathway.[28,29]

Proton pump inhibitors (PPI) and antipsychotic medications are associated with a decrease in diversity in the gut microbiome.[30] In addition, PPI has been linked to dysbiosis caused by a change in the pH and increased susceptibility to *Clostridium difficile* infection.[31] Bahr and colleagues[32] demonstrated that shortly after risperidone use in children, a decreased ratio of Bacteroidetes: Firmicutes in the gut microbiome was associated with an increase in BMI over time, resembling trends seen in obese patients. A possible explanation for the weight gain is that primary bile acids (associated with weight gain) are typically converted into secondary bile acids by healthy microbes in the gut. Gut diversity changes caused by Risperidone prevents the conversion of primary bile acids to secondary bile acids.[33] Primary bile acids stimulate the germination of C. Difficile spores.[34] Thus, weight gain and the resulting insulin resistance due to dysbiosis can be caused by a more desirable environment that promotes the growth of *Clostridium* when PPIs and risperidone are used. PPIs allow this by changing the pH of the gut. Risperidone does this by preventing the conversion of primary bile acids that promote the germination of *Clostridium*. However, primary bile acids also increase weight gain.

For obese subjects, physical activity may reduce the pro-inflammatory effects of cytokines that may link obesity, insulin resistance, and diabetes.[35]

PREVENTING ABERRANT GUT MICROBIOME RELATED TO CHRONIC INFLAMMATION
Protecting Prenatal and Intra-natal Gut Microbiome: Impact of Prenatal Antibiotic Use and Cesarean Section

Cesarean section and prenatal antibiotic use, have a potential impact in causing changes in the maternal offspring microbiome (dysbiosis) and increasing the risk of obesity in children and adolescents. This change in the microbiome may lead to aberrant microbial colonization of the infant's gut and lead to an increased risk of obesity later in life. In a retrospective analysis, based on 436 mother-child dyads followed for 7 years after birth, children exposed to antibiotics in the second or third trimester had an 84% higher risk of obesity. In the same study, delivery via Cesarean Section was associated with a 46% higher risk of obesity. This risk was independent of prenatal antibiotic use. Significant alterations in both gut microbiome due to Cesarean Section delivery and exposure to antibiotics in the second or third trimester were associated with higher offspring obesity risk.[36] This study highlights the importance of a healthy gut microbiome in children and adolescents. Maternal-fetal exchange of gut microbiome may begin before birth and lead to in-utero intestinal seeding in the fetus with a beneficial microbiome that confers protection against child and adolescent obesity. Other meta-analyses have also demonstrated an increased risk of obesity with delivery via cesarean section.[36] Thus, minimizing antibiotics and emphasizing the importance of normal vaginal delivery would be considered an example of universal prevention directed toward a whole population.

SCHOOL-BASED TWELVE-MONTH COGNITIVE-BEHAVIORAL-SKILL BUILDING INTERVENTION IN ADOLESCENTS

A cluster-randomized control intervention was done using the manualized 15-session COPE (Creating Opportunities for Personal Empowerment) program in 779 adolescents over twelve months. COPE was integrated as a health course with 20-min physical activity in each session. Compared with controls, adolescents in the COPE program had a lower BMI at 12 months and a significant decrease in the proportion of overweight and obese adolescents. Of note, adolescents with high depressive symptoms at the beginning of the study had significantly lower depression at 12 months.[37]

SELECTIVE AND INDICATED INTENSIVE LIFESTYLE INTERVENTIONS

These studies include interventions for high-risk/overweight children (selective) or those with signs and symptoms of obesity (indicated).

Mediterranean Style Diet for Children with Obesity, Insulin Resistance, and Metabolic Syndrome

In a comparative study, 49 participants (ages 3–18) were randomly assigned to a Mediterranean style diet (MSD) rich in polyunsaturated fatty acids, fiber, flavonoids, and antioxidants (60% of energy from carbohydrate, 25% from fat, and 15% from protein ($n = 24$); or a standard diet (55% of carbohydrate, 30% from fat and 15% from protein ($n = 25$), the caloric ingest were individualized. At baseline and week 16 of the intervention, the glucose, triglycerides (TG), total cholesterol (TC), high-density lipoprotein cholesterol (HDL-C), and low-density lipoprotein cholesterol (LDL-C) were measured as well as the body composition and anthropometric data. The 24-h recalls determined diet compliance. Paired Student's t and McNemar's tests were used to compare effects in biochemical, body composition, anthropometric, and dietary variables. The MSD group significantly decreased BMI, lean mass, fat mass, glucose, TC, TG, HDL-C, and LDL-C. ($p < 0.05$); the diet compliance increased consumption of omega-three fatty acids, zinc, vitamin E, selenium, and decreased consumption of saturated fatty acids ($p < 0.05$). With regard to metabolic syndrome (MetS), the group following the MSD showed a decrease of 45% in MetS, and as such, a significant difference after week 16 of intervention, ($p < 0.05$). There was no decrease in the standard diet group. The standard diet group decreased glucose levels and frequency of glucose >100 mg/dL ($p < 0.05$). However, weight, media arm circumference (MAC) and lean mass increased in the same period of time in this group.[38]

CHILDREN WITH ABDOMINAL OBESITY AND LIFESTYLE CHANGES

A 2-year family-based lifestyle intervention randomized controlled trial was performed on 107 participants (ages 7–16). The children were assigned either to a usual care group receiving guidance on a healthy diet or an intensive care group that followed a moderate hypocaloric Mediterranean diet. Their parents attended with them. Both received nutritional education on a healthy diet for 8 weeks with follow-up at 22 months. During the 8-week period, usual care subjects received a 30-min individual session with the dietician and five monitoring visits to assess anthropometric parameters. Participants assigned to the intensive care group completed six 30-min individual sessions with the research team. Intake adequacy was evaluated using Dietary Reference Intakes and diet quality through the Diet Quality Index for Adolescents (DQI-A), the Healthy Lifestyle Diet Index (HLD-I), and the Mediterranean Diet Quality Index (KIDMED). The DQI-A is composed of the sum of three categories (quality, diversity, and equilibrium) of bread and cereals, potatoes and grains, vegetables, fruits, milk products, cheese, meat, fish and substitutes, and fats and oils. The HDL-Index is composed of 10 items, eight of which refer to the frequency of consumption of fruit, vegetables, fish and seafood, sweets, regular soft drinks, grain, dairy products, meat, and meat products. Both groups significantly reduced BMI standard deviation scores (BMI-SDS), glucose, and TC levels. The MSD group exhibited a significant increase in the consumption of dietary fiber, proteins, omega 9 fatty acids, zinc, selenium, vitamin E, and flavonoids, furthermore, they consumed fewer saturated fatty acids (p < 0.05) with enhanced compliance with recommendations. Components of metabolic syndrome (MetS) measured were abdominal obesity, dyslipidemia (increase in triglycerides [TG] and low high-density lipoprotein cholesterol [HDL-C] levels), high blood pressure and glucose intolerance. The group following the MSD showed a decrease of 45% in MetS after week 16 of the intervention, (p < 0.05). Intake of calcium, iodine, and vitamin D was higher in the intensive care group, with enhanced compliance with recommendations. DQI-A and HLD-I were significantly higher in the intensive care group vs the usual care group after the treatment.[39]

In conclusion, using the Mediterranean diet was able to reduce BMI-SDS in children with abdominal obesity, improve lipid status, and decrease oxidative stress and nutritional status.

MINDFULNESS FOR OBESITY

An randomized clinical trial (RCT) pilot study used an mindfulness based stress reduction (MBSR)-based program for parents with obesity aimed at preventing obesity in their children ($n = 42$ parent-child dyads), An 8-week mindfulness-based parent stress group intervention (parenting mindfully for health) plus nutrition and physical activity counseling (PMH + N) was aimed at low-income, stressed parents with obesity. The goal was to evaluate weights in their 2–5-year-old children with obesity vs a control group. PMH + N was compared with a control group intervention (C + N), and improvement in parenting was assessed before and after the intervention using the laboratory-based toy wait task (TWT). In addition, nutrition, physical activity, and stress were assessed using a multimethod approach. Eight-week mindfulness-based parent stress group intervention (parenting mindfully for health) plus nutrition and physical activity counseling (PMH + N). Compared with the C + N group, the PMH + N group demonstrated significantly better group attendance ($P < .015$), greater improvement in parental involvement ($P < .05$), and decreased parental emotional eating rating ($P < .011$). Furthermore, C + N, but not PMH + N, was associated with significant increases in child BMI percentile during treatment ($P < .03$) when accounting for the TWT before and after changes in parenting scores.[40]

An RCT pilot study used the Mindfulness-Based Eating Awareness (MB-EAT-A) program. The MB-EAT-A program is an adaptation of the MBSR program for adolescents and has been implemented in some high schools. In the study performed by Barnes and Kristeller on 9th-grade adolescents, (14 males; 35 African Americans, 1 Caucasian, 4 Others; mean age 16.2 ± 1.2 years; BMI $= 32.4 \pm 9.0$, BMI range 19.1 to 58.4) from 6 high school health/physical education classes were randomly assigned to 12-weekly sessions of MB-EAT-A intervention ($n = 18$) or health education control (Control [CTL], $n = 22$). The program increased moderate and intense aerobic exercise and improved consumption of low-calorie and low-fat foods in overweight/obese adolescents in both groups at 3 months, although the positive changes were greater in the MB-EAT-A group. However, at the 6-month follow-up the participants in the MB-EAT-A group continued to improve, whereas the control group lost most of their gains seen during the 3-month post-test. The MB-EAT-A group at 6 months was able to increase the number of servings per week of low-calorie foods (7.7 vs -0.05, $p < 0.02$) and foods low in saturated fats (4.6 vs -2.7, $p < 0.2$) after six months. At 6 mo. follow-up, the MB-EAT-A group increased days/week of moderate exercise by> 30 min/day (0.8 vs -0.7 days/week), and intense aerobic exercise by>20 min/day (1.4 vs -0.5 days/week. A trend was observed whereby the MB-EAT-A group showed a greater decrease in perceived hunger compared with CTLs.[41]

In another study, Shomaker and colleagues[42] randomized overweight/obese adolescent girls at risk for Type 2 Diabetes with depressive symptoms to 6 one-hour weekly group sessions of mindfulness or CBT ($n = 33$, ages 12–17). The mindfulness intervention (Learning to Breathe) was based on MBSR using developmentally appropriate interactive activities and guided discussions to teach standard mindfulness skills. Examples of mindfulness awareness activities include breath awareness, body scanning, mindful eating, sitting meditation, loving-kindness practice, and mindful movement (yoga). Adolescents met for six, one-hour sessions, once per week. Brief (~ 10 min/day) homework was assigned to help adolescents practice skills and apply them to daily life. The cognitive-behavioral group was a manualized depression prevention, the Blues Program, consisting of 1-h session, once per week, for 6 weeks. Content includes psycho-education, cognitive restructuring, pleasant activities, self-reinforcement, and coping skills. At all sessions, adolescents are assigned homework.

Depressive symptoms decreased more in the mindfulness condition at post-treatment (d = .56), and this difference persisted at six months (d = .69). Three adolescents in the cognitive-behavioral condition developed criteria for MDD during the follow-up, and no adolescents did so in mindfulness (P = .24). Accounting for all covariates, anxiety symptoms and perceived stress decreased, with no between-group differences (P > .1). Compared with the cognitive-behavioral intervention, adolescents randomized to mindfulness had greater decreases in fasting insulin at post-treatment (d = .78; P = .04). There were no differences in fasting insulin at six-months (d = .31; P = .34) or fasting glucose at post-treatment (d = .30; P = .34) or six-months (d = .40; P = .21. In addition, at 1-year post-treatment, the mindfulness group showed a slight improvement in BMI and percentage of body fat.

In summary, mindfulness programs are promising for obese children and their families in regard to diet, exercise, eating behavior, insulin resistance in diabetic obese adolescent girls, and prevention of weight gain in children of parents participating in the mindfulness programs. Some studies continued to have positive effects long term. More studies are needed to confirm these results.

EXERCISE FOR OBESE CHILDREN

In a small, randomized control study of 15 obese and 21 lean children, the impact of three months of a physical activity-based lifestyle intervention on inflammatory markers was studied. Alterations in serum retinol-binding protein (RBP4) occur early in the clinical course of obesity and appear to correlate with subclinical inflammation. This lifestyle intervention almost entirely reversed the raised RBP4 levels in obese children and reduced subclinical inflammation markers, including C-reactive protein (CRP) and Interleukin-6 (IL-6). Reduced insulin levels were also correlated with the decrease in serum RBP4 level. Thus, the coordinated reduction of markers of inflammation and serum RBP4 by the lifestyle intervention observed in this study may reflect an amelioration of inflammation.[43]

PROBIOTICS
Obese Children with Non-alcoholic Fatty Liver Disease

A randomized triple-blind trial was conducted among 64 obese children (n = 64, ages 10–18, (BMI) of ≥85th percentile) with sonographic non-alcoholic fatty liver disease (NAFLD). They were randomly allocated to receive probiotic capsules (containing *Lactobacillus acidophilus* ATCC B3208, 3×10^9 colony forming units (CFU); *Bifidobacterium lactis* DSMZ 32269, 6×10^9 CFU; *Bifidobacterium bifidum* ATCC SD6576, 2×10^9 CFU; *Lactobacillus rhamnosus* DSMZ 21690, 2×10^9 CFU) or placebo for 12 weeks. After the intervention, in the probiotic group, the mean levels of alanine aminotransferase decreased from 32.8 (19.6) to 23.1 (9.9) U/L (P = 0.02), and the mean aspartate aminotransferase decreased from 32.2 (15.7) to 24.3 (7.7) U/L (P = 0.02). Likewise, the mean cholesterol, low-density lipoprotein-C, TG, and waist circumference decreased in the intervention group without significant change in weight, BMI, and BMI z score. After the trial, normal liver sonography was reported in 17 (53.1%) and 5 (16.5%) of patients in the intervention and placebo groups, respectively.[44]

Probiotics in Obese Children with Insulin Resistance

The study included 48 obese children (10–15 years old) with insulin resistance. They received dietary advice and were assigned to take the capsules with or without probiotic the probiotic Bifidobacterium pseudocatenulatum (10^{9-10} CFU) daily for

13 weeks. Clinical, biochemical, and gut microbiome measurements were made at baseline and the end of the intervention.

Omentin-1 is thought to be part of the early-defense mechanisms against pathogenic bacteria in the gut, and it has been identified as an adipokine mainly expressed in visceral adipose tissue that can act as a protective factor against cardiovascular disease. Monocyte chemoattractant protein-1 (MCP-1) is a chemokine produced by macrophages and endothelial cells via the activation of the nuclear transcription factor-kB pathway. MCP-1 recruits monocytes, leukocytes, and other inflammatory cells in response to an inflammatory challenge and as a consequence of weight gain. These two adipokines are related to inflammatory processes and endothelial dysfunction. Thus, it could be of interest to evaluate them in the early steps of obesity, such as those that occur in children.

There was a significant improvement in BMI in all children after the intervention, suggesting that weight changes are related to dietary advice. A significant decrease in circulating high-sensitive CRP ($P = 0.026$) and MCP-1 ($P = 0.032$) and an increase in high-density lipoprotein cholesterol ($P = 0.035$) and omentin-1 ($P = 0.023$) in children receiving probiotic supplementation were observed compared with the control group. Regarding gut microbiota, probiotic administration significantly increased the proportion of the Rikenellaceae family members, particularly of the Alistipes genus, which is associated with a lean phenotype. This suggested that B. pseudocatenulatum could favorably modulate the gut ecosystem in obese subjects.[45]

Probiotic VSL3# in Obese Children with Non-alcoholic Steatohepatitis (Non-Alcoholic Fatty Liver Disease)

A double-blind RCT of VSL#3 vs placebo in obese children (ages 9–12 years) with biopsy-proven NAFLD was completed with 48 children, 44 (22 VSL#3 and 22 placebo). The primary outcome was the change in fatty liver severity at four months as detected by ultrasonography. Secondary outcomes were the changes in TG, insulin resistance as detected by the homeostasis model assessment (HOMA), alanine transaminase (ALT), BMI, glucagon-like peptide 1 (GLP-1), and activated GLP-1 (GLP-1). Ordinal and linear models with cluster confidence intervals were used to evaluate the efficacy of VSL#3 vs placebo at 4 months.

A low-calorie diet was prescribed to all patients during the whole study, as recommended by the Italian Recommended Dietary Allowances. Each patient received the following diet: carbohydrate, 50% to 60%; fat, 23% to 30%; fatty acid, two-thirds saturated, one-third unsaturated protein, 15% to 20%; for a total of 25 to 30 Kcal/kg body weight/day. In addition to the prescribed diet, a moderate aerobic exercise program (30–45 min at least three times a week) was also recommended and tailored to individual preferences. One VSL #3 was given for children under age 10 and 2 over age 10. At baseline, moderate and severe NAFLD was present in 64% and 36% of placebo children and 55% and 45% of VSL#3 children. The probability that children supplemented with VSL#3 had none, light, moderate or severe FL at the end of the study was 21%, 70%, 9%, and 0%, respectively, with corresponding values of 0%, 7%, 76%, and 17% for the placebo group ($P < 0.001$). No between-group differences were detected in TG, HOMA, and ALT, whereas BMI decreased and GLP-1 and activated GLP1 (aGLP1) increased in the VSL#3 group ($P < 0.001$ for all comparisons). GLP-1 seems to modulate fatty acid oxidation, decreases lipogenesis, and improves hepatic glucose metabolism. A 4-month supplement of VSL#3 significantly improves NAFLD in children. It was postulated that the VSL#3-dependent GLP-1 increase could be responsible for these beneficial effects.[46]

Synbiotic for Obese Children

An open-label, randomized, controlled study included children with primary obesity ($N = 86$, ages 9–15). The first group was treated with a standard method with a reduced calorie intake and increased physical activity. The second group received add-on daily synbiotic (combination of probiotics and prebiotics) supplementation for one month. This study aimed to evaluate the potential effects of a synbiotic on anthropometric measurements, lipid profile, and oxidative stress parameters. One month of supplementation of the synbiotic resulted in a significant reduction of weight ($P < 0.001$) and BMI ($P < 0.01$). Changes (% reduction compared with baseline) in anthropometric measurements were significantly higher in the children receiving the additional synbiotic supplement ($P < 0.05$). The percentage of children with weight loss was higher in the synbiotic group but not statistically significant (71.4 vs 64.2%, $P > 0.05$). On the 30th day of the synbiotic intervention, total serum cholesterol, low-density lipoprotein cholesterol, and total oxidative stress levels significantly declined ($P < 0.05$). These changes in serum lipid levels were significantly higher in the synbiotic group ($P < 0.05$). Changes in serum total oxidative stress levels before and after the intervention period were significant in the synbiotic group ($P < 0.01$). In the study, changes in weight, BMI, and triceps skinfold thickness were higher in the group receiving the one-month synbiotic supplement than in the standard method group. The supplement tested also had a beneficial profile effect on lipid and total oxidative stress.[47]

Synbiotic in Children with Body Mass Index >85th Percentile

This study was a randomized triple-masked controlled trial among 70 participants aged 6–18 years with BMI equal to or higher than the 85th percentile. The children were randomly assigned to two groups of equal numbers to receive a synbiotic or placebo for 8 weeks. At the end of the trial, the decrease in BMI Z-score, waist circumference, and waist-to-hip ratio were significantly higher in the synbiotic group than in the placebo group. Likewise, the synbiotic group significantly decreased serum TG and total- and low-density lipoprotein-cholesterol levels. The beneficial effects of a synbiotic supplement on controlling excess weight and some cardio-metabolic risk factors among children and adolescents can be considered in clinical practice.[48]

In summary, probiotics in obese children with NAFLD and insulin resistance have promising research in regards to decreasing harmful parameters associated with these diseases. In addition, synbiotics show promise in regards to controlling excess weight, decreasing lipids and decreasing oxidative stress.

MOTIVATIONAL INTERVIEWING IN CHILDREN

MI is a patient-centered communication style that uses specific techniques such as reflective listening, autonomy support, shared decision-making, and eliciting change talk. In a large-scale randomized control trial, 42 practices from the Pediatric Research in Office Settings Network of the American Academy of Pediatrics were randomly assigned to three groups. The primary outcome was the child's BMI percentile at 2–year follow-up. Group one was usual care with measured BMI percentile at baseline and 1- and 2-year follow-up. Group two was a primary care physician (PCP) only intervention in which the PCP delivered four MI counseling sessions to parents over 2 years. Group three was PCP and registered dietician (RD) intervention in which the provider delivered four MI sessions and RD delivered six MI sessions. MI-based sessions used a three-phase model developed by the lead study author that helps clinicians transition from building motivation to planning a course of action. In the usual care group one, PCPs and staff were provided a half-day orientation session that included current treatment guidelines. MI training in groups two and three for PCPs and RDs included two days of in person training and an interactive DVD training system. At 2-year follow-up, the adjusted BMI percentile in group three was significantly lower than in group one. BMI percentile was lower in group two than in group one, but the difference was not significant. Interestingly, PCPs had a much better rate of completing the MI sessions than RDs and seemed more effective even with the modest doses of MI incorporated in the study. This large study demonstrates that MI can significantly reduce obesity in children and could be considered an essential intervention in routine medical care provided to children by PCPs. This study also suggests that motivated PCPs who believe they have the requisite skills to deliver MI can make a huge impact on the trajectory of the child's health[49] We believe this is a remarkable study given the nature of its impact, the low risk associated with an MI session, and the enormous potential benefit in improving health outcomes in children.

Cochrane Review: Lifestyle Intervention for Improving School Achievement in Obese Children

The review is a systematic review based on six studies (14 articles) of 674 overweight and obese children and adolescents in school settings among children aged three to eighteen. The total number of overweight and obese children and adolescents included was 674. Out of the six studies, two studies had only physical activity interventions. The goal was to determine if multicomponent lifestyle interventions targeting physical activity and a healthy diet could improve school achievement in overweight and obese children in high-income countries. In addition, the study wanted to determine if physical activity intervention delivered for weight management could benefit mathematics achievement, executive function, and working memory. The studies included in the review delivered the interventions as part of the school curriculum providing hope that school interventions can make a difference.[50]

Cochrane Review: Lifestyle Interventions in Preschool Children for Obesity

The review is a systematic review based on six randomized control studies in clinical settings representing 1222 overweight and obese children aged 2 to 5 years. Two studies with less intensive intervention in the form of system changes focused on more education, and two to four MI sessions delivered by Nurse Practitioners showed no change in six months. Two studies in parent-child dyads that used a more intensive, multidisciplinary approach with dietary education, physical activity education and coaching, and behavior management in a group setting via in-home individualized intervention for 24 weeks demonstrated significant and sustained effect on obesity at 1-year follow-up. One study testing parent coaching showed a significant reduction in adiposity at six months, and one study with diet intention for education in a dairy-rich diet showed a possible effect on adiposity. This study highlights the intensity of interventions needed to significantly impact and demonstrates the negative impact when only two MI sessions were done.

The preschool age group's focus on physical activity did not seem to have an impact. Thus, combined interventions including a behavioral/MI and coaching component that were both intensive and long-term for parents seemed to have the most impact in the preschool age group.[51]

More or less Study

This study is about the impact of Intensive Lifestyle intervention on behavioral problems in obese preschoolers. This intervention was a randomized control trial in children aged

Table 1
Summary

Treatment	Level of Certainty by USPTF	Strength of Recommendation Based on Benefit and Safety	Evidence Base in Youth	Personal Recommendations of the Reviewer/Passes SECS
I. Motivational Interviewing (MI)				
a. MI, intensive multidisciplinary approach, parent coaching, nutritional education in the clinical setting (Foster et al, 2015[50], n = 1222, ages 2–5, dx overweight or obese)	Moderate	B, but safe	• Cochrane Systematic Review, −6 RCT	• Some evidence for diet counseling, psychological counseling, parent education, coaching, and MI in reducing adiposity in preschool children • Recommend • Possibly expensive but safe, relatively easy, and sensible • Does not pass SECS if too expensive
b. MI by Pediatricians and Registered Dieticians (Resnicow et al, 2015[49], n = 645, 42 pediatric practices, ages 2–8, dx BMI >85th and <97th percentile)	Low No control	C, but safe	• Cluster-randomized, 3-group intervention trial BMI CP and staff (usual care) • Group 2—MI trained PCP did 4 MI sessions in 2 years • Group 3 MI trained PCP did four sessions and Registered Dietitians (RD) did six sessions in 2 years	• MI over 2 years by both providers and RDs (group 3) resulted in statistically significant reductions in BMI percentile. • Recommend • Cheap, safe, relatively easy, and sensible • Passes SECS
II. Lifestyle interventions				
a. Multicomponent lifestyle interventions; six studies, two studies with only physical activity in school setting (Martin et al, 2014[51], n = 674, ages 3–18, dx overweight or obese).	Moderate	B, but safe	• Cochrane, systematic review, −6 RCT	• Could benefit overweight/obese children in school achievement, mathematics, memory, and specific thinking skills. Expensive but safe, relatively easy, and sensible • Recommend • Does not pass SECS if too expensive when designed

Intervention/Study	Level	Rating	Study type	Notes
b. Exposure to maternal microbiota: C-section versus vaginal, in utero antibiotics (Mueller et al, 2015[36], n = 436 dyads, ages 0–7, dx obesity)	Low	C, but safe	Cohort study	• Antibiotics in second/third trimester predicted **84%** higher risk of obesity at age 7. • Birth via C-Section had **46%** higher obesity risk. • Encourage avoidance of oral maternal antibiotics and C-section where possible • Recommend • Passes SECS
c. 18-month therapeutic protocol intensive lifestyle modification (dietary regimen, physical activity, and behavioral interventions) (Rainone et al, 2016[2], n = 20, 18 control ages 5–18, dx obesity 6, months)	Low	C, but safe	• Cross-sectional study with a longitudinal arm	• Successful lifestyle modification is effective in reducing inflammation, suggesting inhibition of the inflammasome. • Recommend • Cheap, safe, relatively easy, and sensible • Passes SECS
d. The parenting program for obesity (10 weekly sessions at 90 min) (Eiffener et al, 2019[52], n = 77, ages 4–6, dx obesity)	Low	C, but safe	RCT	• Obesity treatment may help in reducing emotional distress • Recommend • Cheap, safe, relatively easy, and sensible • Passes SECS
e. Behavioral intervention to promote adherence to diet to reduce LDL-C levels. (Kwiterovich et al, 1995[53], n = 673, ages 8–10, dx LDL-C levels > 80th –<98th)	Low	C, but safe	6 center RCT	• At 3 years, dietary total fat, saturated fat, and cholesterol level decreased significantly as compared with treatment as usual. • Recommend but needs more studies

(continued on next page)

Table 1
(continued)

Treatment	Level of Certainty by USPTF	Strength of Recommendation Based on Benefit and Safety	Evidence Base in Youth	Personal Recommendations of the Reviewer/Passes SECS
f. Three months of physical activity-based lifestyle intervention to evaluate the impact on retinol binding protein (RBP4) levels (Balagopal et al, 2017[43], $n = 33$, ages >14 yr to >18 yr, Dx 21 lean and 15 obese)	Low	C, but safe	RCT	• Lifestyle intervention almost entirely reversed raised RBP4 levels in obese children. • Recommend but needs more studies • Cheap, safe, relatively easy, and sensible • Passes SECS
g. Comparison study of a Mediterranean-style diet (MSD) vs a standard diet (SD) (Velázquez-López et al[38], 2014, $N = 49$, ages 3–18)	Low	C	Randomly assigned comparative study	MSD group significantly decreased BMI, lean mass, fat mass, glucose, TC, TG, HDL-C, and LDL-C. ($p < 0.05$). MSD showed a decrease of 45% in metabolic syndrome (MetS) after 16 weeks ($p < 0.05$). No improvement in MetS was seen in the SD group. Weight, media arm circumference (MAC) and lean mass increased in the SD group. Recommend MSD Passes SECS

The topmost entry (partial, continued from previous page): • Cheap, safe, relatively easy, and sensible • Passes SECS

h. Comparison between a healthy diet (HD) and a hypocaloric Mediterranean diet (MD) (Ojeda-Rodriguez et al[39], 2018, N = 107, ages 7–16)	Low	C	RCT	Both groups were given education for 8 weeks with a 22-month follow-up. Both groups significantly reduced BMI standard deviation score (BMI-SDS), glucose, and total cholesterol levels. Higher dietary scores were associated with lower micronutrient inadequacy. The Diet Quality Index for Adolescents (DQI-A) and Healthy Lifestyle Diet Index (HLD-I) were significantly higher in the intensive care group vs the usual care group after the treatment. Recommend MD over the HD. Passes SECS
III. Cognitive behavioral				
COPE is a cognitive-behavioral skills-building intervention with 20 min of physical activity (Melnyk et al, 2015[37], n = 779, ages 14–16, Dx none high school students)	Low	C, but safe	RCT	• COPE teens had a significantly lower BMI at 12 months • Recommend but needs more studies. • Cheap, safe, relatively easy, and sensible • Passes SECS
IV. Mindfulness Interventions				
a. Mindfulness-Based Stress Reduction (MBSR) vs cognitive behavior therapy (CBT) in diabetics.	Low	C Needs more studies	Pilot RCT	Participants received six 1-h weekly group sessions of mindfulness or CBT. • Depressive symptoms decreased more in the mindfulness

(continued on next page)

Table 1
(continued)

Treatment	Level of Certainty by USPTF	Strength of Recommendation Based on Benefit and Safety	Evidence Base in Youth	Personal Recommendations of the Reviewer/Passes SECS
(Shoemaker et al, 2017[42], ages 12–17, $n = 33$)				condition at post-treatment ($d = .56$), and this difference persisted at six months ($d = .69$). • Adolescents randomized to mindfulness had greater decreases in fasting insulin at post-treatment. • There were no differences in fasting insulin at six-months, or fasting glucose at post-treatment or six-months. • 1-year post-treatment, the mindfulness group showed a slight improvement in BMI and percentage of body fat. • Recommend • (Passes SECS)
b. Mindfulness-Based Eating Awareness (MB-EAT-A). Aimed at low-income, stressed parents with obesity to evaluate weights in their 2–5-year-old children with obesity vs a control group. (Jastreboff et al, 2018[40], $n = 42$ dyads, effect of mindfulness with parents on 2–5-year-old)	Low	C Needs more studies	Pilot RCT	• Eight-week mindfulness program • Mindfulness group had greater improvement in parental involvement and decreased parental emotional eating rating. • The control group was associated with significant increases in child BMI. • Recommend. • (Passes SECS)

Study	Quality	Grade	Study type	Results
c. Mindfulness-Based Eating Awareness (MB- EAT-A) to help adolescent obese individuals (BMI = 32.4 ± 9.0) normalize eating behaviors, and improve exercise and dietary habits (Barnes and Kristell et al, 2016[41], N = 40 adolescents in 9th grade)	Low	C Needs more studies	Pilot RCT	• Randomized to 12 weekly sessions vs education program. • MBSR program • The program increased moderate and intense aerobic exercise and improved consumption of low-calorie and low-fat foods in overweight/obese adolescents in both groups at 3 months, although the changes were greater in the MB-EAT-A group. • However, at 6 months only the MB-EAT-A group continued to improve, whereas the control group decreased the gains that were made. • MB-EAT-A group showed a greater decrease in perceived hunger. • Recommend • (Passes SECS)
V. Probiotics				
a. Effects of Probiotics on Obese Children with Non-Alcoholic Fatty Liver Disease (BMI of ≥85th percentile) (Famouri et al, 2017[44], n = 64, ages 10–18)	Low	C	Triple BPCT	Randomly allocated to receive probiotic capsule (containing Lactobacillus acidophilus; Bifidobacterium lactis; Bifidobacterium bifidum; Lactobacillus rhamnosus or placebo for 12 weeks Probiotic was effective in improving nonalcoholic fatty liver disease and: • improved the lipid profile of obese children.

(continued on next page)

Table 1
(continued)

Treatment	Level of Certainty by USPTF	Strength of Recommendation Based on Benefit and Safety	Evidence Base in Youth	Personal Recommendations of the Reviewer/Passes SECS
				• had a significant effect on improving the level of liver enzymes and sonographic fatty liver. • effects were independent of the weight status Recommend (Passes SECS)
b. Probiotic Bifidobacterium pseudocatenulatum CECT 7765 on cardiometabolic risk factors, inflammatory cytokines and gut microbiota composition in Obese Children with Insulin Resistance (IR) Obese children (Sanchis-Chordà et al, 2019[45], n = 48, ages 10–15)	Low	C	Pilot study	Given daily advice and assigned capsules with or without probiotic (109–10 colony forming units [CFU]) daily for 13 weeks. Compared with the control group, for those receiving Bifidobacterium pseudocatenulatum there was a a. Significant improvement in body mass index b. Significant decrease in circulating high-sensitive C-reactive protein and c. An increase in high-density lipoprotein cholesterol and omentin-1 (thought to be part of the early-defense mechanisms against pathogenic bacteria in the gut) Regarding gut microbiota, probiotic administration significantly increased the proportion of the Alistipes genus, which is associated with a lean phenotype.

				Recommend (Passes SECS)
c. Probiotic VSL3# in Obese Children with Non-Alcoholic Steatohepatitis (NAFLD) (Alisi et al, 2014[46], n = 44, ages 9–12)	Low	C	DBPCT	• Each patient received a low-calorie diet for a total of 25–30 kcal/kg body weight/day. • A moderate aerobic exercise program (30–45 min at least three times a week) was tailored to individual preferences. One VSL #3 was given for children under age 10 and 2 over age 10 for 4 months. • BMI decreased and GLP-1 and activated GLP1 increased in the VSL#3 group ($P < 0.001$) • Probability that children supplemented with VSL#3 had none, light, moderate or severe FL at the end of the study was 21%, 70%, 9%, and 0%, respectively, with corresponding values of 0%, 7%, 76% and 17% for the placebo group ($P < 0.001$). • Recommend • (Passes SECS)
Synbiotic in obese children to study effects of a synbiotic on anthropometric measurements, lipid profile, and oxidative stress parameters (Ipar et al, 2015[47], N = 86, ages 9–15)	Low	C	Open-label RCT	• One group got and increased physical activity. • After 1 month of the synbiotic the percentage of children with weight loss was higher in the synbiotic group but not statistically significant (71.4 vs 64.2%, $P > 0.05$). • Changes in serum total oxidative stress levels and serum lipid

(continued on next page)

Table 1
(continued)

Treatment	Level of Certainty by USPTF	Strength of Recommendation Based on Benefit and Safety	Evidence Base in Youth	Personal Recommendations of the Reviewer/Passes SECS
				levels were significantly higher in the synbiotic group. • On the 30(th) day of synbiotic intervention, serum total cholesterol, low density lipoprotein cholesterol and total oxidative stress levels had significantly declined ($P < 0.05$). • Recommend • Passes SECS
Synbiotic in children with BMI > 85th percentile (Safavi et al, 2013[48], , $n = 70$, ages 6–18)	Low	C	Randomized triple- masked controlled trial	• Randomly assigned to two groups of equal numbers to receive a synbiotic or placebo for 8 weeks. The decrease in BMI Z-score, waist circumference, and waist-to-hip ratio were significantly higher in the synbiotic group than in the placebo group. • The synbiotic group significantly decreased serum triglycerides and total- and low-density lipoprotein- cholesterol levels. • Recommended • (Passes SECS)

Strength of recommendations based on benefit and safety.

A = Recommend strongly. There is a high certainty that the net benefit is substantial *and safe.*

B = Recommend. There is a high certainty that the net benefit is moderate or there is moderate certainty that the net benefit is moderate to substantial *and safe.*

C = Neutral (offer or provide this service for selected patients depending on individual circumstances, based on professional judgment and patient preferences). There is at least moderate certainty that the net benefit is small.

D = Discourage. There is moderate or high certainty that the service has no net benefit or that the harms outweigh the benefits.

I = Insufficient (if the service is offered, patients should understand the uncertainty about the balance of benefits and harms) Current evidence is insufficient to assess the balance of benefits and harms of the service. Evidence is lacking, of poor quality, or conflicting, and the balance of benefits cannot be determined.)

Level of certainty regarding quality.

HIGH Level of evidence with robust positive data meta-analyses or meta-reviews involving two or more RCTs of excellent, robust quality. The available evidence usually includes consistent results from well-designed, well-conducted RCTs in representative child, adolescent or young adult (18–24 years old) populations, assessing the effects on mental health outcomes.

MODERATE Level of evidence with robust positive data involving two or more RCTs of excellent, robust quality. The available evidence usually includes consistent results from well-designed, well-conducted RCTs in representative child, adolescent or young adult (18–24 years old) populations, assessing the effects on mental health outcomes.

LOW Level of evidence with less than two RCTs with good or average quality. The available evidence is insufficient to assess the effects on mental health outcomes.

SECS criteria.

A guide to clinical decisions is that Interventions that are Safe, Easy, Cheap, *and* Sensible (SECS) require less evidence to justify individual trials than those that are Risky, Unrealistic, Difficult, *or* Expensive (RUDE). Because some of the treatments do not have much solid, compelling evidence but would be reasonable to try with a lower bar of evidence, this criterion is also taken into account. Being risky, unrealistic, difficult *OR* expensive (RUDE) disqualifies from SECS. The bolded conjunctions are essential in applying this guide.

4 to 6 diagnosed with obesity. In the intervention, parents were provided a group program of 90 min for ten sessions. The sessions emphasized lifestyle components to support a healthy home environment. Parent-rated scores on the Child Behavioral Checklist (CBCL) improved significantly in the study after obesity treatment, suggesting that obesity treatment can reduce emotional distress among preschoolers.[52]

Dietary Intervention Study

Dietary intervention study (DISC) is a long-term safety and efficacy study of a cholesterol-lowering diet in children with elevated Low-Density Lipoprotein Cholesterol (LDL-C). Six hundred and sixty-three children aged 8 to 10 with elevated LDL-C were randomized to a dietary intervention versus usual care with a mean follow-up of 7.4 years. Dietary intervention promoted a diet with lower fat and cholesterol, and in the study, a dietary fat modification was safely and sustainably attained in actively growing children with elevated LDL-C.[53]

A summary of these studies can be found in **Table 1** using the United States Preventative Services Task Force ratings for the strength of the recommendation and level of certainty for each study. (See **Table 1**).

SUMMARY

Childhood Obesity is a significant global challenge impacting children's health worldwide.[2] Recent research focuses on emerging factors: inflammation, gut microbiome, and environmental influences. Significant alterations in the gut microbiome due to Cesarean Section delivery, exposure to antibiotics in the second or third trimester, and formula feeding were associated with higher offspring obesity risk.[36] In children and adolescents, obesity is characterized by the activation of inflammatory markers and alteration of gut permeability.[2] Emerging evidence indicates prebiotic food and probiotics may favorably alter the gut microbiome, reducing the risk of obesity. A large-scale randomized trial on brief motivational interviewing (MI) by pediatric practices demonstrated reductions in BMI.[52] In addition, successful lifestyle modification is effective in reducing inflammation and BMI.[2] According to a recent Cochrane review, the existing studies suggest that lifestyle interventions could benefit overweight and obese children specifically in overall school achievement, mathematics, memory, and specific thinking skills.[50] Among 2–5-year-old obese children, multi-disciplinary, intensive approaches to treatment have the most evidence of efficacy.[53] In preschool-age children, baseline ADHD symptoms predict poor responses to obesity treatment, but parenting-focused interventions reduce both BMI and externalizing behavioral problems.[36] For children with elevated LDL-C levels, a diet-based intervention focusing on a low-fat diet has been shown effective in modestly reducing LDL-C levels while not negatively impacting the child's psychological well-being.[52] Mindfulness research has some of the most promising results. Mindfulness programs are helpful for obese children and their families in regard to diet, exercise, eating behavior, insulin resistance in diabetic obese adolescent girls, and prevention of weight gain in children of parents participating in the mindfulness programs. Probiotics have striking effects in obese children with NAFLD and insulin resistance and may be extremely effective in targeting harmful parameters associated with these diseases. Synbiotics have shown effectiveness as an adjunct to programs involving diet and exercise in obese children. Finally, for teens, a combination of a short, once-weekly physical activity intervention and CBT skills was found effective in reducing both BMI and depressive symptoms.

In summary, Intensive Lifestyle Interventions, MI-based nutritional coaching for families, physical activity, Mindfulness, synbiotics, and Cognitive behavioral therapy are recommended to help reduce obesity in this age group. Probiotics in obese children with NAFLD and insulin resistance also should be recommended. Including parents is critical to long-lasting effects. In addition, it is becoming increasingly clear that pediatric obesity and youth mental health reciprocally impact each other, and for optimal results, interventions should account for this.

DISCLOSURES

The authors have no conflicts to report.

REFERENCES

1. Ogden CL, Carroll MD, Lawman HG, et al. Trends in obesity prevalence among children and adolescents in the United States, 1988-1994 through 2013-2014. JAMA 2016;315(21):2292–9.
2. Rainone V, Schneider L, Saulle I, et al. Upregulation of inflammasome activity and increased gut permeability are associated with obesity in children and adolescents. Int J Obes 2016;40:1026–33.
3. Bleich SN, Cutler D, Murray C, et al. Why is the developed world obese? Annu Rev Public Health 2008;29:273–95.
4. Aldinger CE, Jones JT. Healthy nutrition: an essential element of a health-promoting school. In Healthy Nutrition: an essential element of a health-promoting school 1998 (pp. 56-56).
5. Weihrauch-Blüher S, Schwarz P, Klusmann JH. Childhood obesity: increased risk for cardiometabolic disease and cancer in adulthood. Metabolism 2019;92:147–52.
6. Simkin DR, Arnold LE. The roles of inflammation, oxidative stress and the gut-brain axis in treatment refractory depression in youth: complementary and integrative medicine interventions. OBM Integr Complement Med 2020;5(4):1–12.
7. Simkin DR. Microbiome and mental health, specifically as it relates to adolescents. Curr Psychiatry Rep 2019;21(9):1–12.
8. Prada PO, Zecchin HG, Gasparetti AL, et al. Western diet modulates insulin signaling, c-Jun N-terminal kinase activity, and insulin receptor substrate-1ser307 phosphorylation in a tissue-specific fashion. Endocrinology 2005;146:1576–87.
9. Pereira MA, Kartashov AI, Ebbeling CB, et al. Fast-food habits, weight gain, and insulin resistance (the CARDIA study): 15-year prospective analysis. Lancet 2005;365(9453):36–42 [Erratum in: Lancet. 2005 Mar 16;365(9464):1030. PMID: 15639678].
10. Meng F, Han Y, Srisai D. New inducible genetic method reveals critical roles of GABA in the control of feeding and metabolism. Proc Natl Acad Sci U S A 2016;113:3645–50.
11. Carvalho BM, Saad MJ. Influence of gut microbiota on subclinical inflammation and insulin resistance. Mediators Inflamm 2013;2013:986734.
12. Rahat-Rozenbloom S, Fernandes J, Cheng J, et al. Acute increases in serum colonic short-chain fatty acids elicited by inulin do not increase GLP-1 or PYY responses but may reduce ghrelin in lean and overweight humans. Eur J Clin Nutr 2017;71:953–8.
13. Mannan M, Mamun A, Doi S, et al. Prospective Associations between depression and obesity for adolescent males and females- a systematic review and meta-analysis of longitudinal studies. PLoS One 2016;11(6):e0157240.
14. Barczyńska R, Litwin M, Sliżewska K, et al. Bacterial microbiota and fatty acids in the faeces of overweight and obese children. Pol J Microbiol 2018;67(3):339–45.
15. Newgard CB. Interplay between lipids and branched-chain amino acids in development of insulin resistance. Cell Metab 2012;15:606–14.

16. Kahn LG, Philippat C, Nakayama SF, et al. Endocrine-disrupting chemicals: implications for human health. Lancet Diabetes Endocrinol 2020;8(8):703–18.

17. De Long NE, Holloway AC. Early-life chemical exposures and risk of metabolic syndrome. Diabetes Metab Syndr Obes 2017;10:101–9.

18. Shehata AA, Schrödl W, Aldin AA, et al. The effect of glyphosate on potential pathogens and beneficial members of poultry microbiota in vitro. Curr Microbiol 2013;66:350–8.

19. Gohil A, Hannon TS. Poor sleep and obesity: concurrent epidemics in adolescent youth. Front Endocrinol (Lausanne) 2018;9:364.

20. Strasburger VC. Children, adolescents, obesity, and the media. Pediatrics 2011; 128(1):201–8 [Erratum in: Pediatrics. 2011 Sep;128(3):594. PMID: 21708800].

21. Fatima Y, Doi SA, Mamun AA. Longitudinal impact of sleep on overweight and obesity in children and adolescents: a systematic review and bias-adjusted meta-analysis. Obes Rev 2015;16(2):137–49.

22. Sanjay PR, Hu FB. Short sleep duration and weight gain: a systematic review. Obesity 2008;16(3):643–53.

23. Suez J, Korem T, Zeevi D. Artificial sweeteners induce glucose intolerance by altering the gut microbiota. Nature 2014;514:181–6.

24. Mitsou EK, Kakali A, Antonopoulou S, et al. Adherence to the Mediterranean diet is associated with the gut microbiota pattern and gastrointestinal characteristics in an adult population. Br J Nutr 2017;117:1645–55.

25. Haro C, García-Carpintero S, Rangel-Zúñiga OA, et al. Consumption of two healthy dietary patterns restored microbiota dysbiosis in obese patients with metabolic dysfunction. Mol Nutr Food Res 2017;61:1700300.

26. Cryan JF, Dinan TG. Mind-altering microorganisms: the impact of the gut microbiota on brain and behaviour. Nat Rev Neurosci 2012;13:701–12.

27. Voreades N, Kozil A, Weir TL. Diet and the development of the human intestinal microbiome. Front Microbiol 2014;5:494.

28. Moloney RD, Desbonnet L, Clarke G, et al. The microbiome: stress, health and disease. Mamm Genome 2014;25(1–2):49–74.

29. Sudo N. Role of gut microbiota in brain function and stress-related pathology. Biosci Microbiota Food Health 2019;38(3):75–80.

30. Lurie I, Yang YX, Haynes K, et al. Antibiotic exposure and the risk for depression, anxiety, or psychosis: a nested case-control study. J Clin Psychiatry 2015;76(11):1522–8.

31. Le Bastard Q, Al-Ghalith GA, Bregoire M, et al. Systematic review: human gut dysbiosis induced by non-antibiotic prescription medications. Aliment Pharmacol Ther 2018;47(3):332–45.

32. Bahr SM, Tyler BC, Wooldridge N, et al. Use of the second-generation antipsychotic, risperidone, and secondary weight gain are associated with an altered gut microbiota in children. Transl Psychiatry 2015;5:e652.

33. Nurmi E. Do microbiome-bile acid interactions explain antipsychotic-induced weight gain. Presented in a symposium on The Life Within: The unconscious contributions of gut microbiota to our lives. American Academy of Child and Adolescent Psychiatry Annual Meeting, Seattle, Washington. October 25th, 2018, unpublished.

34. Sorg JA, Sonenshein AL. Bile salts and glycine as cogerminants for Clostridium difficile spores. J Bacteriol 2008;190:2505–12.

35. Schmidt FM, Weschenfelder J, Sander C, et al. Inflammatory cytokines in general and central obesity and modulating effects of physical activity. PLoS One 2015; 10(3):e0121971.

36. Mueller NT, Whyatt R, Hoepner L, et al. Prenatal exposure to antibiotics, cesarean section and risk of childhood obesity. Int J Obes 2015;39(4):665–70.

37. Melnyk BM, Jacobson D, Kelly SA, et al. Twelve-Month Effects of the COPE Healthy Lifestyles TEEN Program on overweight and depressive symptoms in high school adolescents. J Sch Health 2015;85(12):861–70.
38. Velázquez-López L, Santiago-Díaz G, Nava-Hernández J, et al. Mediterranean-style diet reduces metabolic syndrome components in obese children and adolescents with obesity. BMC Pediatr 2014;14:175.
39. Ojeda-Rodríguez A, Zazpe I, Morell-Azanza L, et al. Improved diet quality and nutrient adequacy in children and adolescents with abdominal obesity after a lifestyle intervention. Nutrients 2018;10(10):1500.
40. Jastreboff AM, Chaplin TM, Finnie S, et al. Preventing childhood obesity through a mindfulness-based parent stress intervention: a randomized pilot study. J Pediatr 2018;202:136–42.e131.
41. Barnes VA, Kristeller JL. Impact of mindfulness-based eating awareness on diet and exercise habits in adolescents. Int J Complement Altern Med 2016;3(2):70.
42. Shomaker LB, Bruggink S, Pivarunas B, et al. Pilot randomized controlled trial of a mindfulness-based group intervention in adolescent girls at risk for type 2 diabetes with depressive symptoms. Complement Ther Med 2017;32:66–74.
43. Balagopal P, Graham TE, Kahn BB, et al. Reduction of elevated serum retinol binding protein in obese children by lifestyle intervention: association with subclinical inflammation. J Clin Endocrinol Metab 2007;92(5):1971–4.
44. Famouri F, Shariat Z, Hashemipour M, et al. Effects of probiotics on nonalcoholic fatty liver disease in obese children and adolescents. J Pediatr Gastroenterol Nutr 2017; 64(3):413–7.
45. Sanchis-Chordà J, del Pulgar EMG, Carrasco-Luna J, et al. Bifidobacterium pseudocatenulatum CECT 7765 supplementation improves inflammatory status in insulin-resistant obese children. Eur J Nutr 2019;58:2789–800.
46. Alisi A, Bedogni G, Baviera G, et al. Randomised clinical trial: the beneficial effects of VSL#3 in obese children with non-alcoholic steatohepatitis. Aliment Pharmacol Ther 2014;39(11):1276–85.
47. Ipar N, Aydogdu SD, Yildirim GK. Effects of synbiotic on anthropometry, lipid profile and oxidative stress in obese children. Benef Microbes 2015;6(6):775–82.
48. Safavi M, Farajian S, Kelishadi R, et al. The effects of synbiotic supplementation on some cardio-metabolic risk factors in overweight and obese children: a randomized triple-masked controlled trial. Int J Food Sci Nutr 2013;64:687–93.
49. Resnicow K, McMaster F, Bocian A, et al. Motivational interviewing and dietary counseling for obesity in primary care: an RCT. Pediatrics 2015;135(4):649–57.
50. Foster BA, Farragher J, Parker P, et al. Treatment interventions for early childhood obesity: a systematic review. Acad Pediatr 2015;15(4):353–61.
51. Martin A, Saunders DH, Shenkin SD, et al. Lifestyle intervention for improving school achievement in overweight or obese children and adolescents. Cochrane Database Syst Rev 2014;(3):CD009728. https://doi.org/10.1002/14651858. CD009728.pub2. Update in: Cochrane Database Syst Rev. 2018 Jan 29;1: CD009728. PMID: 24627300.
52. Eiffener E, Eli K, Ek A, et al. The influence of preschoolers' emotional and behavioural problems on obesity treatment outcomes: secondary findings from a randomized controlled trial. Pediatr Obes 2019;14(11):e12556.
53. Kwiterovich PO, Hartmuller G, Van Horn L, et al. Efficacy and safety of lowering dietary intake of fat and cholesterol in children with elevated low-density lipoprotein cholesterol: the dietary intervention study in children (DISC). JAMA 1995; 273(18):1429–35.

Complementary and Integrative Medicine and Eating Disorders in Youth: Traditional Yoga, Virtual Reality, Light Therapy, Neurofeedback, Acupuncture, Energy Psychology Techniques, Art Therapies, and Spirituality

Aleema Zakers, MD[a],*, Valentina Cimolai, MD[b]

KEYWORDS

- Complementary and integrative medicine • Binge eating disorder • Anorexia nervosa
- Bulimia nervosa • Eating disorders • Yoga • Virtual reality • Light therapy

KEY POINTS

- Overall, eating disorders (EDs) are challenging, and there are no medications or supplements that treat the core symptoms of ED (except lisdexamfetamine for binge eating disorder). The use of medications is primarily to treat comorbid disorders.
- Treatments for ED are primarily therapy-based and require a multidisciplinary approach, and traditional therapeutic approaches are not considered complementary and integrative medicine (CIM) for this disorder. All treatments discussed should be considered part of a comprehensive clinical protocol.
- Yoga for ED has a good to moderate evidence of efficacy on core symptoms in several meta-analyses and RCT. However, the type of yoga, duration, and frequency necessary for efficacy have not been established. Of note, traditional yoga practices that incorporate mindfulness and not just as a form of exercise are programs that show efficacy.
- Technology-based interventions like virtual reality (VR) for EDs focus on eating and body image exposure. During COVID, VR has been increasingly used due to its efficacy and accessibility.

Continued

[a] MPH Georgia Institute of Technology, Moorhouse School of Medicine, Emory School of Medicine, 750 Ferst Drive, Atlanta, GA 30332, USA; [b] Private Practice, Bloom Psychiatry and Wellness and Mindful Healing Group, 1245 Court Street, Clearwater, FL 33756, USA
* Corresponding author.
E-mail address: Azakers3@gatech.edu

Child Adolesc Psychiatric Clin N Am 32 (2023) 421–450
https://doi.org/10.1016/j.chc.2022.08.014
1056-4993/23/© 2022 Elsevier Inc. All rights reserved.

childpsych.theclinics.com

Continued

- Eye movement desensitization and reprocessing (EMDR) and biofeedback/neurofeedback both have moderate–good research and can be used on a VR platform. Biofeedback and neurofeedback increased the ability to tolerate better stress and cope with situations involving food. Whereas EMDR has limited research, it addresses negative memories/trauma associated with body image and eating.
- Music therapy, especially songwriting, as an adjunct can be very helpful due to its ability to elicit issues not shared with the therapeutic team.
- Other therapies mentioned have insufficient evidence.
- Medications: If the proposed mechanism of action of ED is associated with infection/inflammatory reactions. Ketamine and Ayahuasca may work due to extensive bowel prep, eliminating caseinolytic mitochondrial matrix peptidase chaperone subunit B and the possible mental reset they may occur more than the actual medications themselves.
- Relaxations: Spirituality/religious, message, acupuncture, energy psychologies (EMDR and EFT), and art therapies (umbrella of therapies including art therapy, music medicine, dance/movement therapy, and drama therapy) may assist by decreasing the inflammation processes.
- Circadian rhythm balance: Bright light therapy assists by helping regulate circadian rhythm, promoting better sleep/wake, and by extension, regulating the feeding cycle.

INTRODUCTION

In allopathic medicine, we typically use medications to treat, arrest, and ameliorate symptoms of illness. However, in eating disorders (EDs), only one medication (lisdexamfetamine) has robust support for the treatment of the core pathology of binge eating disorder (BED).[1] Although SSRIs and antipsychotics are used in EDs, they do not address core symptoms. Medication treatments have not yielded significant effects on weight-related outcomes or eating pathology, body image, general psychiatric symptoms, obsessions, and compulsivity. One caveat is that SSRIs and antipsychotics, namely olanzapine, have also been helpful in avoidant/restrictive food intake disorder (ARFID).[2] However, overall, pharmacotherapy interventions have a limited evidence base and should not be used as the primary or sole treatment in anorexia nervosa (AN). SSRIs can be used for comorbidities in non-underweight individuals. Olanzapine has the most robust research, which showed no difference from placebo in underweight individuals. In normal weight and overweight individuals, the use of antipsychotics, mainly olanzapine, confers a significant amount of weight gain.

Therefore, the treatment of EDs is fundamentally different from other physical and mental health disorders where the one specialty or one drug/one disorder approach is used. In ED, the standard of care requires several treatment modalities, and collaborative care is the standard of care. No treatment program, out-patient or in-patient, should operate with only one specialty. The current standard of care incorporates individual, group, and family therapy, pediatrics and/or GI, psychiatry, and nutritionists. Interest in the link between AN (AN) and autoimmune disorders has arisen. Of note, region rs4622308 on chromosome 12 has also been linked to autoimmune diseases.[3] This link between EDs and inflammatory processes was further studied, showing a solid bidirectional relationship between ED and autoimmune disease.[4,5] In addition, these studies also discovered an association between ED and the microbiome. These discoveries set the stage for the use of complementary and integrative medicine (CIM) approaches with ED. Micronutrients, vitamins, and probiotics are frequently used as adjunctive treatment in patients with ED to support physical body functioning but do not treat core symptoms.

It is important to note that none of these treatments are used to affect the core pathology of the illness but to support physical body functioning. It is important to note that none of these treatments are used to affect the core pathology of the illness but to support physical body functioning. The recommended treatment for youth is family therapy that addresses the ED. Family-based treatment is a well-established treatment for AN. Compared with nutritional counseling, cognitive behavior therapy (CBT) for 1 year was associated with a significantly higher proportion of participants attaining a good outcome (ie, normal body weight and regular menses). In addition, the CBT group had a lower relapse (22% vs 53%) at 1 year, although this difference was not statistically significant.[6] Furthermore, talk-based therapies such as CBT using mindfulness and embodiment techniques are also widely used and considered a standard of care in ED. Therefore, these therapies will not be included in this CIM article.

ARFID has been separated from other EDs research as it is a relatively new diagnosis that arose after DSM-5 was released. Since that time, research has shown that, unlike other EDs, ARFID presents more in males[7–9] at a young age[10,11] and often with psychiatric comorbidities, such as anxiety (most common), attention-deficit/hyperactivity disorder, and autism spectrum disorder. One systemic review with 3 case studies, and one RCT, using eye movement desensitization and reprocessing (EMDR) in participants suspected to have trauma as the etiology of their eating disorders, demonstrated positive effects one year after follow up but there was not enough evidence to support the efficacy of EMDR.[12] In the past, patients, that would now be known as ARFID, were given the diagnosis of pediatric feeding disorders or failure to thrive with nutritional management and/or behavioral interventions. Since large number of these children have anxiety and the use of self-regulation and anxiety management techniques are used. However, family-based interventions go one step further by empowering parents and have been widely researched. They have consistently shown efficacy, accessibility, and feasibility in several case reports,[13,14] case series,[15] pilot studies,[16,17] clinical trials,[18] and an RTC.[19] Even family interventions using telemedicine are effective.[20] Of note, family interventions/programs vary widely in content, but most seem to be effective and accessible.

In summary, there is no evidence that psychological or pharmacologic interventions used alone to manage ED are warranted. The use of new adjunctive therapies that improve the effectiveness of existing treatments and lead to improved mental health outcomes for this patient group is highly desirable. One of the primary modalities of ED treatment is therapy. This intervention was severely affected during coronavirus (COVID-19), resulting in poor outcomes for ED patients.[21,22] In addition, virtual learning/work (where individuals look at themselves constantly throughout the day) further exacerbated ED.[23] These concerns and the ongoing waxing and waning nature of the pandemic created a space for new evidence-based modalities to emerge. This article aims to identify evidence-based modalities capable of seamless integration into the current multimodal treatment of ED to meet the times.

MODERATE–LARGE EFFECTIVE: FOR CORE SYMPTOMS
Yoga

Yoga is a way of life that teaches balance in living. Movement is only one part of yoga. Yoga guides individuals in controlling their mind, body, and breath and brings them closer to their spiritual body and true divine self. Yoga therapy uses yoga and Ayurveda principles to promote health and balance. Modern lifestyle has influenced the development of many diseases such as EDs. Yoga therapy is postulated to treat EDs by fostering a balanced/yogic lifestyle and encourages individuals to look inward to help build, support, and maintain protective factors. This practice goes beyond the mind and body to affect change in well-being and reduce the risk for disordered eating through use of self-compassion, self-kindness, and the integration of the body by physical practice, and mind through, mindfulness, meditation, and breath work. Yoga allows for a better understanding/control over physical sensations (by increasing the ability to understand bodily cues), emotions, and cognitions. More specifically, yoga focuses on the gut-brain axis to affect change in EDs.

In ancient Indian medicine called Ayurveda, the gut-brain axis has always been a major focus of balance and a key point of intervention in disease processes. The Agni (digestive fire) concept is thought to be a primary source of overall well-being and health and is considered the gatekeeper of life and resides in the gut. In Ayurveda, impaired Agni is at the root of all imbalances and diseases. The gut is known as the second brain in this school of thought. This concept of a second brain makes sense because the gut contains 400 to 600 million neurons.[24] In allopathic medicine, these neurons are known as the enteric nervous system. It is under the direct and indirect influence of the gut microbiota and produces neurotransmitters (serotonin and dopamine) that communicate with the brain. In Ayurveda, a specific diet is used based on what is called a person's Dosha (characteristics) and the Dosha of the illness.

In yoga, these principles are incorporated into movement while focusing on breath work, which helps individuals change perceptions of themselves. For example, a meta-analysis ($n = 2173$; predominantly youth) of mindfulness-based yoga (aka traditional yoga) showed a statistically significant improvement in self-esteem, body image, and body appreciation of participants postintervention.[25]

Precautions for yoga should be used with "yoga" that has been very westernized, is focused on appearance (eg, Beach Body Yoga), and has less focus on core tenets of traditional yoga (mindfulness, body appreciation, self-compassion, and acceptance). A systematic review that included 12 cross-sectional studies demonstrated that none specifically evaluated ED but focused on body image/satisfaction and healthy eating behaviors. In this cross-sectional review, four studies included non-traditional yoga/western exercise practices in study groups (not as controls), and two studies did not specify whether western or eastern exercise was conducted. They found that a high dosage of exercise was associated with a higher prevalence of disordered eating behaviors.[26] Therefore, in severe cases of ED, yoga should only be undertaken by experienced yoga therapy practitioners in conjunction with the individual's treating physician. Hot yoga or other strenuous forms of yoga are not recommended when medical concerns exist. It should be discontinued if yoga interferes with recovery or worsens symptoms.[27] However, several meta-analyses demonstrated that yoga does not negatively affect body mass index (BMI).[28–30] Further, an extensive ($n = 8430$) systematic review and meta-analysis of RCTs included participants from 14 to 84 years of age that indicated yoga seems to be as safe as usual care.[31] Since individuals with ED may misread bodily cues as fullness and may avoid negative feelings they feel they cannot tolerate; yoga may help to correct bodily cues and tolerate feelings by allowing one to recognize when emotions may be affecting one's breathing patterns and how to control for that. Yoga may also reduce negative feelings about body image by allowing the person to look at oneself in a non-judgmental way.

The most significant limitation in reviewing yoga studies is that there is no evidence to guide the specific regimen (eg, duration, frequency, type) of yoga for specific types of EDs. One recent meta-analysis using only RTCs ($n = 754$) identified four types of yoga (Bikram, Hatha, Iyengar, and Viniyoga), at doses of 40 to 90 minutes, and a duration of 5 consecutive days to 12 weeks. Specific treatment regimens were not elucidated.[30] Most studies were small and had predominantly (or only) female participants with no ethnic considerations. One study identified college students included a significant number of males (22.2%) and showed men had a more significant reduction in concern of being overweight and greater body satisfaction than female counterparts' post-yoga intervention.[32] In addition, there is concern about collecting data collected from these nondiverse populations and generalizing to minority populations. However, one study compared minority and white fifth-grade girls ($n = 50$) who were matched for BMI and socioeconomic status. The purpose was to examine ethnic differences in primary prevention programs for ED. They found that minority and white participants were equally responsive to the yoga prevention program.[33] Another concern in studies is that interventions are temporary. Therefore, many RTCs are unable to capture long-term effects as interventions are temporary. Furthermore, many studies do not allow for pooled comparison of long-term data, which was the case in a recent meta-analysis looking at prevention. However, one long-term benefit was noted to be statistically significant: reducing dietary restraint.[25]

Nevertheless, population-based studies, which provide information on how yoga is being practiced in the general public, have shed some light on how yoga may reduce the risk of developing an ED. For instance, body dissatisfaction, a strong risk factor for disordered eating, was the subject of an important, large ($n = 1820$), longitudinal (15 years), population-based study. The study suggested that practicing yoga for more than 30 minutes per week over 1 year can help prevent and treat EDs. The most significant improvement was seen in participants who entered the study in the category of "low body satisfaction."[34]

Several studies have extolled the benefits of yoga on ED in youth in BED and bulimia nervosa (BN). One such RTC compared yoga participants to waitlist controls in an 8-week Kripalu Yoga program. The girls who participated in yoga experienced decreases in binge eating frequency, emotional regulation difficulties, self-criticism, and increases in self-compassion. Yoga participants also experienced increased state mindfulness skills across the 8 weeks of the yoga program.[35] In a recent meta-analysis, participants with BED and BN showed a moderate-to-large effect on core symptoms when yoga interventions were used.[30] Furthermore, EDs have many comorbidities that can influence treatment, and ED can limit the effectiveness of the treatment when individuals are malnourished.

There are two notable small studies in youth that are worth noting. These studies demonstrated that ED symptoms and comorbidities could be treated with yoga interventions. One was a pilot study completed on 20 teenagers between 14 and 18 years of age who met the criteria for AN, BN, and ARFID. The study showed statistically significant decreases in anxiety, depression, and body image disturbance after a 12-week, non-heated Hatha-based, gentle yoga intervention ranging from 60 to 90 minutes.[36] The other study was an RTC conducted in an outpatient population of individuals with AN ($n = 50$) between 11 to 21 years of age. In this study, the yoga group demonstrated more significant decreases in ED symptoms and a similar decline in anxiety and depression as a standard of care. "'Food preoccupation" was measured before and after each yoga session and decreased significantly after all sessions in the treatment group.[28] Overall, it seems that traditional yoga can affect positive change toward the prevention and treatment of EDs in youth. It is essential to understand that yoga is a way of life, not a temporary "fix" to a problem. In utilizing yoga for therapeutic purposes, the goal is to change behaviors through balance, acceptance, and knowledge of one's true self.

Virtual Reality

In virtual reality (VR), ED patients are repeatedly exposed to emotionally provoking eating-related situations and body images that typically result in maladaptive behaviors (eg, binge eating and restricting). Virtual exposure has been considered an alternative for imaginary exposure and an intermediate step for in vivo exposure in combination with embodiment-based procedures and CBT. Psychometric instruments can collect information through patient reporting. VR can produce a sense of "being there" in the middle of the virtual environment where the subject can stay and live a specific experience, evoking emotional responses and a sense of self-reflectiveness as though it was in real time but in a safe environment. VR may allow assessment and treatment to be more accurate.[37]

For clinical use, VR should be part of a comprehensive clinical protocol that supports clinicians and researchers in the implementation.[38] VR uses visual immersive equipment with a head-mounted display. Therapeutic intervention through this modality has shown efficacy in ED since the late 90s. However, more recent advances in technology allow for more feasibility. For example, patients can now get a $20 headset from most stores that sell electronics and use a clinician-controlled app on their phone for an immersive experience. VR has also been studied and successfully used for therapeutic purposes for many mental health comorbidities. VR has been found to be significantly more attractive as a therapy to young adults and teens and demonstrated decreased loss to follow-up in studies.[39]

In reviewing current VR research, two main areas of inquiry emerged from VR studies: virtual work on patients' body image and exposure to virtual food stimuli. We identified two systematic reviews which further elucidated these two areas of interest. In the earlier study, these two areas were highlighted in the context of binge eating in 19 different studies (7 controlled assessment studies, 2 assessment studies, 1 case report, 7 RCTs, and 2 noncontrolled trials). The review found that VR can enhance assessments, psychometric tests, CBT, exposure/experiential treatment, and identification of triggers and treatment. It also demonstrated the potential utility of VR in improving eating-related symptoms, such as binge eating and the urge to eat in different types of ED.[40] The more recent systematic review seemed to build on the earlier one and included 26 studies (8 were RTCs, 12 were nonrandomized studies, and 5 were clinical trials with only 1 participant). One study was used in both systematic reviews. The use of VR techniques by patients with EDs decreased their negative emotional responses to virtual food stimuli or exposure to their body shape.[39] A meta-analysis was also identified, which further supported these findings using the same six RTCs mentioned in the above systematic reviews. The difference in this study was that the meta-analysis included only RCTs totaling 297 participants and showed a more robust effect of VR. The inclusion criteria were more stringent and required VR-enhanced CBT to be compared with treatment as usual (ie, CBT and not waitlist controls or other modalities). In addition, the studies were required to use clinically relevant outcome measures (BMI, frequency of binges/purges, and psychometric assessments). In this meta-analysis, there were statistically significant decreases in binges frequency and situationally induced body dissatisfaction in participants who underwent VR-enhanced CBT compared with CBT alone. No statistically significant changes in purging or BMI were identified.[41]

Recently, there have been even further developments in the use of VR to treat EDs. One RCT was conducted among 35 hospitalized patients receiving treatment of AN. There were 16 patients added to the experimental group (VR), and 19 were in the control group (treatment as usual). The mean age was 18 years old, the mean BMI was 17.48 kg/m, and most were female (31/35). The study demonstrated the efficacy of VR in treating the fear of gaining weight as well as reducing body image disturbances in AN patients. This development has been possible due to advancements in VR technology using embodiment-based procedures.[42] Another advancement in VR was illustrated through a proof-of-concept study wherein inhibitory control training was incorporated to treat binge eating. In this study, 14 participants with once-weekly loss-of-control eating were recruited to use the VR daily, at home, for 2 weeks. They measured feasibility, acceptability, and change in eating at postintervention and 2-week follow-up. Compliance was high, and 86.8% of daily training was completed. Results showed significant decreases in "loss of control" eating postintervention, which was sustained at the 2-week follow-up postintervention.[43] Another RCT conducted at five well-established ED centers with 64 treatment-resistant patients who suffered from BN and BED compared with therapeutic interventions. This study was designed to test if individuals with limited results (after using a structured CBT program) would benefit from an additional-CBT (A-CBT) versus VT using cue exposure therapy. VR was significantly superior to A-CBT at the end of treatment. The number of participants who achieved abstinence from binge eating episodes was 53% in the VR group compared with 25% in the CBT group in patients with BE. In BED, 75% of participants in the VR group achieved abstinence from purging, whereas 31.5% of the A-CBT group reached this goal.[44] In summary, VR seems to be a new approach to the treatment of ED that should be considered in any multifaceted ED treatment program.

MODERATE TO LOW EVIDENCE
Biofeedback and Neurofeedback

These feedback-based techniques are based on operant conditioning and allow individuals to learn how to regulate neurophysiological activity in response to a real-time feedback. They are associated with significant modifications of sympathetic reaction to food-related stimuli and brain activity in several regions of the reward system (eg, insula). These represent immediate and positive reinforcements. The result of feedback-based treatment is to increase motivation, facilitate the learning process, and modify dysfunctional thoughts and behaviors.

Biofeedback

This process helps individuals gain greater awareness of many physiologic functions to be able to manipulate the body systems at will. Individuals are connected to sensors that help monitor physiologic processes such as breathing, heart rate, muscle contractions, temperature, and perspiration. In biofeedback (BF), a large area of focus has been on heart rate, which was implicated as a possible biomarker. A meta-analysis showed the relationship between high-frequency heart rate (HR) variability in BN[45] and a review article demonstrated elevated HR in AN.[46] However, no link between treatment with BF or HR and a reduction of core ED symptoms has been demonstrated in youths in these studies. Therefore, HR cannot be used as a biomarker in youths.

Two studies investigating the use of BF for the treatment of Rumination disorder/ syndrome and regurgitation were performed. One study enrolled 28 patients in a 10-day training and measured outcomes during the 10 days, then 1, 3, and 6 months after treatment. This study showed a drastic decline after treatment intervention and continued progressive improvement of symptoms for 6 months.[47] An RTC followed up this study with 24 participants diagnosed with rumination ranging from 19 to 79 year old in which subjects ($n = 12$) received biofeedback and the control group ($n = 11$) received placebo treatment. These participants were followed 1, 3, and 6 months after receiving three sessions over 10 days. The participants were able to sustain the reduction in rumination activities. Controls were offered treatment after completion of the study and followed for 1, 3, and 6 months and showed similar statistically significant results.[48] This study demonstrated that BF could assist in the treatment of Rumination disorder/syndrome and regurgitation.

Neurofeedback

This process helps individuals voluntarily control their brain activity. It uses *real-time functional MRI* (rt-fMRI) or a *quantitative EEG* (qEEG) that maps out regions that exhibit abnormal activity from normed samples based on age and gender. During neurofeedback (NF) training, the brain receives reinforcement through a visual or auditory stimulus that uses continuous real-time operant conditioning to target deviant brain areas or abnormal EEG biomarkers matched to the impairing symptoms and trains those areas to progress more toward "the norm."[49] Investigators have focused on reduced alpha (calm, relaxed, lucid) activity and increased high beta (awake, efficient information processing, and problem-solving) activity in the frontal lobes. NF targeted in this way is beneficial in reducing depressive[50] and anxiety symptoms.[51] A similar pattern of decreased alpha (9-13 Hz) and increased high beta waves (25-35 Hz) were seen in AN, but no consistent EEG pattern was identified in BN.[52] In a recent feasibility study, 39 participants with BED between the ages of 18 to 60 year old (with BMI more than 25 but <45 kg/m^2) received 10 individual 1-h long EEG-NF sessions. The participants were randomly divided into food-specific EEG-NF ($n = 20$) and general EEG-NF ($n = 19$). Both EEG-NF paradigms significantly reduced objective binge eating episodes, global ED psychopathology, and food craving, which corresponded to a significant reduction of beta activity and medium increase of theta activity from preintervention to postintervention.[53] Alterations in theta wave activity have been consistently found in patients with ED.[54–56] In fact, in one study, AN and controls (CO) were examined during acute starvation T(0) and after weight gain T(1). Theta asymmetry did change from T(0) to T(1) during rest in AN. However, haptic theta symmetry (which records theta asymmetry during active perception-cognitive tasks) was lower in AN patients than in the CO over the right hemisphere and right parietal regions. These results indicated a cortical dysfunction and deficits in somatosensory integration processing of the right parietal cortex in AN patients even after weight gain.[54] Theta waves have been modulated with NF interventions and have been correlated with positive changes in thoughts and actions around eating.[53,57,58]

In addition, a recent RTC found positive effects on eating behaviors after a single day of intense treatment with NF.[57] In this study, 38 overweight and obese participants found high caloric food as less palatable and chose them less frequently postintervention. This group has postulated that NF can support therapeutic interventions to improve self-control.[57] Therefore, NF can be beneficial because overeating is associated with losing control. This loss of control can lead to unhealthy or extreme weight control behaviors, dieting, nonsuicidal self-injury, lower body satisfaction and self-esteem, and higher rates of depression.[59]

Combined studies

Several systematic reviews using BF and NF studies have shown positive efficacy of these techniques on core symptoms of ED after 10 sessions over varying amounts of time.[53,58] One such significant study emerged that focused on core symptoms. In this systematic review of feedback-based ED treatments of EDs, five studies focused on BF and eight on NF; one NF and one BF article were exclusively on children.[60] This review reported that both NF and BF training might decrease food craving severity, overeating episodes, regurgitation and rumination episodes restricting behavior, eating, and weight concerns. Furthermore, this review showed that feedback-based techniques are associated with significant modifications of sympathetic reaction to food-related stimuli and brain activity in several regions of the reward system (eg, prefrontal cortex, amygdala, and insula). NF and BF both improve the ability to tolerate stress and cope with situations involving food, reduction of stressful arousal, and increase top-down control abilities. Different NF protocols achieve this in the following ways: EEG alpha training is to enhance individual alpha frequency, which is usually associated with alert relaxation and also found in meditation in the parietal area; EEG beta training downregulate beta activity, which is positively associated with ruminative states of stressful arousal; alpha/theta training raises posterior theta over alpha amplitude to produce a state of deep relaxation, enhancing top-down mental functions; and rt-fMRI NF has the unique ability to increase functional connectivity between brain areas (ie, dorsolateral prefrontal cortex and ventromedial prefrontal cortex) that regulate the top-down control of appetite for high-calorie foods. *Low-resolution electromagnetic tomography* NF does the same but does not require an fMRI. In summary, this review showed an improved ability to tolerate general stress and cope with situations involving food stressors after the intervention. However, no significant effect on body image disturbance or change in BMI was shown after 10 sessions.

Let us now focus on the 2 articles that only had youth participants. The first study was composed of 76 obese (mean age of 12.75 years) and 27 AN (mean age of 14.25 years) females who were compared with 35 healthy female controls (mean age of 12.5 years). In this study, they hypothesized that stress and maladaptive coping played a role in the etiology of EDs and used BF to mitigate the effects of EDs in these preadolescents. The highest efficacy was demonstrated among the participants with AN.[61] The later study assessed the effects of NF on adolescents (12–18 years) with AN. This study had 22 females randomized into an experimental group ($n = 10$) and a control group ($n = 12$) who received treatment as usual. In addition, the experimental group received 10 sessions of alpha frequency training over 5 weeks in addition to treatment as usual. In this sample, eating behaviors and emotional regulation improved and correlated with theta wave alterations.[58]

In summary, both feedback-based techniques may play a role in reducing core symptoms of ED and have shown efficacy as adjunctive therapy to improve self-control and reduce food-related stress. In addition, BF has promising results to help with rumination, stress and coping related to AN. It seems that the use of NF treatment for ED should be specific to the symptom of ED because this has been where NF has been helpful, but there are several studies where experimental and control groups have not separated. For example, a study[53] used a food-specific EEG NF paradigm versus a general EEG NF paradigm (training the regulation of slow cortical potentials).

Both showed improvement but did not separate from each other. Future research should identify protocols, doses, and frequency of interventions required to treat specific ED symptoms.

Low evidence for core pathology

Acupuncture. Acupuncture is a commonly used integrative treatment characterized by the insertion of needles into specific body points to impact the flow of Qi (vital energy). Acupuncture can have a role in reducing stress, anxiety, and depression in adults [62] and has been studied to treat anxiety and autism in children and adolescents.[63,64]

MOA: Acupuncture works possibly by regulating the hypothalamus–pituitary axis and modulating the limbic-paralimbic-neocortical network; it has been found to affect the release of many neurotransmitters, including beta-endorphins, adrenocorticotropic hormone, serotonin, noradrenaline, and oxytocin, leading to a sense of well-being, and regulation of emotions, memory processing, and autonomic functions.[65] The evidence supporting adjunctive acupuncture for EDs remains scarce and limited to two small randomized trials conducted in Australia by Fogarty and her team.

One randomized cross-over study showed that ten acupuncture sessions added to an outpatient treatment in nine women with EDs (five with AN, four with BN, mean age 23.7) significantly improved quality of life and decrease anxiety and perfectionism. Given the anxiety reduction, acupuncture could help with premeal anxiety, thus increasing energy intake.[66]

In a second RCT, 6 weeks of adjunctive acupuncture was compared with acupressure plus light massage in 26 patients with AN admitted to an inpatient program. The practitioner in both treatments was directed to include expressions of empathy, offer explanations for understanding health, treat participants as individuals, and ensure the interactions were unrushed and pleasant. Participants described both interventions positively and experienced a sense of calmness and relaxation. They developed a strong therapeutic relationship with the study practitioner and perceived a high degree of empathy, which seems to be an essential factor for the recovery from EDs.[67]

Results from these two small trials point toward some benefits from adjunctive acupuncture. Nonetheless, the sample sizes were small and traditional acupuncture can be difficult to implement.

Ear acupuncture (a style developed by the National Acupuncture Detoxification Association) is easier to adopt, because it entails inserting only five needles at specified points in each ear.[68] Two recent qualitative studies, led by Landgren, have focused on the experience of patients using ear acupuncture. Twenty-five patients with AN received the treatment well with an 89% utilization rate. Nine inpatients described the experience as a chance for them to "create a pause, a framework for rest and reflection." Their anxiety decreased, and gaining weight was less difficult to cope with.[69] No severe side effects were reported.[70]

Regarding BED, one retrospective study looked at the use of electroacupuncture, a type of acupuncture that stimulates points by current, in 84 patients aged 18 to 40 years. The study concluded that CBT plus electronic acupuncture is more effective than CBT alone for BED. Participants in the acupuncture and CBT group scored lower in the negative emotion score and had lower total cholesterol, triglycerides, high-density lipoprotein, waist circumference, body weight, BMI, and body fat percentage. The combined therapy group had higher positive emotion scores. There were significant differences in negative emotional scores, TC, waist circumference, and BMI ($P < .05$).[71]

Bright Light Therapy

Bright light therapy (BLT) is a simple-to-deliver and noninvasive biological intervention for disorders with nonnormative circadian features.

MOA: EDs, particularly those with binge eating and night eating features, have documented nonnormative circadian eating and mood patterns, suggesting that BLT may be an efficacious adjunctive intervention that could address the eating core pathology and/or comorbid depressive symptom. BLT is thought to enhance serotonergic transmission, which may also be deregulated in EDs and depression.[72]

A 2016 review on EDs and BLT by Marshall and colleagues included four RCTs, one non-randomized controlled trial, two open-label clinical trials, two case series, and five case studies. The mean age for participants ($n = 175$) was 30.96 years (SD = 10.06) with a majority of females (98.9%, $n = 173$). The study design, lightbox methodology, and treatment duration varied among studies, with the majority being case studies using 10,000 lux in the morning for at least 30 minutes daily for 2 weeks. BLT was generally well tolerated; some recorded side effects included headache, eye fatigue, and feeling "speedy."[73]

- Evidence on core eating pathology

This review concluded that BLT could bring significant improvements in the eating pathology for the duration of the treatment period, with only a select few studies exhibiting null results in one or both of the primary eating outcomes. These improvements were found regardless of the type of ED present. It remains unclear if those effects persist once the treatment ceases, and a boost might be needed.

Two studies examined participants with the AN-restricting subtype. One was an RCT by Janas-Kozik and colleagues, where 24 girls with AN (mean age 17.4) were randomized to receive CBT + BLT (10,000 lux, 30 min daily) or CBT alone with no significant differences in BMI posttreatment in the two groups. However, the group with BLT achieved a significant increase in BMI compared with baseline much sooner than the control group (3 weeks compared with 6 weeks).[74]

Seven studies examined participants with BN (six with purging subtype and one with non-purging subtype) with mixed results. One RCT by Lam[75] found significant decreases in binge eating episodes and purge frequency posttreatment for participants using BLT. Another RCT found more significant reductions in binge eating episodes in the BLT group during treatment than control but no effects on purge frequency. At a 2-week follow-up, binge eating episode reductions were sustained, but there were no significant differences between groups. Finally, another RCT and a case study found no effect of BLT on binge eating or purge frequency.

Three studies investigating night eating syndrome found significant reductions in symptoms (eg, morning anorexia, evening hyperphagia, awakenings during the nighttime that include snacking). However, after completing BLT treatment, two case studies reported that the participants no longer met the criteria for night eating syndrome. In the case of Friedman and colleagues, at a 4-week follow-up, the participant's night eating syndrome symptoms returned but remitted after an additional 12 days of BLT.

- Evidence for effects of BLT on depression in ED

BLT has been used as a treatment of choice for depressive symptoms during seasonal affective disorder.[76] Depression is frequently comorbid with EDs. Hence, much of the research studying BLT in ED looks at depressive symptoms as a secondary outcome.

In a 1998 case study involving a 17-year-old female with ED and worsening symptoms during the winter months, her depression significantly improved after 1 month of BLT.[77] In the RCT by Janas-Kozik discussed above, 24 girls with AN-R had concomitant depressive symptoms and were randomized to CBT plus BLT for 6 weeks (10,000 lux, 30 min daily) versus CBT alone. The improvement of depression was significantly greater in the BLT group, with a significant difference between groups in depression intensity and lower intensity of symptoms posttreatment from baseline.[74]

In the study by Blouin mentioned above, women with BN in the BLT condition showed a significant improvement in depression during exposure, as measured by both the BDI and the SIGH-SAD, with no changes in depression noted in the placebo group. There was a return to pretreatment levels of depression after withdrawal of light exposure (Blouin, 1996). These findings were replicated by another study, not part of the Marshall review, where 24 females with both BN and MDD with a seasonal pattern were treated with an open design, 4-week trial of BLT (10,000 lux, 30–60 minutes per day in the early morning). BLT resulted in significant improvement in mood, with a mean 56% reduction in 29-item Hamilton Depression Rating Scale scores following treatment. Ten of 22 patients met the criteria for remission of depressive symptoms.[78]

All three studies included in the Marshall review on nighttime eating disorder and BLT reported significant reductions in depressive symptoms that in the Friedman study remained in remission at week 4. These studies may suggest that BLT could be an effective non-pharmacological modality for treating depression in patients with AN, bulimia, and night-ED. However, more extended studies with a larger *N* are needed.

Spirituality and Religiosity

Research on the relationship between spirituality and EDs is still limited, although the few studies that have been done suggest it is important.

A 2015 systematic review on spirituality and EDs included 22 studies, of which only four studies were graded as providing reasonably strong evidence, all exploring body image concerns.[79] Participants with strong religious beliefs and a secure and satisfying relationship with God had lower levels of disordered eating, psychopathology, and body image concern when compared with individuals with a superficial faith and an uneasy relationship with God. In addition, prayer and reading body-affirming religious material were powerfully effective as coping strategies.

It is still a question of how to incorporate spirituality and religion in clinical care. A study was done by Richards of 122 women in an inpatient ED treatment (42 with AN, 47 with BN, and 33 with unspecified ED). The study demonstrated that attending to patients' faith (with tools like giving spiritual readings and weekly focused groups) could be slightly more effective than other therapies such as CBT or support groups.[80]

Patients in the spirituality group scored significantly lower on psychological disturbance and ED symptoms and higher on spiritual well-being. In addition, they improved significantly more quickly during the first 4 weeks of treatment with a reduction in depression and anxiety, relationship distress, social role conflict, and ED symptoms.

Art Therapy

Art therapies (AsTs) are an umbrella of therapies including art therapy, music therapy, dance/movement therapy, and drama therapy. They are nonverbal, creative, expressive, and experiential therapies that allow patients to reconnect with their bodies and express their emotions through painting, listening or playing music, movement, or role play. The use of adjunctive AsTs in clinical programs is fairly common. However, most of the published work on the use of art therapy in EDs consists of case studies rather than randomized controlled trials with insufficient or low-quality evidence. One exception is music therapy. Considering that the creative process is unique to the individual, the ability to standardize in AsTs is somewhat difficult but it may be an essential next step to be able to building a strong evidence base for its use.[81]

Art therapy

Art therapies can be used as an adjunctive tool to obtain valuable information for diagnosis, assess the severity and progression of diseases, and understand the patients' psychological states. Moreover, it is well received by patients and not limited by age, language, or illness.

The mechanism through which art therapy might exert its effects remains largely unclear. One hypothesis, in line with the idea of EDs as stress-related immune responses, is that the creative process may lessen defense mechanisms and decrease stress-related reactions.[82]

A mixed-methods unpublished systematic review was presented as a thesis in 2021 and included three case series, one by Chaves that included eight patients aged 12- to 20-year olds.[83] The researcher concluded that there is a lack of evidence for using art therapy as a treatment for ED, primarily as no RCT has been conducted so far. Qualitative findings show that art therapy could promote self-expression, and self-awareness, foster new perspectives, and offer a form of distraction and a sense of pride. Quantitative findings showed the improved quality of life, self-esteem, and slightly reduced anxiety.[84]

Music therapy versus music medicine

Music has been shown to affect different brain areas. Passive listening activates the subcortical (medial geniculate body in the thalamus and amygdala) and the cortical areas (such as the auditory cortex). Active participation stimulates the basal ganglia, cerebellar, and cortical motor areas. Most of the literature is based on music medicine which uses music to accomplish nonmusic objectives, which can be defined as passive listening to prerecorded music provided by medical personnel. Music therapy uses music interventions to accomplish individualized goals within a therapeutic relationship by a credentialed professional who has completed an approved music therapy program.[85]

A 2020 systematic review included 16 articles, of which 2 RCTs involving 3,792 participants suggested that therapeutic application of music may benefit patients with AN and BN, but no information was available on BED. Only three studies involved music therapy. Two were pilot studies. One reduced anxiety and distress in AN ($P < 0.0001$) and the other reduced postmeal anxiety in AN ($P < 0.0001$). The third was a retrospective qualitative analysis of songs written by adolescent inpatients with AN during one-to-one music therapy sessions. Themes arising from the lyrics were categorized in the following six groups: relationship dynamics, aspirations, reference to the disorder and its impact, emotional awareness, accessing support, and identity formation, with the latter being the most dominant theme. Songwriting was a valuable and effective tool in soliciting information often not shared with the multidisciplinary team and ultimately aiding the processing of therapeutic issues. Two RCTs using listening to positive vodcasts changed eating behavior favorably in patients with AN ($P < 0.0001$), but not BN in one study. It helped patients with BN with their anxiety ($P < 0.009$), but not patients with AN. In the other study, patients with AN found that listening to classical music was beneficial to food consumption ($P < 0.001$). Exposure to music altered the estimation of body perception in BN. Listening to a violin concert by Mozart with the induction of happy autobiographical memories resulted in the reduced estimation of body width in patients with BN ($P < 0.01$). Those exposed to the negative mood induction method, reported a larger estimation of their body width. Sessions with a Body Monochord (an instrument shaped like a chair or table that has 64 strings that the clinician plays, whereas the participant sits or lays down to feel the vibrations) helped AN patients verbalize bodily perceptions. No beneficial effect on AN was recorded. However, watching music videos reinforced body dissatisfaction, drive for thinness, bodyweight concerns, preoccupation with physical appearance in pre-teenage and teenage girls, and drive for muscularity in adolescent boys.[86] In summary, music therapy, involving songwriting with a trained music therapist allowed issues not revealed to the multidisciplinary team to be discussed in therapy. Music medicine involving passive listening helped with body perception and anxiety in BN and AN helped with changing eating behaviors.

Dance/movement therapy
The literature on dance and movement therapy (DMT) in ED is scarce.

In a small pilot study including 14 patients (>14-year-old) with ED, seven subjects were assigned via quasi-randomization to a dance–movement group, whereas others continued their treatment as usual. The DMT sessions were based on Chace's model and guided imagery, according to Reddemann. Subjects received the intervention well with improvements in their mood states and increased self-awareness; they felt more positively about their bodies and were less preoccupied with their looks. There was no difference in the alexithymia scores.[87]

Movement per se has always been a controversial topic in ED due to the energy expenditure that can be critical, especially in patients with AN.

A systematic review including eight RCTs involving 213 patients (age: 16–36 years) showed that aerobic and resistance training in AN increases muscle strength, BMI, and body fat percentage. Aerobic exercise and yoga significantly lowered scores of eating pathology and depressive symptoms in both AN and BN, with no adverse effects reported. The study suggests that movement, through supervision of physical therapy and rehabilitation, could be another beneficial adjunctive treatment option for patients with ED.[88]

Drama therapy
Evidence for drama therapy in EDs is limited to case reports with insufficient evidence to support its use.

Pellicciari and his team developed a theater workshop for young patients hospitalized with a 93% satisfaction rate. They suggest that theater can be helpful in decreasing defense mechanisms, mitigating specific symptoms, and improving quality of life during hospitalization.[89]

- Combination of different art therapies

In a recent study, 66 adolescent girls with AN were randomized to music and art therapy coupled with CBT or CBT alone. The combination group had a significantly lower dropout rate, higher treatment satisfaction, lower depression and anxiety scores, and improved cognition regarding food, body shape, and weight. More rigorous trials are needed in the future to see if the use of two or more AsTs can have additive effects.[64]

Massage Therapy

Massage therapy (MT) can increase parasympathetic arousal,[90] produce biochemical changes that are key for ED, and raise patient awareness of their bodies, which some have said that it is critical for resolving body perception dissonance.[91]

Evidence for MT in ED is limited to two small RCTs and case reports. Both RCTs (one in 24 adolescent girls with BN and the second one in 19 individuals with AN) found a decrease in anxiety scores and improvement in mood and ED attitudes on the EDI, including less drive for thinness, bulimia, body dissatisfaction, ineffectiveness, perfectionism, interoceptive awareness, and interpersonal distrust. Higher dopamine and lower cortisol levels were found.[90] Dopamine depletion has been associated with a decrease in food intake and has been implicated in AN and feeding behaviors; although an increase in dopamine was observed in the massage group, there was no weight gain associated with it.[92]

One study by Fogarty, already mentioned in the acupuncture section, showed that women with AN receiving acupressure plus light massage perceived a strong therapeutic relationship with their practitioner as much as the women in the group receiving acupuncture.[67] Interventions that allow a strong therapeutic alliance to form, like MT, could be a beneficial healing adjunct therapy for patients with AN, especially in an inpatient setting, where the necessity of enforcing behavioral change makes the relationship between the medical practitioners and the sufferers of AN often challenging and complex.

Acupressure - Emotional Freedom Technique (EFT)

Although individuals with a previous history of eating disorders were eliminated from an RCT comparing emotional freedom technique (EFT) versus CBT for food cravings, the study indicated that both of these interventions may be useful as an adjunct for the treatment of BED. Eighty-three participants were randomly assigned to either CBT or EFT for 8 weeks (N >18 years of age and had a BMI >25). Food craving scores and the power of food scores (which assesses anticipation (but not consumption) of highly palatable foods) decreased significantly across both groups from pre-intervention to post-intervention ($P<.001$), with this reduction maintained at the 6-month ($P<.001$) and 12-month ($P<.001$). Restraint scores decreased significantly across both groups from pre-intervention to post-intervention ($P<.001$), with an additional significant reduction in restraint scores from the 6- to 12-month follow-up ($P = .005$, d = .005). In a comparison between CBT versus EFT versus community sample, pre-intervention EFT and CBT groups had significantly higher food cravings, power of food scores, and restraint scores than the community sample ($P = .001$, $P<.001$, and $P<.001$, respectively). At post-intervention, no significant differences were found between groups for food cravings, indicating comparable food craving scores to the non-clinical community sample for both CBT and EFT. Only the CBT group obtained significantly higher scores than the community sample ($P = .009$) post-intervention power of food scores, but at 6 and 12 months, there were no differences between any groups. At post-intervention, both the EFT and CBT groups obtained significantly higher restraint scores than the community sample ($P<.001$ and $P = .003$, respectively). Similar results were also observed at the 6-month follow-up, with both the EFT and CBT groups obtaining significantly higher restraint scores than the community sample ($P = .007$ and $P = .003$, respectively). However, at the 12-month follow-up, no significant differences were observed between groups, indicating restraint scores were consistent with the community sample. BMI for the EFT and the CBT groups remained high compared to the community sample. These results indicate that EFT and CBT may be helpful as an adjunct for BED but the treatments should continue for at least 1 year to maintain significant effectiveness.[93]

In a follow-up study,[94] the CBT group did not report any significant changes in anxiety scores over time, but the decrease in depression symptoms pre-to post-intervention was significant and this was maintained at 6-and 12 months. Anxiety and depression scores significantly decreased from pre-to post-intervention for the EFT group and was maintained at 6- and 12-month follow-up. These results suggest that EFT may be more useful for targeting anxiety and depression associated with BED.

After Emerging treatment modalities that currently have limited support

We would be remiss not to discuss microbiome, ketamine, and ayahuasca, the latter two of which were topics heavily covered at the 2021 International Associa-tion of Eating Disorders Professionals (IAEDP) Foundation's annual conference. As discovering the antidepressant effects of dissociative anesthetic Ketamine were elucidated, the search for novel drugs for mental health treatments has increased. During the IAEDP conference, case studies were introduced to practitioners and patients who have successfully used these two treatments. These methods have been most often used as a last resort, after years of very severe illness, most likely due to the increased risk and limited availability of the treatments. Therefore, most research has not been conducted on adolescents and young adults. It should be mentioned that the adolescent brain is not fully developed. Little research has been done on adolescents regarding ketamine and ayahuasca or dose and long-term effects.

Most microbiome research is related to the etiology of EDs and was discussed in the introduction. However, emerging studies use fecal transplants therapeutically for EDs.

The microbiome in AN may be important during treatment in the hospital. AN pa-tients often eat vegetarian or vegan diets low in fat and carbohydrates and high in protein and fiber before therapy. Hospital food is mostly high in calories and rich in carbohydrates and fat and patients requiring oral supplements or nasogastric feeding mostly receive products based on cow's milk. Animal-based foods have been shown to rapidly change the abundance of particular microbial species when previously maintained on a vegetarian diet resulting in an increase in certain inflam-mation-inducing bacteria[95] and a "leaky gut". This inflammatory process may aggra-vate a chronic low-grade inflammation presumed to be present in AN patients. It has been hypothesized that AN is an autoimmune disease caused by changes in the microbiome in which autoantibodies to appetite-regulating neuropeptides, neuro-transmitters, and hypothalamic neurons, disturb appetite and result in decreased intake of food. Therefore, more research must be done to determine what foods eaten during refeeding will not perpetuate the AN, what microbiota would be bene-ficial to prevent the production of these autoantibodies, and how changes in the microbiome (dysbiosis) play a role in depression and anxiety associated with AN.[96,97] In fact, a systemic review of the role of microbiota and ED and treatment revealed microbiota homeostasis seems essential for a healthy communication network between the gut and brain. Dysbiosis may promote intestinal inflammation, alter gut permeability, and trigger immune reactions in the hunger/satiety regulation center contributing to the pathophysiological development of EDs. Lower diversity (alpha diversity) in the microbiome seen in AN leads to dysbiosis. There is an in-crease in auto-antibodies to α-melanocyte stimulating hormone (α-MSH) which af-fects satiety centers to reduce appetite.[98]

A summary of these studies can be found in **Table 1** using the United States Preven-tative Services Task Force ratings for the strength of the recommendation and level of certainty for each study (See **Table 1**).

Table 1
Summary of high-level evidence

Treatment	Level of Certainty	Strength of Recommendation Based on Benefit and Safety	Strength of Recommendation Based on Benefit and Safety	Personal Recommendations of the Reviewer/SECS
I. Yoga				
a. Benefits of Yoga vs waitlist for BN or BED (Brennan et al, 2020[35]. N = 53, >18 yo) 90-min weekly x8 Kripalu Yoga	Low	C	RCT	Improved binge eating frequency, emotional regulation, self-criticism, and self-compassion. Recommend/Passes SECS
b. Yoga for ED (Borden et al, 2020[30]) 43 RCTs, N = 754. Yoga-tested varied widely and included Bikram, Hatha, Iyengar, and Viniyoga without consistent dose or frequency	Moderate	B	Meta-analysis	Moderate/large effect on binge eating and bulimia symptoms, and small effect on body image concerns than controls. Overall effective for prevention and treatment. Recommend/Passes SECS
c. Prevention program meta-analysis (Beccia et al, 2018[25]) 15 RCTs with N = 2173; 5 non-randomized, N = 602	Moderate	B	Meta-analysis 6 studies ages 10–15 y; 11 studies ages 18–24 y, 3 studies 18–60 y.	Mindfulness-based programs more effective than controls in reducing body image concerns, negative affect and promoting body appreciation. Recommend/Passes SECS
d. Yoga vs standard care in AN outpatients (Carei, T., et al 2010[28], N = 54; ages 11–21)	Low	C	RTC	Greater decreases in eating symptoms, maintained on 12-wk f/u. No negative effects on BMI in the yoga group. Recommended/Passes SECS
e. Yoga systematic review and meta-analysis (Vogel et al, 2015[29]) 4 RCTs and 2 OS; N = 209	Moderate	B	Systematic review and meta-analysis	Significant benefit on "drive for thinness and body dissatisfaction compared to usual care (RCTs only). No negative effects on BMI. Recommend/Passes SECS

(continued on next page)

Table 1
(continued)

Treatment	Level of Certainty	Strength of Recommendation Based on Benefit and Safety	Strength of Recommendation Based on Benefit and Safety	Personal Recommendations of the Reviewer/SECS
II. *Virtual Reality (VR)*				
a. VR Eating disorders (Clus et al, 2018[39]) Systematic review, (26 studies, 8 RCTs, 13 nonrandomized studies, 5 clinical trials with 1 participant); N >800	Moderate	B	Systematic review	Decreased negative emotional responses to virtual food and body shape. Significantly more attractive therapy to young adults and teens; decreased loss to f/u. Recommend/Passes SECS
b. VR-enhanced CBT compared to CBT (Low, et al, 2021[41]) 6 RCTs, N = 297.	Moderate	B	Meta-analysis 6 RCTs only (same ones listed in Clus, 2018 study)	Large decrease in frequency of binges and situationally induced body dissatisfaction compared to controls. Recommend/Passes SECS
c. VR cue exposure (VR-CET) vs additional CBT for BN and BED (Ferrer-Garcia et al, 2019[44]) N = 64; ages 34.37 (9.55)	Low	C	Randomized, parallel group study	BE: Abstinence from binge eating episodes 53% in VR and 25% in CBT group BED: Abstinence from purging 75% of in VR group and 31.5% of CBT group. Recommend/Passes SECS
e. VR in patients with BED and BN (Carvalho et al, 2017[40]; N >400; 19 studies (7 controlled assessment studies, 2 assessment studies, 1 case reports, 7 RCT, 2 non-controlled trials	Moderate	B	Systematic review	Can enhance assessment, psychometric testing, identification of triggers, and exposure, experiential and/or CBT treatment. Recommend/Passes SECS
f. VR group vs treatment as usual in hospitalized AN (Porras-Garcia et. al, 2021[42]) N = 35; >13, mean age 18 y/o; mean BMI 17.48 kg/m; mostly F (31/35). Treatment group: 5 additional sessions of VR-based body exposure therapy	Low	C	RTC	Improved efficacy in treating fear of gaining weight and reducing body image disturbances in AN. Recommend/Passes SECS

III. Feedback Based Treatments				
a. ED and related symptoms (Imperatori et al, 2018[60] N >500; 13 studies; 8 RTCs, only 1 double-blind. Only 2 studies were exclusively in youth totaling N = 125. BF in 5 studies and NF in 8 studies. Mean number of sessions per study was 7.42 (range 1–12)	Moderate	B	Systematic Review	BF and NF could help with food cravings, rumination; no changes in body image perception several EDs. Recommend/Passes SECS
b. FMRI neurofeedback left dorsolateral prefrontal cortex (dlPFC) vs visual cortex (controls) (Kohl et al, 2019[57]); N = 38	Low	C	RCT	Both groups showed increase in dlPFC. Positive effects on eating behaviors after a single day in both groups. Recommend/Passes SECS
IV. Acupuncture				
a. Adjunctive acupuncture for ED (AN and BN) vs treatment as usual (Fogarty et al, 2010[66]) N = 9, age 23.7 yo	a. Low	a. C	a. Randomized cross over pilot trial	Improves QoL, decreases anxiety (consider use pre-meals) and expression of perfectionism. No difference in empathy and therapeutic relationship with acupressure plus light massage. Needs more evidence/Passes SECS
b. Acupuncture vs acupressure with light massage for AN (Fogarty et al, 2013[67]) N = 26, age>15 yo.	b. Low	b. C	b. RCT	
V. Expressive Therapies (ArTs)				
a. Music therapy and Music Medicine (Testa et al, 2020[86]; 2 pilots,2 RCTs, N = 3792)	Moderate	B	Systematic review	Recommend listening to classical music, group singing, vodcasts, songwriting, sessions with a Body Monochord. Avoid music videos - reinforces preoccupation with physical appearance. Songwriting with music therapists is the most helpful due to its ability to elicit issues not revealed to the therapeutic team. Passes SECS.

(continued on next page)

Table 1
(continued)

Treatment	Level of Certainty	Strength of Recommendation Based on Benefit and Safety	Strength of Recommendation Based on Benefit and Safety	Personal Recommendations of the Reviewer/SECS
b. Art Therapy (Griffin et al, 2021[84]) 3 case series, N = 100	Low	C	Mixed methods systematic review	No RCT in support. Needs more evidence/Passes SECS
c. Music and Art Therapy combined with CBT in Adolescent with Anorexia vs conventional outpatient treatment once a week (Wang et al, 2021[64]) N = 66, ages 14-19	Low	C	RCT	Improved depression and anxiety, helped establish correct cognition regarding food, body shape, weight. Promising results but unclear if can separate the effects of CBT and ArTs. Low Risk, recommend/Passes SECS
d. Effects of adjunctive dance movement therapy (DMT) vs treatment as usual (Savidaki et al, 2020[87]) N = 14, mean age 20–28.12 sessions over 14 wk	Low	I	Pilot study, quasi randomization	Improved mood states and body image. No difference in alexithymia. Needs more evidence/Passes SECS - it is important to carefully select participants, since movement can be unsafe in AN and other patients with ED
VI. Massage Therapy (MT)				
a. MT vs standard treatment in BN (Field et al, 1998[90]) N = 24, ages 16-21.	a. Low	a. C, not risky	a. RCT	Immediate effects - improved mood, lower anxiety and cortisol level. Long-term - improved eating disorder attitudes on the EDI (eating disorder inventory). Needs more evidence/Passes SECS
b. Adjunctive MT vs standard treatment in AN (Hart et al, 2001[92]) N = 26, age 25.7 yo. 2 massages/wk for 5 wk, total 10 massages	b. Low	b. C, not risky	b. RCT	
VII. Movement				
Physical Therapy (PT) intervention for AN and BN	Moderate	C	Systematic review	Aerobic and resistance training increased muscle strength, BMI, body fat % in AN. Aerobic exercise

Study				
(Vancampfort et al, 2013[88]) N = 213, ages 16–36. 8 RCTs.				improved eating pathology. Passes SECS and depression in AN and BN. Recommend with caution. PT supervision could diminish exercise-related risks in certain ED patients/ Passes SECS
VIII. Bright Light Therapy				
a. Bright light therapy for eating disorders (Beauchamp et al, 2016[73]) N = 175, mean age 30.9 yo. 14 studies, 4 RCTs	Moderate	B but must be followed to see if effect persists	Systemic review	Significant improvement in eating pathology and comorbid depressive symptoms for the treatment period regardless of type of ED. Unclear if effects persist once treatment ceases. Recommend/Passes SECS
IX. Spirituality and Religion				
a. Religiosity, spirituality in relation to disordered eating and body image concerns (Akrawi et al, 2015[79]) N = 6059	Low	I	Systematic review, no RCT	Lower levels of disordered eating, psychopathology and body image concerns with strong religious beliefs. Prayers and body-affirming religious readings effective as coping strategies. Needs more evidence/Passes SECS
b. Spirituality group vs cognitive group vs emotional support group (Richards et al, 2007[80]) N = 122 ages 13-52	Low	C, not risky	RCT	Significantly lower psychological disturbance, ED symptoms and higher spiritual wellbeing in the Spirituality group. Needs more evidence/Passes SECS
X. Energy Psychology				
A. EMDR (Balbo et al, 2017[12]), 4 studies: 1 RTC and 3 case studies; N = 89	Low	C	Systemic review	Positive effects even 1 yr after follow but not enough evidence to support the efficacy of EMDR. Needs more evidence/Passes SECS

(continued on next page)

Table 1 (continued)				
Treatment	Level of Certainty	Strength of Recommendation Based on Benefit and Safety	Strength of Recommendation Based on Benefit and Safety	Personal Recommendations of the Reviewer/SECS
B. EFT vs CBT for food cravings, (Stapleton et al, 2016[98]) Age >18, N = 83 overweight or obese (BMI > 25) in an 8-wk intervention.	Low	C	RCT	Outcome data were collected at baseline, post-intervention (8 wk), and at 6- and 12-mo follow-up. Overall, EFT and CBT demonstrated comparable efficacy in reducing food cravings, one's responsiveness to food in the environment (power of food), and dietary restraint, with Cohen's effect size values suggesting moderate to high practical significance for both interventions. BMI did not change F/U study- Anxiety and depression scores significantly decreased from pre-to post-intervention for the EFT group, only depression scores did the same for CBT. Both were maintained at 6- and 12-mo follow-up. Somatoform scores significantly decreased from pre-intervention to all follow-up points for the CBT group. EFT did not have this effect. Recommend as adjunct for BED

A systematic review on the role of microbiota in the pathogenesis and treatment of eating disorders. (Carbone, et al, 2020[103]) ages young adults and older, total N not given	Moderate	B	Systemic Review – 17 studies (2 RCTs)	Sixteen studies were included, mostly regarding AN. Alpha diversity (lower diversity) and lower short-chain fatty acid (SCFA) levels were found in patients with AN. Lower alpha diversity and SCFAs causes dysbiosis this promotes intestinal inflammation, alters gut permeability, and triggers immune reactions in the hunger/satiety regulation center contributing to the pathophysiological development of EDs. Microbial richness increased in AN after weight regain on fecal microbiota transplantation.

Strength of Recommendations based on benefit and safety:

A = Recommend Strongly. There is a high certainty that the net benefit is substantial and safe.

B = Recommend. There is a high certainty that the net benefit is moderate or there is moderate certainty that the net benefit is moderate to substantial and safe.

C = Neutral (offer or provide this service for selected patients depending on individual circumstances, based on professional judgment and patient preferences). There is at least moderate certainty that the net benefit is small.

D = Discourage. There is moderate or high certainty that the service has no net benefit or that the harms outweigh the benefits.

I = Insufficient (if the service is offered, patients should understand the uncertainty about the balance of benefits and harms). Current evidence is insufficient to assess the balance of benefits and harms of the service. Evidence is lacking, of poor quality, or conflicting, and the balance of benefits cannot be determined).

Level of certainty regarding quality:

HIGH: Level of evidence with robust positive data meta-analyses or meta-reviews involving two or more RCTs of excellent, robust quality. The available evidence usually includes consistent results from well-designed, well-conducted RCTs in representative child, adolescent or young adult (18–24 year old) populations, assessing the effects on mental health outcomes.

MODERATE: Level of evidence with robust positive data involving two or more RCTs of excellent, robust quality. The available evidence usually includes consistent results from well-designed, well-conducted RCTs in representative child, adolescent or young adult (18–24 year old) populations, assessing the effects on mental health outcomes.

LOW: Level of evidence with less than two RCTs with good or average quality. The available evidence is insufficient to assess the effects on mental health outcomes.

SECS Criteria: A guide to clinical decisions is that Interventions that are Safe, Easy, Cheap, *and Sensible* (SECS) require less evidence to justify individual trials than those that are Risky, Unrealistic, Difficult, *or* Expensive (RUDE). Because some of the treatments do not have much solid, compelling evidence but would be reasonable to try with a lower bar of evidence, this criterion is also taken into account. Being risky, unrealistic, difficult OR expensive (RUDE) disqualifies from SECS. The bolded conjunctions are essential in applying this guide.

SUMMARY

In ED, the standard of care requires interdisciplinary collaboration and the adoption of several treatment modalities.[99,100] With the exception of lisdexamfetamine (Vyvanse) for BED, medication has not yielded significant effects.[1] Hence, the importance of examining complementary and integrative modalities that can elevate the efficacy of standard treatment. Several other modalities have been used historically for wellness for centuries, like traditional yoga and acupuncture. These interventions have been recognized and are now being researched. Others include spirituality/religion, the arts (art therapy, music therapy, DMT, and drama therapy), and massage. Music therapy seems to hold the most promise due to its ability to elicit issues not normally shared with the therapeutic team. Massage has only two small RCTs; interestingly, both showed physiologic changes with improvements in depression, anxiety, and eating pathology. It has been challenging to prescribe these modalities as standardized interventions. The different delivery of that these modalities have made it difficult to do comparative studies. Outcomes are difficult to study due to the individual nature of how these modalities are experienced. However, it is worth harnessing the benefits of these modalities when people have a particular interest in them.

With younger generations, technology-based interventions have been shown to increase retention in treatment and have good efficacy with core symptoms of EDs.[39] The best thing about VR is its versatility of it. It increased the ability to tolerate stress and cope with situations involving food. It is very good for eating and body image exposure and has allowed patients to continue treatment during COVID quarantines. In addition, VR is accessible, and other modalities can be utilized via this platform, such as BLT[101] EMDR and biofeedback[102] EMDR has limited research but addresses negative memories/trauma associated with body image and eating, and use in VR and in-person was not statistically different.[103] BLT can be a safe adjunctive therapy for ED core symptomatology and depressive symptoms.[73] Other technologies such as NF continue to be expensive and are often used more as a last resort. Overall, the trends in ED treatment are the combination of old methods with modern delivery modalities, which have shown to be effective and evidence-based to support their use.

DISCLOSURE

Nothing to disclose; no commercial or financial conflicts of interests to disclose.

REFERENCES

1. Schneider E, Higgs S, Dourish CT. Lisdexamfetamine and binge-eating disorder: a systematic review and meta-analysis of the preclinical and clinical data with a focus on mechanism of drug action in treating the disorder. Eur Neuropsychopharmacol 2021;53:49–78.

2. Brewerton TD, D'Agostino M. Adjunctive use of olanzapine in the treatment of avoidant restrictive food intake disorder in children and adolescents in an eating disorders program. J child Adolesc Psychopharmacol 2017;27(10):920–2.

3. Duncan L, Yilmaz Z, Gaspar H, et al. Eating Disorders Working Group of the Psychiatric Genomics Consortium. Thornton, L, Hinney, A, Daly, M, Sullivan, PF, Zeggini, E, Breen, G, & Bulik CM. 2017:850-858.

4. Zerwas S, Larsen JT, Petersen L, et al. Eating disorders, autoimmune, and autoinflammatory disease. *Pediatr* Dec 2017;140(6). https://doi.org/10.1542/peds. 2016-2089.

5. Hedman A, Breithaupt L, Hübel C, et al. Bidirectional relationship between eating disorders and autoimmune diseases. J Child Psychol Psychiatry 2019; 60(7):803–12.

6. Pike KM, Walsh BT, Vitousek K, et al. Cognitive behavior therapy in the posthospitalization treatment of anorexia nervosa. Am J Psychiatry 2003;160(11): 2046–9.

7. Bryson AE, Scipioni AM, Essayli JH, et al. Outcomes of low-weight patients with avoidant/restrictive food intake disorder and anorexia nervosa at long-term follow-up after treatment in a partial hospitalization program for eating disorders. Int J Eat Disord 2018;51(5):470–4.

8. Nicely TA, Lane-Loney S, Masciulli E, et al. Prevalence and characteristics of avoidant/restrictive food intake disorder in a cohort of young patients in day treatment for eating disorders. J Eat Disord 2014;2(1):21.

9. Norris ML, Robinson A, Obeid N, et al. Exploring avoidant/restrictive food intake disorder in eating disordered patients: a descriptive study. Int J Eat Disord 2014;47(5):495–9.

10. Fisher MM, Rosen DS, Ornstein RM, et al. Characteristics of avoidant/restrictive food intake disorder in children and adolescents: a "new disorder" in DSM-5. J Adolesc Health 2014;55(1):49–52.

11. Schöffel H, Hiemisch A, Kiess W, et al. Characteristics of avoidant/restrictive food intake disorder in a general paediatric inpatient sample. Eur Eat Disord Rev 2021;29(1):60–73.

12. Balbo M, Zaccagnino M, Cussino M, et al. Eye Movement Desensitization and Reprocessing (EMDR) and eating disorders: a systematic review. Clinical Neuropsychiatry:J Treatment Evaluation 2017;14(5):321–9.

13. Rosania K, Lock J. Family-based treatment for a preadolescent with avoidant/ restrictive food intake disorder with sensory sensitivity: a case report. Front Psychiatry 2020;11:350.

14. Brown M, Hildebrandt T. Parent-facilitated behavioral treatment for avoidant/ restrictive food intake disorder: a case report. Cogn Behav Pract 2020;27(2): 231–51.

15. Spettigue W, Norris ML, Santos A, et al. Treatment of children and adolescents with avoidant/restrictive food intake disorder: a case series examining the feasibility of family therapy and adjunctive treatments. J Eat Disord 2018;6:20.

16. Breiner CE, Miller ML, Hormes JM. ARFID Parent Training Protocol: a randomized pilot trial evaluating a brief, parent-training program for avoidant/restrictive food intake disorder. Int J Eat Disord 2021;54(12):2229–35.

17. Shimshoni Y, Silverman WK, Lebowitz ER. SPACE-ARFID: a pilot trial of a novel parent-based treatment for avoidant/restrictive food intake disorder. Int J Eat Disord 2020;53(10):1623–35.

18. Knatz Peck S, Towne T, Wierenga CE, et al. Temperament-based treatment for young adults with eating disorders: acceptability and initial efficacy of an intensive, multi-family, parent-involved treatment. J Eat Disord 2021;9(1):110.

19. Lock J, Sadeh-Sharvit S, L'Insalata A. Feasibility of conducting a randomized clinical trial using family-based treatment for avoidant/restrictive food intake disorder. Int J Eat Disord 2019;52(6):746–51.

20. Applewhite B, Cankaya Z, Heiderscheit A, et al. A systematic review of scientific studies on the effects of music in people with or at risk for autism spectrum disorder. Int J Environ Res Public Health 2022;(9):19. https://doi.org/10.3390/ ijerph19095150.

21. Castellini G, Cassioli E, Rossi E, et al. The impact of COVID-19 epidemic on eating disorders: a longitudinal observation of pre versus post psychopathological features in a sample of patients with eating disorders and a group of healthy controls. Int J Eat Disord 2020;53(11):1855–62.

22. Sideli L, Lo Coco G, Bonfanti RC, et al. Effects of COVID-19 lockdown on eating disorders and obesity: a systematic review and meta-analysis. Eur Eat Disord Rev 2021;29(6):826–41.

23. Pikoos TD, Buzwell S, Sharp G, et al. The Zoom effect: exploring the impact of video calling on appearance dissatisfaction and interest in aesthetic treatment during the COVID-19 pandemic. Aesthet Surg J 2021;41(12):NP2066–75.

24. Furness JB. The enteric nervous system and neurogastroenterology. Nat Rev Gastroenterol Hepatol 2012;9(5):286–94.

25. Beccia AL, Dunlap C, Hanes DA, et al. Mindfulness-based eating disorder prevention programs: a systematic review and meta-analysis. Ment Health Prev 2018;9:1–12.

26. Domingues RB, Carmo C. Disordered eating behaviours and correlates in yoga practitioners: a systematic review. Eat Weight Disorders-Studies Anorexia, Bulimia Obes 2019;24(6):1015–24.

27. Couturier J, Isserlin L, Norris M, et al. Canadian practice guidelines for the treatment of children and adolescents with eating disorders. J Eat Disord 2020; 8(1):1–80.

28. Carei TR, Fyfe-Johnson AL, Breuner CC, et al. Randomized controlled clinical trial of yoga in the treatment of eating disorders. J Adolesc Health 2010;46(4): 346–51.

29. Vogel H, Cramer H, Ostermann T. Effects of Yoga on eating disorders–A systematic review and meta-analysis. Eur J Integr Med 2015;7:26.

30. Borden A, Cook-Cottone C. Yoga and eating disorder prevention and treatment: a comprehensive review and meta-analysis. Eat Disord 2020;28(4):400–37.

31. Cramer H, Ward L, Saper R, et al. The safety of yoga: a systematic review and meta-analysis of randomized controlled trials. Am J Epidemiol 2015;182(4): 281–93.

32. Kramer R, Cuccolo K. Yoga practice in a college sample: associated changes in eating disorder, body image, and related factors over time. Eat Disord 2020; 28(4):494–512.

33. Cook-Cottone C, Jones LA, Haugli S. Prevention of eating disorders among minority youth: a matched-sample repeated measures study. Eat Disord 2010; 18(5):361–76.

34. Watts AW, Rydell SA, Eisenberg ME, et al. Yoga's potential for promoting healthy eating and physical activity behaviors among young adults: a mixed-methods study. Int J Behav Nutr Phys Activity 2018;15(1):1–11.

35. Brennan MA, Whelton WJ, Sharpe D. Benefits of yoga in the treatment of eating disorders: results of a randomized controlled trial. Eat Disord 2020;28(4): 438–57.

36. Hall A, Ofei-Tenkorang NA, Machan JT, et al. Use of yoga in outpatient eating disorder treatment: a pilot study. J Eat Disord 2016;4(1):1–8.

37. North MM, North SM. A comparative study of sense of presence of traditional virtual reality and immersive environments. Australas J Inf Syst 2016;20.

38. Brown T, Vogel EN, Adler S, et al. Bringing virtual reality from clinical trials to clinical practice for the treatment of eating disorders: an example using virtual reality cue exposure therapy. J Med Internet Res 2020;22(4):e16386.

39. Clus D, Larsen ME, Lemey C, et al. The use of virtual reality in patients with eating disorders: systematic review. J Med Internet Res 2018;20(4):e7898.

40. De Carvalho MR, Dias TRdS, Duchesne M, et al. Virtual reality as a promising strategy in the assessment and treatment of bulimia nervosa and binge eating disorder: a systematic review. Behav Sci 2017;7(3):43.

41. Low TL, Ho R, Ho C, et al. The efficacy of virtual reality in the treatment of binge-purging eating disorders: a meta-analysis. Eur Eat Disord Rev 2021;29(1):52–9.

42. Porras-Garcia B, Ferrer-Garcia M, Serrano-Troncoso E, et al. A randomized controlled trial for reducing fear of gaining weight and other eating disorder symptoms in anorexia nervosa through virtual reality-based body exposure. J Clin Med 2021;10(4):682.

43. Manasse SM, Lampe EW, Juarascio AS, et al. Using virtual reality to train inhibitory control and reduce binge eating: a proof-of-concept study. Appetite 2021; 157:104988.

44. Ferrer-Garcia M, Pla-Sanjuanelo J, Dakanalis A, et al. A randomized trial of virtual reality-based cue exposure second-level therapy and cognitive behavior second-level therapy for bulimia nervosa and binge-eating disorder: outcome at six-month followup. Cyberpsychology, Behav Social Networking 2019; 22(1):60–8.

45. Peschel SK, Feeling NR, Vogele C, et al. A meta-analysis on resting state high-frequency heart rate variability in bulimia nervosa. Eur Eat Disord Rev Sep 2016; 24(5):355–65.

46. Peyser D, Scolnick B, Hildebrandt T, et al. Heart rate variability as a biomarker for anorexia nervosa: a review. Eur Eat Disord Rev 2021;29(1):20–31.

47. Leake I. Functional gastrointestinal disorders: biofeedback therapy reduces regurgitation episodes in rumination. Nat Rev Gastroenterol Hepatol 2014; 11(6):331.

48. Barba E, Accarino A, Soldevilla A, et al. Randomized, placebo-controlled trial of biofeedback for the treatment of rumination. Official J Am Coll Gastroenterol ACG 2016;111(7):1007–13.

49. Simkin DR, Thatcher RW, Lubar J. Quantitative EEG and neurofeedback in children and adolescents: anxiety disorders, depressive disorders, comorbid addiction and attention-deficit/hyperactivity disorder, and brain injury. Child Adolesc Psychiatr Clin 2014;23(3):427–64.

50. Fernández-Álvarez J, Grassi M, Colombo D, et al. Efficacy of bio-and neuro-feedback for depression: a meta-analysis. Psychol Med 2022;52(2):201–16.

51. Russo GM, Balkin RS, Lenz AS. A meta-analysis of neurofeedback for treating anxiety-spectrum disorders. J Couns Dev 2022.

52. Bartholdy S, Musiat P, Campbell IC, et al. The potential of neurofeedback in the treatment of eating disorders: a review of the literature. Eur Eat Disord Rev 2013; 21(6):456–63.

53. Blume M, Schmidt R, Schmidt J, et al. EEG neurofeedback in the treatment of adults with binge-eating disorder: a randomized controlled pilot study. Neurotherapeutics 2021;1–14.

54. Grunwald M, Weiss T, Assmann B, et al. Stable asymmetric interhemispheric theta power in patients with anorexia nervosa during haptic perception even after weight gain: a longitudinal study. J Clin Exp Neuropsychol 2004;26(5): 608–20.

55. Rodriguez G, Babiloni C, Brugnolo A, et al. Cortical sources of awake scalp EEG in eating disorders. Clin Neurophysiol 2007;118(6):1213–22.

56. Tóth E, Túry F, Gáti Á, et al. Effects of sweet and bitter gustatory stimuli in anorexia nervosa on EEG frequency spectra. Int J psychophysiology 2004; 52(3):285–90.

57. Kohl SH, Veit R, Spetter MS, et al. Real-time fMRI neurofeedback training to improve eating behavior by self-regulation of the dorsolateral prefrontal cortex: a randomized controlled trial in overweight and obese subjects. Neuroimage 2019;191:596–609.

58. Lackner N, Unterrainer HF, Skliris D, et al. EEG neurofeedback effects in the treatment of adolescent anorexia nervosa. Eat Disord 2016;24(4):354–74.

59. Goldschmidt AB, Loth KA, MacLehose RF, et al. Overeating with and without loss of control: associations with weight status, weight-related characteristics, and psychosocial health. Int J Eat Disord 2015;48(8):1150–7.

60. Imperatori C, Mancini M, Della Marca G, et al. Feedback-based treatments for eating disorders and related symptoms: a systematic review of the literature. Nutrients Nov 2018;10(11). https://doi.org/10.3390/nu10111806.

61. Pop-Jordanova N. Psychological characteristics and biofeedback mitigation in preadolescents with eating disorders. Pediatr Int 2000;42(1):76–81.

62. Arvidsdotter T, Marklund B, Taft C. Effects of an integrative treatment, therapeutic acupuncture and conventional treatment in alleviating psychological distress in primary care patients-a pragmatic randomized controlled trial. BMC Complement Altern Med 2013;13(1):1–9.

63. Leung B, Takeda W, Holec V. Pilot study of acupuncture to treat anxiety in children and adolescents. J Paediatr Child Health Aug 2018;54(8):881–8.

64. Wang C, Xiao R. Music and art therapy combined with cognitive behavioral therapy to treat adolescent anorexia patients. Am J Transl Res 2021;13(6):6534–42.

65. Fang J, Jin Z, Wang Y, et al. The salient characteristics of the central effects of acupuncture needling: limbic-paralimbic-neocortical network modulation. Hum Brain Mapp 2009;30(4):1196–206.

66. Fogarty S, Harris D, Zaslawski C, et al. Acupuncture as an adjunct therapy in the treatment of eating disorders: a randomised cross-over pilot study. Complement Therapies Med 2010;18(6):233–40.

67. Fogarty S, Smith CA, Touyz S, et al. Patients with anorexia nervosa receiving acupuncture or acupressure; their view of the therapeutic encounter. Complement Therapies Med 2013;21(6):675–81.

68. Stuyt EB, Voyles CA. The National Acupuncture Detoxification Association protocol, auricular acupuncture to support patients with substance abuse and behavioral health disorders: current perspectives. Subst Abuse Rehabil 2016; 7:169–80.

69. Hedlund S, Landgren K. Creating an opportunity to reflect: ear acupuncture in anorexia nervosa - inpatients' experiences. Issues Ment Health Nurs 2017; 38(7):549–56.

70. Landgren K. Ear acupuncture as an adjunct in a treatment protocol for anorexia nervosa: utilization rate and nurses' experience. Acupunct Med 2021;40(4): 322–32.

71. Cheng C, Liu X, Zhu S, et al. Clinical study on electroacupuncture for obese patients with binge eating disorder: a retrospective study. Medicine 2020;99(49): e23362.

72. Krysta K, Krzystanek M, Janas-Kozik M, et al. Bright light therapy in the treatment of childhood and adolescence depression, antepartum depression, and eating disorders. J Neural Transm (Vienna) 2012;119(10):1167–72.

73. Beauchamp MT, Lundgren JD. A systematic review of bright light therapy for eating disorders. Prim Care Companion CNS Disord 2016;18(5):26718.

74. Janas-Kozik M, Krzystanek M, Stachowicz M, et al. Bright light treatment of depressive symptoms in patients with restrictive type of anorexia nervosa. J Affect Disord 2011;130(3):462–5.

75. Lam RW, Goldner EM, Solyom L, et al. A controlled study of light therapy for bulimia nervosa. Am J Psychiatry 1994;151(5):744–50.

76. Terman M, Terman JS. Light therapy for seasonal and nonseasonal depression: efficacy, protocol, safety, and side effects. CNS Spectr 2005;10(8):647–63, quiz 672.

77. Ash JB, Piazza E, Anderson JL. Light therapy in the clinical management of an eating-disordered adolescent with winter exacerbation. Int J Eat Disord 1998; 23(1):93–7.

78. Lam RW, Lee SK, Tam EM, et al. An open trial of light therapy for women with seasonal affective disorder and comorbid bulimia nervosa. *J Clin Psychiatry* Mar 2001;62(3):164–8.

79. Akrawi D, Bartrop R, Potter U, et al. Religiosity, spirituality in relation to disordered eating and body image concerns: a systematic review. J Eat Disord 2015;3(1):29.

80. Richards PS, Berrett ME, Hardman RK, et al. Comparative efficacy of spirituality, cognitive, and emotional support groups for treating eating disorder inpatients. Eat Disord 2006;14(5):401–15.

81. Frisch MJ, Franko DL, Herzog DB. Arts-based therapies in the treatment of eating disorders. *Eat Disord* Mar-apr 2006;14(2):131–42.

82. Bucharová M, Malá A, Kantor J, et al. Arts therapies interventions and their outcomes in the treatment of eating disorders: scoping review protocol. Behav Sci 2020;10(12):188.

83. Chaves E. The creation of art books with adolescents diagnosed with an eating disorder: effectiveness, self-esteem, and related factors. University of Denver; 2011.

84. Griffin C, Fenner P, Landorf KB, et al. Effectiveness of art therapy for people with eating disorders: a mixed methods systematic review. Arts in Psychotherapy 2021;76:101859.

85. Yinger OS, Gooding L. Music therapy and music medicine for children and adolescents. Child Adolesc Psychiatr Clin N Am 2014;23(3):535–53.

86. Testa F, Arunachalam S, Heiderscheit A, et al. A systematic review of scientific studies on the effects of music in people with or at risk for eating disorders. Psychiatria Danubina 2020;32(3–4):334–45.

87. Savidaki M, Demirtoka S, Rodriguez-Jimenez RM. Re-inhabiting one's body: a pilot study on the effects of dance movement therapy on body image and alexithymia in eating disorders. J Eat Disord 2020;8:22.

88. Vancampfort D, Vanderlinden J, De Hert M, et al. A systematic review of physical therapy interventions for patients with anorexia and bulemia nervosa. Disabil Rehabil 2014;36(8):628–34.

89. Pellicciari A, Rossi F, Iero L, et al. Drama therapy and eating disorders: a historical perspective and an overview of a Bolognese project for adolescents. J Altern Complement Med 2013;19(7):607–12.

90. Field T, Schanberg S, Kuhn C, et al. Bulimic adolescents benefit from massage therapy. *Adolescence* Fall 1998;33(131):555–63.

91. Meerman R, Vandereycken W. Some considerations on the behavioral treatment of chronic weight disorders. Cogn Behav Ther 1985;14(2):73–80.

92. Hart S, Field T, Hernandez-Reif M, et al. Anorexia nervosa symptoms are reduced by massage therapy. *Eat Disord*. Winter 2001;9(4):289–99.

93. Stapleton P, Bannatyne AJ, Urzi KC, et al. Food for thought: a randomised controlled trial of emotional freedom techniques and cognitive behavioral therapy in the treatment of food cravings. Appl Psychol Health Well Being 2016; 8(2):232–57. Epub 2016 May 3. PMID: 27140673.

94. Stapleton P, Bannatyne A, Chatwin H, et al. Secondary psychological outcomes in a controlled trial of emotional freedom techniques and cognitive behaviour therapy in the treatment of food cravings. Complement Ther Clin Pract 2017; 28:136–45. Epub 2017 Jun 8. PMID: 28779921.

95. Herpertz-Dahlmann B, Seitz J, Baines J. Food matters: how the microbiome and gut–brain interaction might impact the development and course of anorexia nervosa. Eur Child Adolesc Psychiatry 2017;26:1031–41. https://doi.org/10.1007/s00787-017-0945-7.

96. Roubalová R, Procházková P, Papežová H, et al. Anorexia nervosa: gut microbiota-immune-brain interactions. Clin Nutr 2020;39(3):676–84. Epub 2019 Mar 23. PMID: 30952533.

97. Sirufo MM, Magnanimi LM, Ginaldi L, et al. Anorexia nervosa and autoimmune comorbidities: a bidirectional route? CNS Neurosci Ther 2022;28(12):1921–9. Epub 2022 Sep 16. PMID: 36114699; PMCID: PMC9627382.

98. Carbone EA, D'Amato P, Vicchio G, et al. A systematic review on the role of microbiota in the pathogenesis and treatment of eating disorders. Eur Psychiatry 2020;64(1):e2. PMID: 33416044; PMCID: PMC8057489.

99. Dalle Grave R, Eckhardt S, Calugi S, et al. A conceptual comparison of family-based treatment and enhanced cognitive behavior therapy in the treatment of adolescents with eating disorders. J Eat Disord 2019;7(1):1–9.

100. UK NGA. Eating disorders: recognition and treatment. London: National Institute for Health and Care Excellence (NICE); 2017. PMID: 28654225.

101. Li C, Sun C, Sun M, et al. Effects of brightness levels on stress recovery when viewing a virtual reality forest with simulated natural light. Urban Forestry & Urban Greening 56:126865 doi:10.1016/j.ufug.2020.126865.

102. Liou H, Lane C, Huang C, et al. Eye movement desensitization and reprocessing in a primary care setting: assessing utility and comparing efficacy of virtual versus in-person methods. Telemed J E Health 2022;28(9):1359–66. Epub 2022 Feb 8. PMID: 35133887.

103. Rockstroh C, Blum J, Göritz AS. Virtual reality in the application of heart rate variability biofeedback. Intz J Human Computer Stud 2019;130:209–20.

Iron Deficiency in Attention-Deficit Hyperactivity Disorder, Autism Spectrum Disorder, Internalizing and Externalizing Disorders, and Movement Disorders

Dimitri Fiani, MD[a], Solangia Engler, MS[b], Sherecce Fields, PhD[b], Chadi Albert Calarge, MD[a,c],*

KEYWORDS

- Iron deficiency • Brain development • Depression • Anxiety • ADHD

KEY POINTS

- Iron is an essential nutrient for normal brain development and function, including memory, attention, and emotion regulation.
- The impact of iron deficiency (ID) on the brain varies depending on the time it occurs during development. Notably, certain deficits may be irreversible when ID occurs early in life.
- ID is associated with increased risk for neuropsychiatric disorders, notably attention-deficit hyperactivity disorder, internalizing disorders, and restless leg syndrome.
- Treatment with psychotropic medication, in particular risperidone, can affect iron homeostasis and increase the risk of ID.
- Iron supplementation has not been thoroughly examined but may be beneficial in iron-deficient children with psychopathology.

INTRODUCTION

Iron is a micronutrient essential for various bodily functions, including erythropoiesis and immune response.[1] In the brain, iron is not uniformly distributed, with the basal

[a] Menninger Department of Psychiatry and Behavioral Sciences, Baylor College of Medicine, 8080 N Stadium Dr. Ste 180.35, Houston, TX 77054, USA; [b] Department of Psychological & Brain Sciences, Texas A&M University, College Station, TX 77843, USA; [c] Department of Pediatrics, Baylor College of Medicine, 1102 Bates Avenue, Ste 790, Houston, TX 77030, USA
* Corresponding author.
E-mail address: chadi.calarge@bcm.edu
Twitter: @dimitrifiani (D.F.)

Child Adolesc Psychiatric Clin N Am 32 (2023) 451–467
https://doi.org/10.1016/j.chc.2022.08.015
1056-4993/23/© 2022 Elsevier Inc. All rights reserved.

Abbreviations	Expansion
ADHD	Attention-deficit hyperactivity disorder
ASD	Autism spectrum disorder
ID	Iron deficiency
MRI	Magnetic resonance imaging
QSM	Quantitative susceptibility mapping
RLS	Restless leg syndrome
RCT	Randomized controlled trial
sF	Serum ferritin concentration

ganglia storing a disproportionately larger amount of iron compared with other regions.[2] This is also true at the cellular level, with oligodendrocytes, astrocytes, and microglia having a larger iron content compared with neurons.[2] Iron is critical for multiple brain processes, including neurotransmitter synthesis, myelination, energy metabolism, and cellular respiration.[3–5] Moreover, iron has been shown to play an important role in higher-order cognitive functions, like attention and memory.[6–8]

Given iron's essential role in normal brain development and function and given that iron deficiency (ID) is the most common nutritional deficiency in the world, affecting upward of a billion people,[9] mental health providers should be familiar with the potential neuropsychiatric sequelae of ID. This is particularly relevant to infants, children, and adolescents given that rapid physical growth characteristic of childhood and adolescence increases the risk for ID to emerge.[10] This, in turn, could jeopardize the critical changes the brain undergoes during development.[11] Moreover, minority populations are at a particularly heightened risk, as ID is about twice as prevalent in Black and Mexican American female adolescents compared with their non-Hispanic White counterparts.[12]

DEFINING IRON DEFICIENCY

Based on the World Health Organization (WHO), ID is present when serum ferritin concentration (sF) is < 15 µg/L in adults and children more than five years of age and when sF is < 12 µg/L in children under five years old.[13] Nutritional deficiencies are usually diagnosed when the nutrient's blood concentration is below a threshold considered necessary for normal physiological functions. A couple particularities exist regarding Iron. First, because serum iron concentration is relatively variable, ID is defined based on other iron-related markers, including sF (**Table 1**). Ferritin is a storage protein, and its low concentration is considered the most sensitive and specific noninvasive marker of ID, in the absence of infection or inflammation.[14] Second, the threshold to define ID has been established based on levels below which anemia would ensue (ie, when the bone marrow is deficient in iron).[14,15] However, during a state of iron insufficiency, iron is prioritized for hematopoiesis, at the expense of other organs, in a hierarchical manner.[16] In fact, when the need for iron exceeds intake, iron is initially diverted from the liver, then the muscles, etc. Eventually, even brain iron is tapped, to protect the organism against anemia. As a result, concerns have been raised that the current threshold to establish the presence of ID might be too conservative[17,18] as it does not account for the role iron plays in maintaining other essential physiological functions outside hematopoiesis, particularly in the brain.[19] Consequently, the sF cutoff to define ID varies across studies, laboratories, and health authorities worldwide.[20]

Although low sF is specific for ID, sF increases in certain conditions associated with infections or immune activation, potentially masking ID.[21] As such, several laboratory

Table 1
Laboratory tests in iron deficiency and iron deficiency anemia

	Normal Values (in Children and Adolescents[a])	Iron Deficiency	Iron Deficiency Anemia
Serum iron (μg/dL)	3–11 years: 53–119 >12 years: 59–158 (M); 37–145 (F)	↓	↓
Serum ferritin (μg/L)	<5 years: >12 in the absence of infection >5 years: 15–200 (M); 15–150 (F)	↓	↓↓
Transferrin saturation (%)	1–10 years: 22–39 11–17 years: 27–44	↓	↓↓
Serum transferrin (mg/dL)	200–360	↑	↑
Serum hepcidin (μg/L)		↓	↓
Hemoglobin (g/dL)	1–5 years: 10.9–15 5–11 years: 11.9–15 11–18 years: 12.7–17 (M); 11.9–15.5 (F)	Normal	↓
Mean corpuscular volume (fl)	1–6 years: 75–90 6–12 years: 77–90 12–18 years: 79–95	Normal	↓

[a] Normal values are sex and age dependent. Only the normal ranges for children and adolescents are listed, given this article's scope.

tests are helpful to evaluate for ID (see **Table 1**). Transferrin is a protein that transfers iron in the blood. Its value is typically estimated by measuring the Total Iron Binding Capacity, the maximum amount of iron that the blood can carry. Dividing serum iron by TIBC provides Transferrin Saturation. Unlike ferritin, TIBC is not affected by inflammation. Hepcidin is a major regulator of iron homeostasis, inhibiting its intestinal absorption.[14,22–25]

IRON AND BRAIN DEVELOPMENT AND FUNCTION

Novel methods, using MRI, have been used to quantify changes in iron content during development and examine its association with cognitive function. Using quantitative susceptibility mapping (QSM), Carpenter and colleagues[7] estimated brain iron content in healthy preteens, finding that iron content in the basal ganglia increased with age and that higher levels of iron in the right caudate were associated with higher spatial IQ. Peterson and colleagues[26] repurposed functional MRI scans from 12- to 21-year-old healthy youth, confirming the increase with age in subcortical nuclei iron content and finding it to plateau by early adulthood. They further showed larger iron concentrations in females and in the right hemisphere compared with males and the left hemisphere, respectively. Moreover, left dentate nucleus and substantia nigra iron content was positively associated with lower working memory speed.[26] Building on this work, Larsen and colleagues[2] observed in 8- to 26-year-old healthy volunteers that the magnitude and tempo of the increase in iron content over time varied between subregions of the basal ganglia, with the globus pallidus and putamen having the biggest magnitude and the most prolonged periods of iron accumulation. They further confirmed the presence of sex differences and found that performers in the top 5% on complex cognitive tasks had had a significantly larger increase in putamen iron concentration during follow-up. Importantly, another longitudinal study in 18- to 30-year-old healthy participants found that the increase in nucleus accumbens iron content was positively correlated with the increase in presynaptic vesicular dopamine storage, captured using positron emission tomography (PET) with [11C] dihydrotetrabenazine.[27]

The nature and extent of ID's impact on the brain varies depending on its timing during development. For instance, early-life ID, even without anemia, has been associated with neural structural abnormalities that are irreversible, disrupting brain function and impacting performance across multiple areas in adulthood.[6] Specifically, prenatal ID has been associated with an increased risk of schizophrenia and autism spectrum disorder (ASD)[28] and ID in utero and up to 2 years of age can lead to inattention, cognitive problems, and poor executive control, even in adulthood.[29] In contrast, the sequelae of ID in school-age children and young adults appear to be reversible with the replenishment of iron stores.[30,31] Overall, the long-term implications of ID on academic performance, functioning, and productivity can be staggering, estimated to amount to over 400 age- and disability-adjusted life-years per 100,000 population globally, with a bigger impact on women and young boys compared with men and young girls.[32,33]

EXTERNALIZING DISORDERS

As noted earlier, ID in infancy and the toddler years has been associated with the later onset of attention-deficit hyperactivity disorder (ADHD) and disruptive behavior. This includes an increased prevalence of the oppositional defiant disorder, aggression, and delinquency.[34] Notably, these difficulties have emerged in school-age children despite attempts to replenish body iron stores early in life, denoting the potentially irreversible nature of the brain changes associated with ID when it develops in infancy.

The exact mechanism implicating ID in externalizing disorders is unknown but is thought to be related to iron's role in dopaminergic signaling, given that dopamine pathways dysfunction has been found in ADHD.[35] Iron is necessary for dopamine metabolism as it is a cofactor for tyrosine hydroxylase and monoamine oxidase.[36,37] Moreover, ID has been associated with reduced density of dopamine D_1 and D_2 receptors and of the dopamine transporter in the basal ganglia.[1,38]

Several studies have found children with ADHD to have lower sF and a higher prevalence of ID.[39–44] Moreover, ID has been associated with more severe ADHD symptoms.[40,41] As for other externalizing conditions, ID in infancy has been associated with excessive alcohol use in adolescence and elevated rates of ID have been found in adolescents involved in the juvenile justice system.[45,46]

Some have attributed the association between ADHD and ID to malnutrition due to psychostimulants-induced anorexia.[47] This contention, however, may be challenged by several observations: (1) This association has been observed in treatment-naïve children with ADHD[41]; (2) MRI studies have found lower iron content in several brain regions (eg, thalamus, striatum, caudate nucleus, hippocampus, substantia nigra, anterior cingula, olfactory gyrus, and the right lingual gyrus) in unmedicated children with ADHD[48–51]; (3) ID in infancy is associated with increased risk for ADHD in children and adolescents[52]; (4) low mean cell volume, a marker of ID, in the toddler years is associated with decreased sensitivity to ADHD treatment later during childhood[53]; (5) sF at the initiation of amphetamine treatment is inversely related to response to psychostimulants[41]; and (6) preliminary evidence suggests that iron supplementation might alleviate ADHD symptom severity (**Table 2**).[31,54–56] In particular, Konofal and colleagues[55] randomized 5- to 8-year-old French children with ADHD and

Table 2
Iron supplementation studies in youth with attention-deficit hyperactivity disorder and iron deficiency

First Author, Year of Publication	Treatment	Study Design	ADHD Assessment	Findings After Iron Supplementation
Pongpitakdamrong et al.,[31] 2022	12 weeks of 2–4 mg/kg/day of elemental iron.	Placebo-controlled parallel-group RCT in ADHD, 19% of whom with anemia (N = 52, age 6–18 yr).	Vanderbilt ADHD Diagnostic Rating Scales (Informant: parents and teachers).	Significant improvement in parents' but not teachers' ratings, even in the absence of anemia.
El-Baz et al.,[51] 2019	6 months of 6 mg/kg of iron and 55 mg/kg of zinc	Open-label iron and zinc supplementation in ADHD with iron and zinc deficiency (N = 50, age 6–16 yr).	Parents Conners Rating Scale and Wechsler Intelligence Scale for Children.	Iron and zinc supplementation resulted in improvement in ADHD symptoms and in verbal and total IQ, but not in performance IQ.
Konofal et al.,[55] 2008	12 weeks of 80 mg/day of elemental iron.	Placebo-controlled parallel-group double-blind RCT in non-anemic ADHD (N = 23, age 5–8 yr).	Parents Conner's Rating Scale, Clinical Global Impression Scale, ADHD Rating Scale	Improvement in ADHD symptom severity, particularly inattention, on the ADHD Rating Scale, but not on the Conner's scale.
Sever et al.,[56] 1997	30 days of 5 mg/kg/day of elemental iron.	Open-label in non-anemic ADHD (N = 14, age 7–11 yr).	Connors Rating Scale (Informant: parent and teacher).	Significant increase in serum ferritin levels and decrease in Parents' ratings, though not correlated with change in ferritin concentration. No change in teachers' ratings.

Abbreviation: RCT, randomized controlled trial.

sF < 30 μg/L but without anemia to 80 mg/day of elemental iron (*N* = 17) vs. placebo (*N* = 5). Although 12 weeks later sF had increased to an average 55.7 μg/L in the iron supplementation arm, no significant effect was found on the Conner's Parent Rating Scale (the primary outcome variable in the study) or the Conner's Teacher Rating Scale. On the other hand, a significant reduction in the investigator-completed ADHD Rating Scale score was observed.[55] Similarly, 6- to 18-year-old Thai children with ADHD and ID (defined as sF < 30 μg/L or transferrin saturation < 16%) and who were on a stable dose of methylphenidate for at least one month were randomized to placebo (*N* = 26) or 2 to 4 mg/kg/day of elemental ferrous iron (*N* = 26) for 12 weeks.[31] Significant improvement in ADHD symptom severity was reported by parents but not teachers. Two small open-label supplementation studies in children with ADHD also showed some promising findings.[54,56]

INTERNALIZING DISORDERS

The impact of ID on brain development and function may increase the proclivity of youth to develop internalizing disorders, including anxiety and depressive disorders.[57–65] As reviewed earlier, iron is relevant to several neurotransmitter signaling pathways, including monoaminergic, implicated in emotional processing and regulation.[34,59,65,66] Moreover, ID has been shown to disrupt normal brain development, resulting in emotional dysregulation and neurocognitive impairments as observed in internalizing symptoms.[67–69] In fact, children and adolescents with ID anemia were more than twice as likely to have anxiety disorders, depressive disorders, or bipolar disorders compared with those without anemia.[39] However, because anemia is associated with several manifestations that overlap with internalizing symptoms (eg, irritability, apathy, fatigue, low mood, concentration difficulties), investigators have also sought to examine the psychiatric effects of ID without anemia. Much of this work has involved women of reproductive age,[70–78] showing improvement in internalizing symptoms with iron supplementation in women with postpartum depression.[79]

Mirroring the observations in adults, a few studies have found ID to be associated with worse internalizing symptoms in children and adolescents.[80] For example, sF was inversely correlated with both anxiety and depressive symptom severity in a study of unmedicated 12- to 17-year-old females.[81] Notably, the symptoms were more severe in participants with sF < 15 μg/L compared with those with sF > 15 μg/L. Similarly, the symptoms were significantly higher in participants with sF < 20 μg/L compared with those with sF> 20 μg/L, supporting the contention that the sF cutoff to define ID may be too conservative when it comes to psychiatric sequelae. Moreover, sF was inversely correlated with the volume of the left caudate, left putamen, and right putamen, revealing the potential impact of ID on brain structure.[81] Additionally, in a retrospective study of 6- to 15-year-old Japanese children referred for a psychiatric evaluation, those whose sF decreased below 50 μg/L following iron supplementation showed a reduction in internalizing symptom severity.[82] Finally, one of two small-scale, controlled studies in adolescent girls showed iron supplementation to improve mood, energy, and concentration (**Table 3**).[83,84]

AUTISM SPECTRUM DISORDER AND SLEEP DISORDERS

Compared with neurotypical children, ID is more frequent in those with ASD, particularly when intellectual disability is present.[11,39,85–88] In fact, up to 30% of children with ASD may have ID.[89,90] Several reasons could explain this association, including restricted dietary intake due to limited food preferences,[91,92] prevalent gastrointestinal concerns,[93] and medication side effects (see below). ID in children with ASD has been

Table 3
Iron supplementation studies in youth with internalizing symptoms and iron deficiency

First Author, Year of Publication	Treatment	Study Design	Internalizing Symptom Assessment	Findings After Iron Supplementation
Ballin et al.,[83] 1992	8 weeks of 105 mg elemental ferrous iron.	Placebo-controlled parallel-group RCTs in girls with ID ($N = 59$, age 16–17 yr).	Questionnaire containing items about lassitude, fatigue, concentration, and mood.	Significant improvement in lassitude, ability to concentrate, and mood.
Bruner et al.,[84] 1996	8 weeks of 260 mg elemental ferrous iron.	Placebo-controlled parallel-group RCTs in girls with ID, without anemia ($N = 81$, age 13–18 yr).	Brief questionnaire about changes in energy, attention, memory, and mood.	No significant difference was observed.
Mikami[82] 2019	12 weeks of 50 to 100 mg of elemental ferrous iron.	Observational, in participants with sF <50 µg/L ($N = 10$, age 6–15 yr).	Clinical Global Impression Severity, Japanese shortened version of the Profile of Mood States, the Pittsburgh Sleep Quality Index (Informant: parent and child)	Significant improvement in anxiety ratings at 6 weeks and in depression, anger, fatigue, and confusion ratings at 12 weeks.

Abbreviation: RCT, randomized controlled trial.

associated with sleep disturbances such as restless sleep, which can improve after iron supplementation.[94]

Although current evidence is limited, ID might also be associated with pediatric sleep disorders, including general sleep disturbances, periodic limb movement disorder, sleep-disordered breathing, and restless sleep disorder.[95]

MOVEMENT DISORDERS

One of the most widely known neuropsychiatric effects of ID is its association with restless leg syndrome (RLS) which has been reported in 25 to 35% of patients with ID anemia.[96] Moreover, lower sF are associated with a more severe presentation.[97] Notably, in adults with RLS, sF is decreased and transferrin concentration increased in the cerebrospinal fluid despite a lack of difference in serum levels of these markers.[98] Furthermore, imaging studies have also found a reduction in Substantia Nigra iron content in patients with RLS, a finding replicated in autopsy studies.[99] These findings converge to implicate ID and associated dopaminergic dysfunction in RLS.[100]

Iron supplementation is currently standard of care in patients with RLS with a target sF of at least 50 µg/L in children and 75 µg/L in adults.[97] This target is substantially higher than the threshold used to diagnose ID, again suggesting that the threshold developed based on hematological parameters is likely too conservative and does not account for the physiological needs of the brain.

Other movement disorders that are possibly associated with ID include akathisia following treatment with second-generation antipsychotics, although the exact pathophysiology remains poorly elucidated.[101]

IRON HOMEOSTASIS AND PSYCHOTROPICS

Because both ID and many psychotropic medications alter dopaminergic signaling, the authors have examined how the two might interact in children and adolescents. As reviewed above, lower mean cell volume in the toddler years and baseline sF appeared to predict relative resistance to psychostimulants.[41,53]

During short- and long-term treatment with risperidone, a potent antagonist of the dopamine D_2 receptor, weight gain was inversely associated with sF in three independent samples.[87,102,103] Although the exact mechanism is unknown, haloperidol and chlorpromazine have been shown to reduce liver nonheme iron stores in iron-replete rats.[104] Chlorpromazine has iron-chelating properties.[105] In children and adolescents, one study suggested low iron stores during risperidone treatment could be due in part to obesity-induced inflammation.[102] Inflammation is known to stimulate the release of hepcidin, a potent inhibitor of iron absorption.[14,106] However, another prospective study suggested that the effect may be specific to risperidone, compared with other antipsychotics, inhibiting iron repletion even in the absence of weight gain.[87] Consistent with the findings that ID reduces the density of the dopamine D_2 receptor in the basal ganglia,[38] our group also found that sF was inversely related to prolactin concentration, even after accounting for several factors, including serum risperidone concentration.[102] A more recent study, however, failed to replicate this association.[103] Of note, sF was not associated with extrapyramidal signs in risperidone-treated children and adolescents.[103]

Other psychotropics have also been shown to affect iron homeostasis. For instance, lithium use has been associated with reduced iron levels in rat erythrocytes.[107] Finally, although iron's role in neurotransmitter signaling extends beyond dopamine[1] and despite the possibility that ID may affect the efficacy of other classes of psychotropic medications (eg, antidepressants), to our knowledge this has not been examined.

Table 4
Quality of randomized controlled trials of iron supplementation in youth with iron deficiency and externalizing or internalizing disorders

Treatment	Strength of Recommendation Based on Benefit and Safety	Level of Certainty by USPTF Definitions	Evidence Base in Youth	Evidence-Based or Passes SECS Criteria	Personal Recommendations of the Reviewer
Iron Supplementation Studies					
ADHD					
12 weeks of 80 mg/day of elemental ferrous iron (Konofal, 2008, N = 23, age 5–8 yr)	I, but favorable risk/benefit ratio	Low	One small placebo- controlled parallel- group RCT in non-anemic	SECS	Await further research but replenish iron stores if iron deficiency is present, with or without anemia
12 weeks of 2–4 mg/kg/day of elemental ferrous iron (Pongpitakdamro, 2022, N = 52, age 6–18 yr)	I, but favorable risk/benefit ratio	Low	One small placebo- controlled parallel- group RCT in ADHD, 19% of whom with anemia	SECS	Await further research but replenish iron stores if iron deficiency is present, with or without anemia
Mood/Well being					
8 weeks of 105 mg elemental ferrous iron (Ballin, 1992, N = 59, age 16–19 yr)	I, but favorable risk/benefit ratio	Low	One placebo- controlled parallel- group RCTs in healthy girls	SECS	Await further research but replenish iron stores if iron deficiency is present, with or without anemia
8 weeks of 260 mg elemental ferrous iron (Bruner, 1996, N = 81, age 13–18 yr)	I, but favorable risk/benefit ratio	Low	One placebo- controlled parallel- group RCTs in girls with iron deficiency, without anemia	SECS	Await further research but replenish iron stores if iron deficiency is present, with or without anemia

Abbreviation: RCT, randomized controlled trial.
Strength of recommendations based on benefit and safety.
A = *Recommend strongly.* There is a high certainty that the net benefit is substantial *and safe.*
B = *Recommend.* There is a high certainty that the net benefit is moderate or there is moderate certainty that the net benefit is moderate to substantial *and safe.*

(continued on next page)

Table 4
(continued)

C = *Neutral* (offer or provide this service for selected patients depending on individual circumstances, based on professional judgment and patient preferences). There is at least moderate certainty that the net benefit is small.

D = *Discourage*. There is moderate or high certainty that the service has no net benefit or that the harms outweigh the benefits.

I = *Insufficient* (if the service is offered, patients should understand the uncertainty about the balance of benefits and harms) Current evidence is insufficient to assess the balance of benefits and harms of the service. Evidence is lacking, of poor quality, or conflicting, and the balance of benefits cannot be determined.

Level of certainty regarding quality.

HIGH Level of evidence with robust positive data meta-analyses or meta-reviews involving 2 or more RCTs of excellent, robust quality. The available evidence usually includes consistent results from well-designed, well-conducted RCTs in representative child, adolescent or young adult (18–24 years old) populations, assessing the effects on mental health outcomes.

MODERATE Level of evidence with robust positive data involving two or more RCTs of excellent, robust quality. The available evidence usually includes consistent results from well-designed, well-conducted RCTs in representative child, adolescent or young adult (18–24 years old) populations, assessing the effects on mental health outcomes.

LOW Level of evidence with less than two RCTs with good or average quality. The available evidence is insufficient to assess the effects on mental health outcomes.

SECS criteria.

A guide to clinical decisions is that Interventions that are Safe, Easy, Cheap, *and* Sensible (SECS) require less evidence to justify individual trials than those that are Risky, Unrealistic, Difficult, *or* Expensive (RUDE). Because some of the treatments do not have much solid, compelling evidence but would be reasonable to try with a lower bar of evidence, this criterion is also taken into account. Being risky, unrealistic, difficult *OR* expensive (RUDE) disqualifies from SECS. The bolded conjunctions are essential in applying this guide.

SUMMARY

Iron is essential for brain development and function. Children, particularly females and those from minority backgrounds, are among the most vulnerable populations to developing ID. Before anemia becomes manifest, low body iron stores may alter brain structure and function, causing a variety of neuropsychiatric symptoms. In fact, ID is frequently found in patients with ADHD, where it is associated with more severe symptoms and possibly poorer response to psychostimulants. ID has also been associated with the severity of internalizing symptoms, ASD, movement disorders, and sleep disorders. These findings are important to bear in mind as they are telling of a potentially reversible risk factor for psychopathology.

Treating ID can have important clinical ramifications, with regard to reducing the severity of certain psychiatric conditions and/or optimizing treatment efficacy and tolerability. However, iron supplementation may be associated with certain risks, including dysbiosis and increased infection risk.[108] Therefore, research is urgently needed to determine what threshold may be optimal for preventing brain iron insufficiency or depletion, rather than merely preventing anemia. To that end, advances in neuroimaging will help shed light on factors that modulate brain iron content and its impact on brain structure and function, in children and adolescents with and without psychopathology. The public health impact of such work can be substantial.

For a summary of quality of research and benefits based on randomized controlled trial, please see **Table 4**.

CLINICS CARE POINTS

- Iron deficiency (ID) is a prevalent nutritional deficiency that disproportionately affects vulnerable populations and minorities. Even in the absence of anemia, ID is associated with psychopathology in children.

- It may be advisable to check serum ferritin concentration in children with risk factors for ID and those with psychiatric problems such as attention-deficit hyperactivity disorder, internalizing disorders, autism spectrum disorder, and movement disorders. Obtaining a C-reactive protein measurement concurrently would help rule out acute inflammation.

- If the presence of ID is confirmed, 325 mg of ferrous sulfate every other day is indicated, preferably taken with orange juice and without dairy products. This schedule is as effective as more frequent dosing, but with greater adherence and fewer adverse effects.[109] Children with ID unresponsive to 2 to 3 months of iron supplementation at this dosage should have their scheduled changed to daily supplementation for another 2 to 3 months, before a referral to hematology is considered.

- Certain medications, such as proton pump inhibitors and H2 receptor antagonists, inhibit iron absorption. Conversely, iron may inhibit the absorption of several medications, including minocycline (used for acne treatment).

- Future research should examine whether revisiting the current cutoff to diagnose ID is necessary to optimize brain development and function.

DISCLOSURE

The Authors have no conflict of interest to disclose.

REFERENCES

1. Beard JL. Iron biology in immune function, muscle metabolism and neuronal functioning. J Nutr 2001;131(2S-2):568S–79S [discussion: 580S].

2. Larsen B, Bourque J, Moore TM, et al. Longitudinal development of brain iron is linked to cognition in youth. J Neurosci 2020;40(9):1810–8.

3. Beard JL, Connor JR, Jones BC. Iron in the brain. Nutr Rev 1993;51(6):157–70.

4. Connor JR, Menzies SL. Relationship of iron to oligodendrocytes and myelination. Glia 1996;17(2):83–93.

5. Weiland A, Wang Y, Wu W, et al. Ferroptosis and its role in diverse brain diseases. Mol Neurobiol 2019;56(7):4880–93.

6. Bastian TW, Rao R, Tran PV, et al. The effects of early-life iron deficiency on brain energy metabolism. Neurosci Insights 2020;15. 2633105520935104.

7. Carpenter KLH, Li W, Wei H, et al. Magnetic susceptibility of brain iron is associated with childhood spatial IQ. Neuroimage 2016;132:167–74.

8. Lozoff B, Georgieff MK. Iron deficiency and brain development. Semin Pediatr Neurol 2006;13(3):158–65.

9. GBD 2016 Disease and Injury Incidence and Prevalence Collaborators. Global, regional, and national incidence, prevalence, and years lived with disability for 328 diseases and injuries for 195 countries, 1990-2016: a systematic analysis for the Global Burden of Disease Study 2016. Lancet 2017;390(10100):1211–59.

10. Seyoum Y, Humblot C, Nicolas G, et al. Iron deficiency and anemia in adolescent girls consuming predominantly plant-based diets in rural Ethiopia. Sci Rep 2019;9(1):17244.

11. Pivina L, Semenova Y, Doşa MD, et al. Iron deficiency, cognitive functions, and neurobehavioral disorders in children. J Mol Neurosci 2019;68(1):1–10.

12. Gupta PM, Hamner HC, Suchdev PS, et al. Iron status of toddlers, nonpregnant females, and pregnant females in the United States. Am J Clin Nutr 2017; 106(Suppl 6):1640S–6S.

13. WHO, World Health Organization. Serum ferritin concentrations for the assessment of iron status and iron deficiency in populations. 2011. Available at: http://www.who.int/vmnis/indicators/serum_ferritin.pdf. Accessed March 31, 2022.

14. Pasricha S-R, Tye-Din J, Muckenthaler MU, et al. Iron deficiency. Lancet 2021; 397(10270):233–48.

15. Foy BH, Li A, McClung JP, et al. Data-driven physiologic thresholds for iron deficiency associated with hematologic decline. Am J Hematol 2020;95(3):302–9.

16. Zamora TG, Guiang SF, Widness JA, et al. Iron is prioritized to red blood cells over the brain in phlebotomized anemic newborn lambs. Pediatr Res 2016; 79(6):922–8.

17. Musallam KM, Taher AT. Iron deficiency beyond erythropoiesis: should we be concerned? Curr Med Res Opin 2018;34(1):81–93.

18. Pratt JJ, Khan KS. Non-anaemic iron deficiency - a disease looking for recognition of diagnosis: a systematic review. Eur J Haematol 2016;96(6):618–28.

19. Camaschella C, Girelli D. The changing landscape of iron deficiency. Mol Aspects Med 2020;75:100861.

20. Garcia-Casal MN, Peña-Rosas JP, Pasricha S-R. Rethinking ferritin cutoffs for iron deficiency and overload. Lancet Haematol 2014;1(3):e92–4.

21. Cullis JO, Fitzsimons EJ, Griffiths WJ, et al, British Society for Haematology. Investigation and management of a raised serum ferritin. Br J Haematol 2018; 181(3):331–40.

22. Mattiello V, Schmugge M, Hengartner H, et al, SPOG Pediatric Hematology Working Group. Diagnosis and management of iron deficiency in children with or without anemia: consensus recommendations of the SPOG Pediatric Hematology Working Group. Eur J Pediatr 2020;179(4):527–45.

23. Camaschella C. Iron deficiency: new insights into diagnosis and treatment. Hematol Am Soc Hematol Educ Program 2015;2015:8–13.
24. Weiss G, Goodnough LT. Anemia of chronic disease. N Engl J Med 2005; 352(10):1011–23.
25. Hershko C. Assessment of iron deficiency. Haematologica 2018;103(12): 1939–42.
26. Peterson ET, Kwon D, Luna B, et al. Distribution of brain iron accrual in adolescence: evidence from cross-sectional and longitudinal analysis. Hum Brain Mapp 2019;40(5):1480–95.
27. Larsen B, Olafsson V, Calabro F, et al. Maturation of the human striatal dopamine system revealed by PET and quantitative MRI. Nat Commun 2020;11(1):846.
28. Georgieff MK. Iron deficiency in pregnancy. Am J Obstet Gynecol 2020;223(4): 516–24.
29. East P, Doom JR, Blanco E, et al. Iron deficiency in infancy and neurocognitive and educational outcomes in young adulthood. Dev Psychol 2021;57(6): 962–75.
30. Houston BL, Hurrie D, Graham J, et al. Efficacy of iron supplementation on fatigue and physical capacity in non-anaemic iron-deficient adults: a systematic review of randomised controlled trials. BMJ Open 2018;8(4):e019240.
31. Pongpitakdamrong A, Chirdkiatgumchai V, Ruangdaraganon N, et al. Effect of iron supplementation in children with attention-deficit/hyperactivity disorder and iron deficiency: a randomized controlled trial. J Dev Behav Pediatr 2022; 43(2):80–6.
32. Wang M, Gao H, Wang J, et al. Global burden and inequality of iron deficiency: findings from the Global Burden of Disease datasets 1990-2017. Nutr J 2022; 21(1):16.
33. Sørensen LB, Damsgaard CT, Dalskov S-M, et al. Diet-induced changes in iron and n-3 fatty acid status and associations with cognitive performance in 8-11-year-old Danish children: secondary analyses of the optimal well-being, development and health for Danish children through a healthy new nordic diet school meal study. Br J Nutr 2015;114(10):1623–37.
34. Doom JR, Richards B, Caballero G, et al. Infant iron deficiency and iron supplementation predict adolescent internalizing, externalizing, and social problems. J Pediatr 2018;195:199–205.e2.
35. Del Campo N, Chamberlain SR, Sahakian BJ, et al. The roles of dopamine and noradrenaline in the pathophysiology and treatment of attention-deficit/hyperactivity disorder. Biol Psychiatry 2011;69(12):e145–57.
36. Lu H, Chen J, Huang H, et al. Iron modulates the activity of monoamine oxidase B in SH-SY5Y cells. Biometals 2017;30(4):599–607.
37. Ramsey AJ, Hillas PJ, Fitzpatrick PF. Characterization of the active site iron in tyrosine hydroxylase. Redox states of the iron. J Biol Chem 1996;271(40): 24395–400.
38. Burhans MS, Dailey C, Beard Z, et al. Iron deficiency: differential effects on monoamine transporters. Nutr Neurosci 2005;8(1):31–8.
39. Chen M-H, Su T-P, Chen Y-S, et al. Association between psychiatric disorders and iron deficiency anemia among children and adolescents: a nationwide population-based study. BMC Psychiatry 2013;13:161.
40. Percinel I, Yazici KU, Ustundag B. Iron deficiency parameters in children and adolescents with attention-deficit/hyperactivity disorder. Child Psychiatry Hum Dev 2016;47(2):259–69.

41. Calarge C, Farmer C, DiSilvestro R, et al. Serum ferritin and amphetamine response in youth with attention-deficit/hyperactivity disorder. J Child Adolesc Psychopharmacol 2010;20(6):495–502.

42. Oner O, Oner P, Bozkurt OH, et al. Effects of zinc and ferritin levels on parent and teacher reported symptom scores in attention deficit hyperactivity disorder. Child Psychiatry Hum Dev 2010;41(4):441–7.

43. Cortese S, Konofal E, Bernardina BD, et al. Sleep disturbances and serum ferritin levels in children with attention-deficit/hyperactivity disorder. Eur Child Adolesc Psychiatry 2009;18(7):393–9.

44. Konofal E, Cortese S, Marchand M, et al. Impact of restless legs syndrome and iron deficiency on attention-deficit/hyperactivity disorder in children. Sleep Med 2007;8(7–8):711–5.

45. East P, Delker E, Lozoff B, et al. Associations among infant iron deficiency, childhood emotion and attention regulation, and adolescent problem behaviors. Child Dev 2018;89(2):593–608.

46. Rosen GM, Deinard AS, Schwartz S, et al. Iron deficiency among incarcerated juvenile delinquents. J Adolesc Health Care 1985;6(6):419–23.

47. D'Amato TJ. Is iron deficiency causative of attention-deficit/hyperactivity disorder? Arch Pediatr Adolesc Med 2005;159(8):787–8.

48. Chen Y, Su S, Dai Y, et al. Quantitative susceptibility mapping reveals brain iron deficiency in children with attention-deficit/hyperactivity disorder: a whole-brain analysis. Eur Radiol 2022. https://doi.org/10.1007/s00330-021-08516-2.

49. Adisetiyo V, Jensen JH, Tabesh A, et al. Multimodal MR imaging of brain iron in attention deficit hyperactivity disorder: a noninvasive biomarker that responds to psychostimulant treatment? Radiology 2014;272(2):524–32.

50. Cortese S, Azoulay R, Castellanos FX, et al. Brain iron levels in attention-deficit/hyperactivity disorder: a pilot MRI study. World J Biol Psychiatry 2012;13(3):223–31.

51. Tang S, Zhang G, Ran Q, et al. Quantitative susceptibility mapping shows lower brain iron content in children with attention-deficit hyperactivity disorder. Hum Brain Mapp 2022. https://doi.org/10.1002/hbm.25798.

52. East PL, Doom JR, Blanco E, et al. Iron deficiency in infancy and sluggish cognitive tempo and ADHD symptoms in childhood and adolescence. J Clin Child Adolesc Psychol 2021;1–12. https://doi.org/10.1080/15374416.2021.1969653.

53. Turner CA, Xie D, Zimmerman BM, et al. Iron status in toddlerhood predicts sensitivity to psychostimulants in children. J Atten Disord 2012;16(4):295–303.

54. El-Baz FM, Youssef AM, Khairy E, et al. Association between circulating zinc/ferritin levels and parent Conner's scores in children with attention deficit hyperactivity disorder. Eur Psychiatry 2019;62:68–73.

55. Konofal E, Lecendreux M, Deron J, et al. Effects of iron supplementation on attention deficit hyperactivity disorder in children. Pediatr Neurol 2008;38(1):20–6.

56. Sever Y, Ashkenazi A, Tyano S, et al. Iron treatment in children with attention deficit hyperactivity disorder. A preliminary report. Neuropsychobiology 1997;35(4):178–80.

57. Beard JL, Chen Q, Connor J, et al. Altered monamine metabolism in caudate-putamen of iron-deficient rats. Pharmacol Biochem Behav 1994;48(3):621–4.

58. Beard JL, Erikson KM, Jones BC. Neurobehavioral analysis of developmental iron deficiency in rats. Behav Brain Res 2002;134(1–2):517–24.

59. Carlson ES, Stead JDH, Neal CR, et al. Perinatal iron deficiency results in altered developmental expression of genes mediating energy metabolism and neuronal morphogenesis in hippocampus. Hippocampus 2007;17(8):679–91.

60. Fretham SJB, Carlson ES, Wobken J, et al. Temporal manipulation of transferrin-receptor-1-dependent iron uptake identifies a sensitive period in mouse hippo-campal neurodevelopment. Hippocampus 2012;22(8):1691–702.

61. Golub MS, Hogrefe CE, Germann SL. Iron deprivation during fetal development changes the behavior of juvenile rhesus monkeys. J Nutr 2007;137(4):979–84.

62. Kennedy BC, Dimova JG, Siddappa AJM, et al. Prenatal choline supplementa-tion ameliorates the long-term neurobehavioral effects of fetal-neonatal iron defi-ciency in rats. J Nutr 2014;144(11):1858–65.

63. Mohamed WMY, Unger EL, Kambhampati SK, et al. Methylphenidate improves cognitive deficits produced by infantile iron deficiency in rats. Behav Brain Res 2011;216(1):146–52.

64. Schmidt AT, Waldow KJ, Grove WM, et al. Dissociating the long-term effects of fetal/neonatal iron deficiency on three types of learning in the rat. Behav Neuro-sci 2007;121(3):475–82.

65. Tran PV, Kennedy BC, Pisansky MT, et al. Prenatal choline supplementation di-minishes early-life iron deficiency-induced reprogramming of molecular net-works associated with behavioral abnormalities in the adult rat hippocampus. J Nutr 2016;146(3):484–93.

66. Barks A, Hall AM, Tran PV, et al. Iron as a model nutrient for understanding the nutritional origins of neuropsychiatric disease. Pediatr Res 2019;85(2):176–82.

67. Suveg C, Morelen D, Brewer GA, et al. The emotion dysregulation model of anx-iety: a preliminary path analytic examination. J Anxiety Disord 2010;24(8):924–30.

68. Weems CF, Silverman WK. An integrative model of control: implications for un-derstanding emotion regulation and dysregulation in childhood anxiety. J Affect Disord 2006;91(2–3):113–24.

69. Mennin DS, Heimberg RG, Turk CL, et al. Preliminary evidence for an emotion dysregulation model of generalized anxiety disorder. Behav Res Ther 2005;43(10):1281–310.

70. Beard JL, Hendricks MK, Perez EM, et al. Maternal iron deficiency anemia af-fects postpartum emotions and cognition. J Nutr 2005;135(2):267–72.

71. Corwin EJ, Murray-Kolb LE, Beard JL. Low hemoglobin level is a risk factor for postpartum depression. J Nutr 2003;133(12):4139–42.

72. Kim J, Wessling-Resnick M. Iron and mechanisms of emotional behavior. J Nutr Biochem 2014;25(11):1101–7.

73. Fordy J, Benton D. Does low iron status influence psychological functioning? J Hum Nutr Diet 1994;7(2):127–33.

74. Karl JP, Lieberman HR, Cable SJ, et al. Randomized, double-blind, placebo-controlled trial of an iron-fortified food product in female soldiers during military training: relations between iron status, serum hepcidin, and inflammation. Am J Clin Nutr 2010;92(1):93–100.

75. Low MSY, Speedy J, Styles CE, et al. Daily iron supplementation for improving anaemia, iron status and health in menstruating women. Cochrane Database Syst Rev 2016;4:CD009747.

76. Rangan AM, Blight GD, Binns CW. Iron status and non-specific symptoms of fe-male students. J Am Coll Nutr 1998;17(4):351–5.

77. Vahdat Shariatpanaahi M, Vahdat Shariatpanaahi Z, Moshtaaghi M, et al. The relationship between depression and serum ferritin level. Eur J Clin Nutr 2007; 61(4):532–5.

78. Yi S, Nanri A, Poudel-Tandukar K, et al. Association between serum ferritin concentrations and depressive symptoms in Japanese municipal employees. Psychiatry Res 2011;189(3):368–72.

79. Wassef A, Nguyen QD, St-André M. Anaemia and depletion of iron stores as risk factors for postpartum depression: a literature review. J Psychosom Obstet Gynaecol 2019;40(1):19–28.

80. Lozoff B, Jimenez E, Hagen J, et al. Poorer behavioral and developmental outcome more than 10 years after treatment for iron deficiency in infancy. Pediatrics 2000;105(4):E51.

81. Abbas M, Gandy K, Salas R, et al. Iron deficiency and internalizing symptom severity in unmedicated adolescents: a pilot study. Psychol Med 2021;1–11. https://doi.org/10.1017/S0033291721004098.

82. Mikami K, Okazawa H, Kimoto K, et al. Effect of oral iron administration on mental state in children with low serum ferritin concentration. Glob Pediatr Health 2019;6. 2333794X19884816.

83. Ballin A, Berar M, Rubinstein U, et al. Iron state in female adolescents. Am J Dis Child 1992;146(7):803–5.

84. Bruner AB, Joffe A, Duggan AK, et al. Randomised study of cognitive effects of iron supplementation in non-anaemic iron-deficient adolescent girls. Lancet 1996;348(9033):992–6.

85. Sidrak S, Yoong T, Woolfenden S. Iron deficiency in children with global developmental delay and autism spectrum disorder. J Paediatr Child Health 2014; 50(5):356–61.

86. Bener A, Khattab AO, Bhugra D, et al. Iron and vitamin D levels among autism spectrum disorders children. Ann Afr Med 2017;16(4):186–91.

87. Calarge CA, Ziegler EE, Del Castillo N, et al. Iron homeostasis during risperidone treatment in children and adolescents. J Clin Psychiatry 2015;76(11): 1500–5.

88. Gunes S, Ekinci O, Celik T. Iron deficiency parameters in autism spectrum disorder: clinical correlates and associated factors. Ital J Pediatr 2017;43(1):86.

89. Latif A, Heinz P, Cook R. Iron deficiency in autism and Asperger syndrome. Autism 2002;6(1):103–14.

90. Hergüner S, Keleşoğlu FM, Tanıdır C, et al. Ferritin and iron levels in children with autistic disorder. Eur J Pediatr 2012;171(1):143–6.

91. Tsujiguchi H, Miyagi S, Nguyen TTT, et al. Relationship between autistic traits and nutrient intake among Japanese children and adolescents. Nutrients 2020;12(8). https://doi.org/10.3390/nu12082258.

92. Castro K, Faccioli LS, Baronio D, et al. Feeding behavior and dietary intake of male children and adolescents with autism spectrum disorder: a case-control study. Int J Dev Neurosci 2016;53:68–74.

93. Madra M, Ringel R, Margolis KG. Gastrointestinal issues and autism spectrum disorder. Child Adolesc Psychiatr Clin N Am 2020;29(3):501–13.

94. Dosman CF, Brian JA, Drmic IE, et al. Children with autism: effect of iron supplementation on sleep and ferritin. Pediatr Neurol 2007;36(3):152–8.

95. Leung W, Singh I, McWilliams S, et al. Iron deficiency and sleep - a scoping review. Sleep Med Rev 2020;51:101274.

96. Trenkwalder C, Allen R, Högl B, et al. Restless legs syndrome associated with major diseases: a systematic review and new concept. Neurology 2016; 86(14):1336–43.
97. Allen RP, Picchietti DL, Auerbach M, et al. Evidence-based and consensus clinical practice guidelines for the iron treatment of restless legs syndrome/Willis-Ekbom disease in adults and children: an IRLSSG task force report. Sleep Med 2018;41:27–44.
98. Earley CJ, Connor JR, Beard JL, et al. Abnormalities in CSF concentrations of ferritin and transferrin in restless legs syndrome. Neurology 2000;54(8): 1698–700.
99. Earley CJ, Connor J, Garcia-Borreguero D, et al. Altered brain iron homeostasis and dopaminergic function in restless legs syndrome (Willis-Ekbom disease). Sleep Med 2014;15(11):1288–301.
100. Trotti LM. Restless legs syndrome and sleep-related movement disorders. Continuum (Minneap Minn) 2017;23(4, Sleep Neurology):1005–16.
101. Schoretsanitis G, Nikolakopoulou A, Guinart D, et al. Iron homeostasis alterations and risk for akathisia in patients treated with antipsychotics: a systematic review and meta-analysis of cross-sectional studies. Eur Neuropsychopharmacol 2020;35:1–11.
102. Calarge CA, Ziegler EE. Iron deficiency in pediatric patients in long-term risperidone treatment. J Child Adolesc Psychopharmacol 2013;23(2):101–9.
103. Calarge CA, Murry DJ, Ziegler EE, et al. Serum ferritin, weight gain, disruptive behavior, and extrapyramidal symptoms in risperidone-treated youth. J Child Adolesc Psychopharmacol 2016;26(5):471–7.
104. Ben-Shachar D, Youdim MB. Neuroleptic-induced supersensitivity and brain iron: I. Iron deficiency and neuroleptic-induced dopamine D2 receptor supersensitivity. J Neurochem 1990;54(4):1136–41.
105. Rajan KS, Manian AA, Davis JM, et al. Studies on the metal chelation of chlorpromazine and its hydroxylated metabolites. Adv Biochem Psychopharmacol 1974;9(0):571–91.
106. Ganz T, Nemeth E. Hepcidin and iron homeostasis. Biochim Biophys Acta 2012; 1823(9):1434–43.
107. Kiełczykowska M, Kopciał E, Kocot J, et al. Lithium disturbs homeostasis of essential microelements in erythrocytes of rats: selenium as a protective agent? Pharmacol Rep 2018;70(6):1168–72.
108. Georgieff MK, Krebs NF, Cusick SE. The benefits and risks of iron supplementation in pregnancy and childhood. Annu Rev Nutr 2019;39:121–46.
109. Rimon E, Kagansky N, Kagansky M, et al. Are we giving too much iron? Low-dose iron therapy is effective in octogenarians. Am J Med 2005;118(10):1142–7.

Autism Spectrum Disorder and Complementary-Integrative Medicine

Pankhuree Vandana, MD[a],*,
Deborah R. Simkin, MD, DFAACAP ABIHM, BCN[b,1],
Robert L. Hendren, DO[c], L. Eugene Arnold, MEd, MD[d]

KEYWORDS

- Autism treatment • Vitamins/minerals/diet • Essential fatty acids

KEY POINTS

- Many families use CIM treatment for their children with an autism spectrum disorder and perceive that their physicians have limited knowledge of various available CIM treatments.
- Practitioners should routinely review all treatment modalities the family may be receiving and be prepared to discuss risk, benefits, and interactions with other treatments in a non-judgemental and supportive manner.
- Treatments that might be safely recommended include melatonin, omega-3 fatty acids, & multivitamin/minerals in doses below the upper recommended limit. Evidence for any benefits of medical marijuana exceeding its risk does not yet exist.
- Probiotics might be helpful in specific cases of comorbid gastrointestinal symptoms. Folinic acid (d,l-leucovorin)may be helpful in improving communication, attention, and stereotypy in some autistic individuals with Cerebral Folate Deficiency or low folate levels.
- N-acetyl cysteine in dosages of 1800 to 2400 mg/d may be beneficial as augmentation to risperidone for hyperactivity, and irritability.
- Animal-assisted therapy and music therapy have limited evidence for improving core symptoms of autism.

[a] Division of Child & Adolescent Psychiatry, Columbia University Valegos College of Physicians and Surgeons, Center for Autism and the Developing Brain, 21 Bloomingdale Road, White Plains, NY 10605, USA; [b] Department of Psychiatry, Emory University School of Medicine; [c] University of California San Francisco, Pritzker Building, 675 18th Street, San Francisco, CA 94143-3132, USA; [d] Department of Psychiatry and Behavioral Health, Ohio State University, McCampbell 395E, 1581 Dodd Drive, Columbus, OH 43210, USA
[1] Present address: 4641 Gulfstarr Drive, Suite 106, Destin, FL 32541.
* Corresponding author.
E-mail address: pv2359@cumc.columbia.edu

Child Adolesc Psychiatric Clin N Am 32 (2023) 469–494
https://doi.org/10.1016/j.chc.2022.08.004
1056-4993/23/© 2022 Elsevier Inc. All rights reserved.

BACKGROUND
The Rationale for the Use of Complementary-Integrative Medicine in Autism Spectrum Disorder

Recent studies have suggested "gene-by- environment" interaction as a likely etiology of ASD.[1–6] Several environmental factors such as exposure to toxins, certain viral infections, maternal metabolic conditions, environmental pollution, and advanced paternal age have been identified to increase the risk of ASD in the offspring.[7] This explains the interest in ameliorating potential triggers through improvement in nutrition, reducing exposure to toxins in utero, and other factors.[8] In essence, autism can be looked at from a neurophysiological and metabolic aspect. Decreased pruning resulting in the overabundance of synapses in infancy, excessive local and reduced long-range neuronal connectivity and increased excitatory/inhibitory ratio of neurotransmitter provides a basis for neurophysiological abnormalities in the etiology of ASD. This may explain the higher rates of seizures (20%–50%) classically seen in autism compared with the normal population.[9]

Metabolically, autistic children have been found to have more mitochondrial dysfunction than their neurotypical counterparts.[10] Exposure to certain medications, heavy metals, toxic chemicals, and infections as well as gene mutations can lead to increased oxidative stress responsible for mitochondrial damage. Oxidative stress can be caused by an abnormality in folate and DNA methylation cycles which in turn can lead to epigenetic aberrations. A deficiency of folic acid activity due to either poor diet, poor absorption, or methylenetetrahydrofolate reductase (MTHFR) deficiency (mutation) resulting in lower methylenetetrahydrofolate (MTHF) levels can interfere with DNA methylation, resulting in damaged neural cells and reduced catechol-O-methyltransferase (COMT) activity resulting in deficient neurotransmitter metabolism. Oxidative stress in genetically predisposed individuals can lead to neuronal damage resulting in autistic symptomatology.

The presence of ASD phenotype in metabolic abnormalities involving glutathione synthesis, folate metabolism, and other steps support the use of antioxidants to reduce symptom severity of ASD.[11] There is ample opportunity to use CIM to benefit all these processes.

There are 3 major categories of CIM per NCCIM (1) natural products, (2) Mind-body practices, (3) other traditional medicine, including Chinese Traditional, Ayurveda & homeopathy. Due to the lack of pharmacologic interventions targeting core symptoms of ASD, there is an ongoing search for an agent that may be able to do so.

This article attempts to discuss the most used CIM treatments, the rationale for interest in ASD, the strength of current evidence for its efficacy in this population, and pertinent adverse effects.

Clinical Assessment and Biomarkers

Assessment is based on understanding the elements of gene expression, including metabolic issues, not only DNA and symptoms. Integrative treatment is based on targeting processes leading to health rather than only diagnosed pathology, and interest is increasing in studying biomarker targets.[12] Significant subsets of children with ASD have an endophenotype of intestinal inflammation, digestive enzyme abnormalities, metabolic impairments, oxidative stress, mitochondrial dysfunction, and immune problems, which range from immune deficiency through hypersensitivity to autoimmunity.

The strongest evidence for the use of biomarkers in the assessment of ASD continues to be routine laboratory testing, most of which have a low rate of abnormalities.[13] These include a metabolic panel that includes glucose, liver function tests, and a complete blood count with differential and platelet count. The following have been identified but are not routinely tested: physiologic biomarkers of neuroimmune and metabolic abnormalities; neurologic biomarkers, including abnormalities in brain structure, function, and neurophysiology; subtle behavioral biomarkers including the atypical development of visual attention; genetic biomarkers; and gastrointestinal biomarkers.

Increasingly, practitioners interested in taking an integrative medicine approach (especially when supported by the history and physical) will include magnesium, selenium, zinc/copper, vitamin C, vitamin D3 (usually 1,25-dihydroxyvitamin D), other fat-soluble vitamins, ferritin, total iron, total iron binding capacity, percent iron saturation, lead screening, serum amino and urine organic acids, lipid panel, lactate/pyruvate/ubiquinone, carnitine (free and total), cytokines, red blood cell folate, and vitamin B12 tests, especially if indicated by a biomarker. Homocysteine, methylenetetrahydrofolate (MTHF), and S-adenosylmethionine/S-adenosylhomocysteine (SAM/SAH) are suggested as useful markers for folate and methyl B12 function.[14] Genomics, proteomics, metabolomics, and transcriptomes hold promise for identifying treatment targets but as yet no replicable tests for these parameters are identified.[15]

INDIVIDUAL TREATMENTS
Melatonin

Melatonin (N-acetyl-5-methoxytryptamine) is a neurohormone secreted by the pineal gland that establishes circadian rhythms. Low melatonin levels have been reported in autism, possibly due to the absence of the Acetylserotonin O-methyltransferase (ASMT) gene, which encodes the last enzyme in melatonin synthesis. Melke (2008)[16] showed significantly low ASMT activity and melatonin levels in about 250 individuals with ASD compared with controls. Many individuals with neurodevelopmental disorders, including ASD, struggle with sleep disorders. Melatonin levels in patients with ASD and their relatives are significantly lower than in those without ASD.[17] Patients with decreased melatonin levels complained of sleep-related problems more frequently.

Sleep disorders affect 50% to 60% of patients with ASD, and unlike the neurotypical population, they do not improve as children get older.[18] Poor sleep is associated with more significant behavioral difficulties and higher caregiver fatigue. Lower nocturnal melatonin excretion is associated with the severity of social communication impairments.[19] Several well-conducted RCTs and systematic reviews have established the benefits of melatonin supplementation for sleep disturbances in children with ASD. Melatonin increased total sleep duration by 73 min and decreased sleep latency by 66 min in a systematic review and meta-analysis of 5 randomized, placebo-controlled trials involving 57 participants.[20] Both short-acting and long-acting formulations of melatonin have established efficacy in children with ASD to treat insomnia. A prospective, open-label 522-week follow-up study of prolonged-release melatonin (doses of 2, 5, or 10 mg) was effective in 95 children and adolescents with neurogenetic disorders; minimal side effects were found.[21] Reported side effects included nightmares, morning fatigue, enuresis, headache, dizziness, diarrhea, and hypothermia. Decreases in blood pressure and serum glucose were noted, so it is prudent to monitor individuals on antihypertensive or hypoglycemic agents. CYP1A2 and CYP2C19 primarily metabolize melatonin, so enzyme inhibitors and inducers can impact levels of this hormone.

Melatonin can be used to target sleep-onset insomnia with dosages of 1 to 3 mg about 30 min before bedtime. When used as a chronobiotic, melatonin can adjust the phase and/or period of disrupted circadian rhythm via the melatonin receptors in the suprachiasmatic nucleus. Anecdotally, autistic children seem sensitive to sleep disruption during seasonal changes in the light/dark cycle. A dose of 0.2 to 0.5 mg can be used about 3 to 4 hours before bedtime. Long-term studies on melatonin usage in ASD do not exist, so it is prudent to attempt to taper/withdraw it every 6 to 8 months to assess its ongoing need and utility.

Omega-3 fatty acids

Omega-3 (N-3) fatty acids (eicosapentaenoic acid, EPA; docosahexaenoic acid, DHA) are a type of PUFA (polyunsaturated fatty acids) and one of the most used CIM treatments by families of individuals with ASD.[22] PUFAs are an essential component of neuronal membrane phospholipids and are necessary for synaptic plasticity, neuro-protection, and growth.[23] About 1/5th of the brain's dry weight consists of PUFA containing DHA, EPA, and AA. Besides the importance of brain structure, EPA is the precursor for series 3 anti-inflammatory eicosanoids. The human body depends on diet and essential dietary precursors linoleic acid and alpha-linolenic acid (ALA) to synthesize these PUFAs.[24] In addition, deficiency of fatty acid desaturase or competition from dietary omega-6 fatty acids can bottleneck the anabolism of EPA and DHA from ALA. Parletta and colleagues (2016) found lower levels of EPA & DHA; AA (arachidonic acid, an omega-6 fatty acid) was also low despite high omega-6/omega-3 ratio in ASD (n = 85) compared with ADHD (n = 401) and controls (n = 79).[25] In this study, Childhood Autism Rating Scales (CARS) scores correlated significantly negatively with DHA, EPA, and AA levels. A meta-analysis of 15 case-control studies (N = 1193) confirmed these results.[26] Compared with typically developed children, ASD populations had lower DHA (-2.14 [95% CI -3.22 to -1.07]; $P < .0001$; $I^2 = 97\%$), EPA (-0.72 [95% CI -1.25 to -0.18]; $P = .008$; $I^2 = 88\%$), and AA (-0.83 [95% CI, -1.48 to -0.17]; $P = .01$; $I^2 = 96\%$) and higher total n-6 LCPUFA to n-3 LCPUFA ratio (0.42 [95% CI 0.06–0.78]; $P = .02$; $I^2 = 74\%$). In a meta-analysis of four RCTs (N = 107) omega-3 PUFAs improved social interaction (-1.96 [95% CI -3.5 to -0.34]; $P = .02$; $I^2 = 0$) and repetitive and restricted interests and behaviors (-1.08 [95% CI -2.17 to -0.01]; $P = .05$; $I^2 = 0$) more than placebo.

At least 8 double-blind randomized controlled trials (DBRCTs) have studied the impact of Omega 3 on core symptoms and other ASD behavior. In a meta-analysis of dietary interventions, Omega 3 was more effective than the placebo for affective disturbances, hyperactivity, language, and social autistic symptoms; however, the effect size was small.[27] In a 2X2 DBRPCT VIDOMA trial, 73 individuals 2.5 yrs.−8 yrs. old with ASD were randomized to Vitamin D3 (2000 IU/day) versus Vitamin D + Omega 3 (VIDOM) versus Omega-3 LCPUFA (722 mg DHA/d; OM) versus double placebo for 12 months.[28] VIDOM combination was associated with significant positive effects on the social awareness domain of the Social Responsiveness Scale (SRS) (OM -2.4, $P = .03$, VIDOM -2.9 $P = .03$), with a nonsignificant trend for greater improvement in SRS total score in the OM ($P = .09$) than placebo. The rate of positive response (define as at least 30% improvement in SRS total score) was 20%-25% in all active treatment groups as compared with placebo. The same group studied the reduction in irritability and hyperactivity on the Aberrant Behavior Checklist in 111 children and found that after 12 months, OM (-5.0, $P = .001$) and VID (-4.0, $P = .01$) groups had greater reduction in irritability than placebo.[29] However, this study did not include baseline inflammatory states in the analysis. Therefore, in exploratory analysis of the data from the Vitamin D and Omega-3 LCPUFA in Autism (VIDOMA) trial, 77 children with ASD (2.5–8.0 years) were randomized to vitamin D (VID, 2000 IU/day), omega-3 LCPUFA; (722 mg/d docosahexaenoic acid), both, or placebo.[30] Non-fasting baseline plasma interleukin-1β (IL-1β) was measured in 67 children (Mazahery and colleagues 2020). Children were categorized as having undetectable/normal IL-1β (<3.2 pg/mL, n = 15) or elevated IL-1β ($\geq$3.2 pg/mL, n = 52) There was evidence for an effect of interaction (with baseline inflammatory state) on treatment response for SRS-total (P = .06), SRS-social communicative functioning (P = .04), SRS-awareness (P = .006), and SRS-communication (P = .09). Of 21 outcome measure comparisons (interventions vs placebo), 4 (2 significant and 2 borderline significant) showed greater improvements when all children (regardless of the presence/absence of inflammation at baseline) were included, and 10 (5 significant and 5 borderline significant) showed greater improvements when only children with elevated IL-1β were included. In the first mixed model analysis, when all children were included, VID was associated with no effect on behavioral outcomes (all P > .1 and negligible effect sizes), OM was associated with a greater improvement in SRS-awareness (P = .01 and ηp 2 = 11) and a trend for greater improvement in SRS-total (P = .06 and ηp 2 = 0.07), and VIDOM with a greater improvement in SRS-awareness (P = .01 and ηp 2 = 0.11) and a trend for greater improvement in SRS-social communicative functioning (P = .05 and ηp 2 = 0.07) compared with placebo (not adjusted for multiple outcome measure comparisons). However, in the second mixed model analysis, when only children with elevated IL-1β at baseline were included, VID was associated with a greater improvement in SRS-awareness (P = .01 and ηp 2 = 0.14) and a trend for greater improvement in SRS-total (P = .07 and ηp 2 = 0.08), SRS-communication (P = .07 and ηp 2 = 0.07) and SRS-social communicative functioning (P = .09 and ηp 2 = 0.07), OM was associated with a greater improvement in SRS-awareness (P = .003 and ηp 2 = 0.18), SRS-total (P = .01 and ηp 2 = 0.14), SRS-social communicative functioning (P = .03 and ηp 2 = 0.11) and a trend for greater improvement in SRS-motivation (P = .05 and ηp 2 = 0.09), VIDOM with a greater improvement in SRS-awareness (P = .01 and ηp 2 = 0.14) and a trend for greater improvement in SRS-social communicative functioning (P = .05 and ηp 2 = 0.09) compared with placebo (not adjusted for multiple outcome measures comparisons). Due to the small sample size, no subgroup analysis was performed for those with undetectable/normal IL-1β. In this exploratory analysis of data from the VIDOMA trial, the authors found that both vitamin D and omega-3, either individually or together, were significantly superior to placebo in improving several domains of social and communicative functioning when pretreatment blood IL-1β concentrations were elevated.

In a 6-week randomized controlled trial with 57 children aged 5 to 8 yrs. with ASD, Omega-3 at 1.3 g/d showed a nominally (not significant) greater reduction in hyperactivity (−5.3) than placebo (−2.6).[31] With 1.5 gm/d Ω 3 fatty acids in thirteen 5 to 17 yr. old with ASD accompanied by severe tantrums and aggression, Amminger and colleagues, found a trend toward improvement for hyperactivity (0.71, P = .098) in the OM group.[32] Thus, evidence suggests a possible modest effect. Failure to find significance consistently may be secondary to small study sizes and low dosages in some studies of EPA/DHA combination. Most studies in ASD have used 1.3 to 1.5 gm/d, but one dipped as low as 722 mg/d and included only DHA. Weight-based dosing has not been used. Considering the current data on efficacy and adverse effects, a subset of individuals with ASD may respond to this intervention. In an open-label trial by Posar and Visconti 2016, 41 participants showed significant improvement on all subscales of SRS and Social and Attention Problems scales of CBCL. In this study, baseline fatty acid levels were predictive of response to omega −3 treatment.[22] Treatment guidelines based on RCT's and systematic reviews were recommended[33]: (1) ADHD: a combination of eicosapentaenoic acid (EPA) + docosahexaenoic acid (DHA) $\geq$ 750 mg/d, and a higher dose of EPA (1200 mg/d) for those with inflammation or allergic diseases for 16−24 weeks; (2) Major Depression: a combination of a EPA + DHA of

1000–2000 mg/d, with EPA:DHA ratio of 2 to 1, for 12–16 weeks; (3) ASD: a combination of EPA + DHA of 1300–1500 mg/d for 16–24 weeks as add-on therapy targeting lethargy and hyperactivity. The dose recommendations were based on available studies. However, given that ASD children have a high ratio of n-6 LCPUFA to n-3 LCPUFA and anti-inflammatory effect of EPA, the 2/1 ratio of EPA/DHA may be better in ASD children with obvious inflammation.[34] Nevertheless, optimal doses and ratios have not been established. Adverse effects of Omega 3 are mild and include nausea, diarrhea, and increased risk of bleeding on greater than 3 gm/d of fish oil. A fishy taste may make it less palatable, particularly for those with sensory sensitivities. The authors recommend that Omega 3 fatty acids be stopped 1 to 2 days before any surgeries as a precautionary measure against bleeding; the surgeon's advice should be sought.

To summarize, both short- and long-term studies support low rates of adverse events, good tolerability, and acceptance of omega-3 supplements. In general, omega-3 may reduce hyperactivity, irritability, lethargy, and language impairment in a subset of children, especially those with low levels of omega-3 fatty acids and increased inflammatory markers like IL-1β. More studies using weight-based dosing, different ratios of EPA to DHA, and a longer duration of treatment are needed.

N-Acetylcysteine

N-Acetylcysteine (NAC) is an antioxidant derived from the amino acid L-cysteine. It is a glutamatergic modulator and modulates apoptosis, neuroinflammation, glutamate, and dopamine dysregulation. Individuals with ASD have lower plasma GSH (glutathione) and higher glutathione disulfide than controls.[35] It has attracted attention in the treatment of ASD because glutamate-GABA abnormalities in the corticostriatal circuitry are proposed. At least 4 double-blind RCTs have studied its efficacy and tolerability in children/adolescents with ASD. In 40 autistic children ages 4 to 12 yrs. NAC (600–900 mg daily) added to risperidone reduced the irritability & hyperactivity subscales of the ABC significantly more than risperidone alone (P = .02, .01).[36] This finding replicated an 8-week DBRPCT of 40 children with autism whereby NAC + risperidone was superior to risperidone alone for irritability.[37]

Hardan and colleagues (2012) published a 12-week DBRPCT of NAC with 33 autistic children aged 3 to 10 yr. randomized to NAC 3600 mg/d titrated over 4 weeks. NAC showed significantly greater improvement on the ABC irritability subscale than placebo (d = 0.6) and was well tolerated.[38] In a 6-month long RCT of 102 prepubertal children (3–9.9 yr), NAC did not separate from placebo on SRS, Vineland, or ADOS, but conclusions were limited by the low dosing of 500 mg/d 39 However, Wink and colleagues (2016) in a DBRPCT of 31 children 4 to 12 yrs. od using NAC at 60 mg/kg/d found no significant difference in CGI severity scores.[40] Nevertheless, glutathione levels did increase, which may be useful for decreasing oxidative stress.

To summarize, NAC can be a well-tolerated augmentation agent to target residual irritability and hyperactivity in children with ASD, specifically in situations whereby first- and second-line agents to treat hyperactivity (psychostimulants, alpha agonists, atomoxetine) have failed or have been poorly tolerated, and side effects limit dose increase of risperidone. Studies showed limited effect on core symptoms of autism. Mild gastrointestinal side effects can be expected at daily doses of 1800 to 2400 mg.

FOLATE, METHYLATION, AND TRANSSULFURATION CYCLES
Methyl B12

Methyl B12 is an essential cofactor in the transsulfuration and transmethylation pathway, which is necessary to maintain the levels of critical antioxidants cysteine and glutathione. Some children with ASD exhibit impaired methylation capacity and increased oxidative stress.[41] Based on this finding, Bertoglio K, et al (2010) completed a 12-week double-blind, placebo-controlled cross-over trial of 30 patients who were randomized to receive methyl B12 injections of 64.5 mcg/kg every 3 days.[42] B12 injections were well tolerated, but no statistically significant difference was found on means for behavioral or glutathione endpoints overall. However, a subset of 30% did show significant improvement in the CGI- Improvement scale and 2 behavioral measures only when on active treatment, particularly if they had a high glutathione redox status (GSH/GSSG). Side effects included hyperactivity and increased mouthing behaviors. In a larger study, Hendren and colleagues (2016) found considerable improvement in clinician-rated CGI- I in 50 children (average age 5.3 yrs.) after receiving methlyb12 injections (75 mcg/kg) versus saline every 3 days for 8 weeks.[43] More extended and larger studies with adequate dosing are needed to assess possible benefits for core symptoms of autism.

Oxidative Stress in the Folate and Methylation Cycles in Autism

However, methyl B12 alone may not be sufficient; other factors also play a role in the folate, methylation, and transsulfuration cycles (**Fig. 1**). Interventions may have to be multi-modal and specific to the individual child. The folate, methylation, and trans-sulfuration cycles are important to (A) the formation of neurotransmitters, (B) the methylation of DNA, affecting epigenetic events, and (C) the diversion of homocysteine in the methyl cycle to form glutathione in the transsulfuration cycle to neutralize reactive oxygen species (see **Fig. 1**).[44] To focus on the methylation cycle, a decrease in the active form of vitamin B9, 5-methyltetrahydrofolate or L methyl-folate (5-MTHF) would increase homocysteine and decrease S-adenosylmethionine (SAMe), necessary for the methylation of DNA. Low DNA methylation has been associated with autism.[45] Likewise, decreased absorption of B 12, which donates a methyl group to homocysteine and joins L-methylfolate to produce SAM-e, would

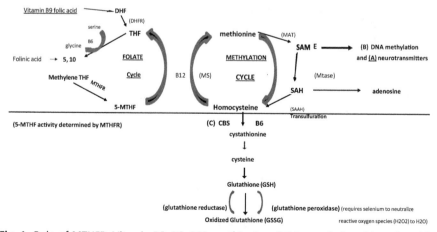

Fig. 1. Role of MTHFR, Vitamin B9, B6, B12, methionine, SAM-e, and glutathione in oxidative stress and MTHFR. 5-MTHF, 5- methyl tetrahydrofolate (L-methyl folate); CBS, cystathionine beta-synthase; DHF, dihydrofolate; DHFR, DHF reductase; MAT, methionine adenosyltransferase; MS, methionine synthase; Mtase, methyltransferase; SAH, S-adenosyl-homocysteine; SAHH, S-adenosyl-L-homocysteine hydrolase-transsulfuration; SAM-E, S-adenosylmethionine; THF, Tetrahydrofolate.

decrease the methylation of DNA, as well as decrease absorption of vitamin B6 needed to convert the tetrahydrofolate (THF) to. N5, N10 methylene THF via dihydrofolate reductase (DHFR). Thus, decreased absorption of B12, B6, and/or folate due to such things as dysbiosis could disrupt this process even when there is no genetic risk associated with MTHFR.[44]

As discussed by Steluti and colleagues (2017), the folate cycle also supports the formation of DNA by 2 other processes.[46] First, N5, N10 Methylene Tetrahydrofolate (THF) is used to form pyrimidines for the synthesis of cytosine and thymine bases of DNA (**Fig. 2**). N5, N10 Methylene THF is then cycled back to dihydrofolate (DHF). Second, THF also can be converted to 10 Formyl THF to form purines for the synthesis of adenine and guanine bases of DNA (**Fig. 3**). 10, Formyl THF can be recycled back to N5, N10 Methyl THF directly or to THF where it can form 5, 10 Methylene THF. A byproduct of the formation of purines is guanosine triphosphate (GTP) (see **Fig. 3**).

Folate deficiencies can result in DNA damage and serious pathologies, such as neural tube defects, megaloblastic anemia, acceleration of arteriosclerosis, changes in the central nervous system, and certain types of cancer[47] and autism.[48] In addition, oxidative stress, with reactive oxygen species (ROS), can damage both membrane lipid and embedded folate transporting proteins and hence impair net folate transport to the CNS.[49] Hence, reducing oxidative stress and preventing folate deficiency can decrease the risk of autism.

Oxidative stress may decrease folate transport, but it can also hinder the folate/methylation cycle in 2 other ways. First, GTP is converted to tetrahydrobiopterin (BH4). Although DHF is converted to tetrahydrofolate (THF) by the enzyme dihydrofolate reductase (DHFR), DHFR can also convert dihydrobiopterin (BH2) to tetrahydrobiopterin (BH4). BH2 can also be converted to BH4 by dihydropteridine reductase (QPDR). DHFR is used as a backup system when there is a defect in QPDR (**Fig. 4**). If Folic acid or BH4 is low, nitric oxide synthetase (NOS) coupled with BH2 promotes the formation of superoxides and hydrogen peroxide, 2 highly toxic reactive oxygen species (ROS). BH4 is needed to assure that ROS are not produced. DHFR will convert BH2 to BH4 to try to circumvent the formation of ROS while decreasing the conversion of DHF to THF thus decreasing the amount of 5-MTHF available for the methylation cycle (see **Fig. 4**).[50] Second, As BH4 is used as a co-factor for tyrosine hydroxylase to convert tyrosine to dopamine and for tryptophan hydroxylase to convert tryptophan to serotonin, if BH4 is low secondary to oxidative stress, those neurotransmitter levels may decrease (see **Fig. 4**). BH4 is also used as a co-enzyme for nitric oxide synthetase to convert arginine to Nitric oxide (NO), which dilates blood vessels. When ROS levels

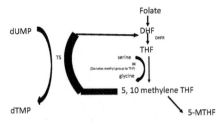

Fig. 2. N5, N10 methylene THF is used to produce pyrimidines for cytosine and thymine bases of DNA. DHF, dihydrofolate; DHFR, Dihydrofolate reductase; dTMP, deoxythymidine monophosphate; dUMP, deoxyuridine monophosphate; THF, tetrahydrofolate; TS, thymidylate synthase.

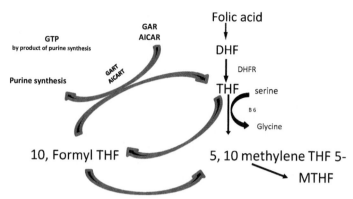

Fig. 3. THF can be used to form 10, formyl tetrahydrofolate (THF) which is used to form purine synthesis of adenine and guanine DNA bases. AICAR, 5-aminoimidazole-4-carboxamide ribonucleotide; AICARFT, 5-aminoimidazole-4-carboxamide ribonucleotide formyltransferase; DHF, dihydrofolate; DHFR, Dihydrofolate reductase; dTMP, deoxythymidine monophosphate; dUMP, deoxyuridine monophosphate; GAR, glycinamide ribonucleotide; GART, glycinamide ribonucleotide transformylase; GTP, Guanosine triphosphate; THF, tetrahydrofolate; TS, thymidylate synthase.

rise, S-adenosylmethionine (SAMe) may be diverted to S-adenosylhomocysteine (SA) to produce homocysteine if glutathione is needed to neutralize hydrogen peroxides produced during oxidative stress (see **Fig. 1**). In either of these cases, one would expect to see a decreased ratio of glutathione (GSH) to oxidized glutathione (GSSH). One might also suspect that folic acid and BH4 are low.

FOLINIC ACID

Folinic acid (a reduced form of Folic acid) can easily be converted to 5, 10 methylene THF which can then be directly converted to 5-MTHF by MTHFR (see **Fig. 1**). In a

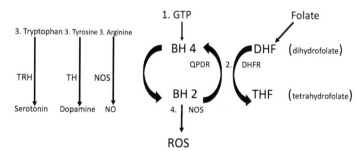

Fig. 4. When 10, formyl THF is formed from THF to produce purines for DNA synthesis, a by-product is GTP. 1. Guanosine triphosphate (GTP) is used to produce tetrahydrobiopterin (BH4), which is the co-factor for enzymes producing dopamine, serotonin, and Nitric oxide (NO). 2. Dihydrofolate reductase (DHFR) can convert DHF to THF, and dihydrobiopterin (BH2) to tetrahydrobiopterin (BH4) or BH2 can be converted to BH4 by dihydropteridine reductase (QPDR). 3. BH 4 is a co-factor used to form serotonin, dopamine, and nitric oxide (NO), by way of the enzymes tryptophan hydroxylase (TRH), tyrosine hydroxylase (TH), and nitric oxide synthetase (NOS). 4. If BH 4 is unavailable, BH 2 will form reactive oxygen species (ROS) like superoxides and hydrogen peroxides using NOS, thereby increasing oxidative stress.

DBPCT, 55 children with ASD mean age of 13.4 ± 2.0 yrs. (35 men) were randomized to 10 weeks of folinic acid (2 mg/kg vs placebo up to 50 mg/d). Repeated measures analysis showed significant time × treatment interaction on Aberrant Behavior Checklist inappropriate speech (F = 3.51; df = 1.61; P = .044), stereotypic behavior (F = 4.02; df = 1.37; P = .036), and hyperactivity/noncompliance (F = 6.79; df = 1.66; P = .003) subscales. In contrast, no significant effect was found on lethargy/social withdrawal (F = 1.06; df = 1.57; P = .336) or irritability (F = 2.86; df = 1.91; P = .064) subscales.[51] A meta-analysis showed that MTHFR 677C > T and 1298A > C polymorphisms are involved in genetic susceptibility to autism by ethnicity. MTHFR 677 C > T polymorphism is associated with increased ASD risk overall and by ethnicity, while MTHFR 1298A > C was significantly associated with ASD risk only in Caucasians.[52] Either way, an MTHFR defect may be addressed by using folinic acid.

ROLE OF FOLATE, FOLATE RECEPTOR α (FRα), AND FRα AUTOANTIBODIES

Cerebral folate deficiency, a disorder in which folate concentrations are below normal in the cerebrospinal fluid (CSF) but not in the blood, has been linked to autism. Folate is primarily transported across the choroid plexus epithelium attached to the folate receptor α (FRα). FRα dysfunction was linked to FRα autoantibodies (FRAAs). There are 2 types of FRAAs. Blocking FRAA interferes with the binding of folate to the FRα; binding FRAA binds to the FRα and triggers an antibody-mediated immune reaction. Folinic acid can cross the blood-brain barrier by using the reduced folate carrier (RFC) when the FRα is blocked by FRAAs or is nonfunctional due to a mitochondrial dysfunction and/or genetic mutations.[53] In an RDBPCT, 48 children (mean age 7.3 years; 82% male) with ASD and language impairment were randomized to 12 weeks of high dose folinic acid (2 mg kg/d, maximum 50 mg/d; n23) or placebo (n = 25).[54,55] Children were subtyped by glutathione and folate receptor-α autoantibody (FRAA). For FRAA-positive participants, improvement in verbal communication was significantly greater in those receiving folinic acid than in those receiving placebo (Cohen's d = 0.91). Improvements in subscales of the Vineland Adaptive Behavior Scale, the Aberrant Behavior Checklist, the Autism Symptom Questionnaire, and the Behavioral Assessment System for Children were significantly greater in the folinic acid group than with placebo. There was no significant difference in adverse events.

Vargasen and colleagues (2018) compared 3 clinical trials: 1. Methylcobalamin (methyl B12, met B12, or MeCbL) (75 mcg/kg every 3 days) + oral low dose folinic acid (LDFA) (400 mcg b.i.d.) to 40 children with autism 2 to 7 years old for 12-weeks in an open trial; 2. High dose folinic acid (HDFA)-2 mg/kg/d up to 50 mg/d for 12 weeks to 23 children 3 to 14 year old in a DBPCT; 3. Tetrahydrobiopterin (BH4) (20 mg/kg once daily) in an open label trial for 16 weeks to 10 children 2 to 6 years old.[5] Concentrations and ratios of metabolites in the folate-dependent one-carbon metabolism (FOCM) and transsulfuration (TS) pathways were measured in each study, with 15 measurements in each (the 3 above and placebo or typically developing children) data set. Six of these measures were associated with DNA methylation: methionine, S-adenosylmethionine (SAM), S-adenosylhomocysteine (SAH), the SAM/SAH ratio (an indicator of DNA methylation capacity), homocysteine, and adenosine. The remaining 9 measures were precursors of glutathione or markers of redox metabolism: total cysteine, glutamylcysteine (Glu-Cys), cysteinylglycine (Cys-Gly), total and free reduced glutathione (tGSH and fGSH, respectively), oxidized glutathione (GSSG), the ratios of total and free reduced glutathione to oxidized glutathione (tGSH/GSSG and fGSH/GSSG, respectively, indicators of intra-cellular oxidative stress), and percent oxidized glutathione [a derived measure calcu-lated as 2GSSG/(GSH + 2GSSG)]. The study attempted to predict changes in adaptive behavior, as quantified by the Vineland Adaptive Behavior Scales (VABS) Composite score, from changes in FOCM/TS measurements. Treatment with MeCbl with or without LDFA significantly shifted the metabolites toward the values of the control group. Contrary to this, treatment with HDFA had a smaller, though still noticeable, effect while the placebo group showed marginal, but not clinically insig-nificant, variations in metabolites. A second analysis was then performed to predict changes in adaptive behavior, quantified by the Vineland Adaptive Behavior Com-posite, from changes in (FOCM) and transsulfuration (TS). The 6 FOCM/TS biochem-ical measurements with the highest cross-validated response to treatment were 1-methionine, 1-Glu-Cys, 1-Cys-Gly, 1-tGSH, 1-tGSH/GSSG, and 1-fGSH/GSSG, all of which are measures of percent oxidized glutathione. The Vineland Adaptive Behavior Composite improvements were negatively associated with percent oxidized glutathione, which was related to oxidative stress. Despite the improve-ments, however, no treatment came close to offering complete normalization of FOCM/TS metabolism; the highest ASD misclassification rate was 49.5% in the HDFA treatment group. In another study, Li and colleagues (2018) did find that the measure of percent DNA methylation has even greater importance to the ASD/TD (typically developing) classification than percent oxidized glutathione.[56] However, this study was not able to measure the link to DNA methylation that has also been related to improvements on the VABS.

A systematic review identified studies reporting folate receptor alpha antibodies (FRAAs) in association with ASD, or the use of d,l-leucovorin (folinic acid) in the treatment of ASD.[57] D,l,-leucovorin is reduced folate that can bypass the blockage at the folate receptor alpha by using the reduced folate carrier. A meta-analysis found that the pooled prevalence of ASD in individuals with cerebral folate defi-ciency (CFD) was 44%, while the pooled prevalence of CFD in ASD was 38% (with cross-study heterogeneity). The etiology of CFD in ASD was attributed to FRAAs in 83% of the cases and mitochondrial dysfunction in 43%. A significant in-verse correlation was found between FRAA serum titers and 5-MTHF CSF concen-trations in 2 studies. The prevalence of FRAA in ASD was 71%. Children with ASD were 19-fold more likely to have an FRAA compared with typically developing chil-dren without an ASD sibling. For individuals with ASD and CFD, meta-analysis also found improvements with d,l-leucovorin in overall ASD symptoms (67%), irritability (58%), ataxia (88%), pyramidal signs (76%), movement disorders (47%), and epi-lepsy (75%). Twenty-one studies (including 4 placebo-controlled and 3 other pro-spective, controlled) Found d,l-Leucovorin to significantly improve communication with medium-to-large effect sizes and have a positive effect on core ASD symp-toms and associated behaviors (attention and stereotypy). Significant adverse ef-fects across studies were generally mild, the most common being aggression (9.5%), excitement or agitation (11.7%), headache (4.9%), insomnia (8.5%), and increased tantrums (6.2%). Taken together, d,l-leucovorin (folinic acid) seems to improve core and associated symptoms of ASD and seems safe and generally well-tolerated, with the strongest evidence from the blinded, placebo-controlled studies.

DAIRY EXCLUSION DIET: There seems to be a correlation between dairy and FRAAs. FRA blocked per ml of serum significantly decreased after 3 to 13 months on a milk-free diet. In 7 of the 12 patients, FR autoantibody titers decreased below detectable limits, and all enjoyed a significant decrease in the antibody titer. The antibody titer did not decrease in a comparison group of 12 patients maintained on folinic acid and a regular diet containing milk products. During the 3 to 13 months on a milk-free diet, signs of ataxia improved or disappeared completely in all except the oldest patient, who had been diagnosed at age 19 years. One patient with severe ataxia, who had remained nonambulatory during treatment with folinic acid, started to walk. The diet also led to complete seizure control in 2 patients. One autistic patient who had partly improved with folinic acid showed a marked further improvement with milk-free diet in communication skills with fewer stereotypies. The onset of the disorder during the first 3 to 6 months of life, after the switch to bovine milk, suggests a delayed or disrupted synergy between the adaptive and innate immune systems in the gut.[58]

To summarize, the role of the folate and methylation cycles may play a substantial role in the risk of developing autism and the severity of the symptoms. For children with MTHFR defects, the use of folinic acid (leucovorin) may be a way to address 5-MTHF deficiencies as folinic acid can directly enter the folate cycle as N5, N10, Methylene THF, especially when children carry the FRAAs. Eliminating bovine milk from the diets of these children, especially early in life, may deter the possible harmful effects that FRAAs may have on the folate and methylation cycles. Correlations to these treatments, improvements on the Vineland Applied Behavior Scale and improvements in normalizing the FOCM/TS components in regard to oxidized glutathione and the link to DNA methylation should be included in future research.

Probiotics

A systemic review identified studies that attempted to ameliorate behavioral manifestations of ASD via modifying the gut microbiome to modulate the gut-brain-microbiome axis.[59] Autistic children are known to manifest many GI problems. Gut dysbiosis may increase intestinal permeability, leading to more severe GI symptoms and a systemic inflammatory response, which can alter permeability across the blood-brain barrier and synaptogenesis in the brain. Eleven RCTs were identified. The most effective probiotics supplemented multiple species, such as the VIS-BIOME probiotic (4 strains of lactobacilli, 3 strains of bifidobacteria, and one strain of S. thermophiles) and the Microbiota Transfer Therapy (MTT). These supplements significantly decreased GI distress, particularly constipation, and significantly improved certain aspects of behavior such as repetitive and oppositional/defiant behaviors. In the visbiome study,[60] GI distress significantly correlated with the abundance of Lactobacillus; however, there were no discernible changes in microbiota composition. These results were not significant, although PedsQL did have a medium effect size (d = 0.49). Notably, the effects of the probiotic were carried over through the 3-week washout period. The strength of this study was using a probiotic supplement that contained diverse microbial species (8 different species of bacteria).

In an intensive probiotic therapy, a study used microbiota transfer therapy (MTT) to completely replace the gut microbiome in children.[61] The MTT procedure involved a 2-week antibiotic treatment (oral vancomycin), a bowel cleanse, and then an extended fecal microbiota transplant (FMT), which consisted of a high initial dose followed by daily and maintenance doses for 7 to 8 weeks. The successful microbial colonization was confirmed via NGS sequencing. The overall bacterial diversity and the abundance of Bifidobacterium, Prevotella, and Desulfovibrio, among others, increased following MTT, and these changes persisted even after the cessation of treatment (followed for 8 weeks). MTT increased diversity in children with ASD ($P = .001$) and remained higher than baseline 8 weeks posttreatment. Overall, there was an 80% reduction in

GI symptoms by the end of treatment and a 72% reduction after 8 weeks posttreatment ($P < .001$). The childhood Autism Rating Scale (CARS), which rates core ASD symptoms, decreased by 22% from the beginning to the end of the treatment and remained decreased by 24% (relative to baseline) 8 weeks after treatment was discontinued ($P < .001$). Furthermore, the average developmental age increased by 1.4 years during the 18 weeks ($P < .001$) across all subdomain areas.

Three prebiotic studies indicated auspicious results. All 3 studies had positive outcomes after prebiotic supplementation, particularly improving GI complaints. These associations are especially promising as the highest prebiotic dose contained only 4.8 g of prebiotic, while the lowest contained just 0.319 to 0.675 g per day. These dosages are particularly low considering that the recommended daily value of fiber is 30 g per day, and children with ASD typically consume around half of that dose. In 2 studies bacterial diversity decreased despite improvements in symptoms. However, the prebiotic supplementation significantly altered fecal and urine metabolites, by increasing short-chain fatty acids (SCFAs), particularly butyrate, which maintains gut integrity and is known to be significantly lower in children with autism. Dysbiosis is associated with an increase in lipopolysaccharides (LPS) from gram-negative bacteria which increase in numbers as healthy bacteria that produced SCFA decrease in numbers. LPS induces an inflammatory process that increases inflammatory cytokines (g TNF-α, IL-1β, and IL-13).and a corresponding increase of neuroinflammation in the brain occurs.[62]

It is critically important to note that many of these benefits were temporary, lasting only as long as the probiotic/prebiotic was administered. There were no discernible changes in microbiota composition or diversity longer than the washout period. MTT is a notable exception to this observation. Administering a standard microbiome extract ameliorated ASD symptoms and microbial diversity for 2 years postadministration. Overall, the most promising results were seen with complex, sustained interventions involving more than one treatment modality such as MTT and combined prebiotic-probiotic supplementation. It seems that eliminating pathogenic species, reseeding the gut with a diverse combination of bacteria, followed by sustained, meaningful prebiotic use is more likely to establish a lasting therapeutic microbiome. Although this approach is supported by mouse studies, especially for Lactobacillus reuteri, further human research is needed to confirm clinical utility with details.

OTHER EXCLUSION DIETS

Gluten and casein-free diet are among the most popular dietary interventions that families of children with ASD attempt, due to the popular hypothesis that gut inflammation leads to increased gut permeability, leading to excessive opioid activity and core symptoms of ASD. Interest in the link between gluten and ASD started around 1969 when studies looked at the prevalence of Celiac disease (CD) in autism and schizophrenia and found it higher than in the general population.[63] These studies were limited by a lack of diagnostic confirmation of either condition. Since then, several larger studies have indicated that ASD does appear comorbid with CD. Additionally, the heightened rate of gastrointestinal symptoms in children with ASD has also contributed to ongoing interest in the use of dietary modification to target ASD symptoms.[64] These findings related to the autoimmunity theory of autism have led to ongoing interest in exclusion diets to reduce the presence of dietary proteins that may increase immune reactive intermediary substances with opioid activity.[65]

Studies showing increased gut permeability, inflammation caused by oxidative stress, and shared genetic factors between CD and a sub-set of the ASD population supported continued interest in these interventions.[66] About 13 RCTs to date have studied the impact of gluten and casein-free diets on behavioral and social symptoms of autism. half showed some improvement while 6 had negative results. Study limitations include the high risk of the placebo/nocebo effect due to studies being unblinded. Additionally, the short length of the studies possibly missed the time required for physiologic adjustments to different dietary regimens and hence, potential clinical impact on symptoms. In a crossover design, 37 children without gluten/casein allergies with autism were randomized to 6 months GFCFD (gluten-free and casein-free diet) or regular diet first, then crossed over to the opposite diet. No significant difference in behavioral symptoms or urinary beta-casomorphin concentration was found.[67]

Due to the lack of adequately sized, adequate duration, placebo-controlled trials, and considering the nutritional impact, a GF/CF diet is currently not recommended except dairy-free for proven cases of FRAAs as outlined above. For families interested in trying these exclusion diets, clinicians should recommend the supervision of a nutritionist/dietician.

Multivitamins

The severity of autism has been related to the severity of nutritional deficiencies. There are very few trials of micronutrient (vitamins & minerals) supplementation in children. A placebo-controlled pilot of 20 children aged 3 to 8 years found micronutrient supplements associated with better sleep and fewer gastrointestinal symptoms.[68] An RCT of oral vitamin and mineral supplementation of 141 children and adults with autism showed significantly more improvement in hyperactivity and melt downs than with placebo.[69] Due to the limited number of studies, this treatment has not routinely been recommended unless there are concerns for nutritional deficiencies, which are likely with the idiosyncratic diets many children with autism restrict themselves to. However, in a large systematic review and meta-analysis of 5 articles, 9 independent trials, 231,163 children, and 4459 cases, prenatal multivitamin was associated with decreased risk of autism in offspring (RR, 0.62; 95% CI, 0.45–0.86; $P = .003$).[70] Based on the low risk, ease, low expense, and logical sense, it passes the SECS criterion.

Cannabinoids/Cannabidiol

Imbalance in the cannabinoid systems has been reported in children with ASD. Anandamide, an endocannabinoid, is at a lower concentration in children with autism versus neurotypical peers.[71] Increased expression of CB2 receptors is found in mononuclear cells of autistic children.[72] Epidiolex is the first cannabinoid compound that has been FDA approved for use in children, those with seizures such as Dravet Syndrome/Lenox Gastaut Syndrome, which has high rates of autism-like symptoms (FDA announcement 2020).[73] To date, no large placebo-controlled trials establishing the efficacy of cannabinoids, CBD or Tetrahydrocannabinol (THC) in treating core symptoms of autism or behavioral problems have been completed. Open-label trials are primarily observational. In a double-blind randomized crossover study of 150 children with autism, 2 oral cannabidiol solutions (whole plant extract & purified form of cannabis) with 20:1 CBD: THC ratio produced insignificant differences from placebo on outcome scales such as the CGI, HSQ-ASD, and SRS.[74] Despite several well-designed trials underway to study the efficacy and tolerability of cannabis in autism spectrum disorder, the data needed to guide clinical treatment are currently absent and this does not yet pass the SECS criterion, given the known risks.

MIND-BODY THERAPEUTICS
Music Therapy

Per the American Music Therapy Association, Music Therapy is the clinical and evidence-based use of music interventions to accomplish individualized goals within a therapeutic relationship by a credentialed professional who has completed an approved music therapy program. Recent years have seen several case studies and narrative and systematic reviews on this topic, reporting mixed results.

In an RCT of 51 children aged 6 to 12 years Sharda and colleagues (2018), children were randomized to musical versus nonmusical intervention, a structurally matched behavioral intervention.[75] Both interventions were 45-min-long weekly sessions by the same accredited Music Therapist who used musical instruments and rhythmic cues to target social communication skills. Postintervention, communication scores (Children's Communication Checklist) were higher in the music group ($P = .01$). In the music group, compared with the behavioral treatment, post-intervention resting-state brain functional connectivity was greater between auditory and subcortical regions ($z = 3.94$, P,0.0001) and between auditory and frontal-motor regions ($z = 3.16$, P, 0.0001), and lower between auditory and visual regions ($z = 4.01$, $P<.00001$). Postintervention brain connectivity change in the music group was related to communication improvement ($z = 3.57$, $P<.0001$). Overall, pragmatic language skills seemed to be most affected by this intervention, while the impact on core symptoms of ASD was minimal. A limitation was that the outcome measures were parent-reported, and not all parents were blinded to the intervention arm of their children. In summary, music seems to improve social communication and auditory-motor connectivity in children with autism.

In a review of 10 controlled trials in 165 children with ASD comparing music therapy alone to music therapy + standard care to placebo found that music therapy may improve social-emotional reciprocity, social adaptation skills, and verbal and nonverbal communication skills within the therapy context.[76] However, The Trial of Improvisational Music Therapy's Effectiveness for Children with Autism (TIME-A) RCT with 364 children comparing improvisational music therapy to "enhanced standard care," which included usual local care, parent counseling and ASD psychoeducational psychotherapy, did not find any significant difference in ASD symptom severity based on ADOS social effect. This study's limitations include the importance of assessing the quality of life and adaptive functioning in addition to the severity of ASD symptoms.[77]

Current data show little improvement in core ASD symptomatology with music therapy except pragmatic speech based on one trial.[75] However, this intervention may pass SECS in a particular context, to increase involvement/participation in community activities[78] –but the time/resource burden of balancing other therapies with more robust evidence should be considered.

Acupuncture
Acupuncture involves the insertion of needles into the skin and tissues for therapeutic purposes. It is currently widely used for pain, nausea, and anxiety. Its use in ASD families varies based on demographics. A survey of caregivers in a neurodevelopmental pediatric clinic at Children's Hospital in Hong Kong established prevalence rates as high as 40%, compared with 1% in families in the US and Canada.[79] The possible mechanism of action is unclear.

At least 16 RCTs have examined the safety and efficacy of acupuncture for ASD. Results have been mixed/inconclusive. A systematic review and meta-analysis of 27 studies with 1736 patients showed that this treatment, when complemented with behavioral and educational interventions, significantly decreased overall scores on the CARS (MD-8.10, 95% CI -12.80—3.40) and the Autism Behavioral Checklist (MD -8.92 95%C −11.29 – to −6.54) and was well tolerated, with some efficacy in targeting symptoms of ASD.[80] This analysis found no significant difference between acupuncture + Behavioral and Education Interventions (BEI) groups versus BEI alone on communication skills, stereotypy, and language abilities. The authors cautioned against generalizing results due to heterogeneity in treatment modalities, performance biases, and location bias. The feasibility of this treatment of children has often been questioned due to the need to restrict limb activity during treatment. A systematic review and meta-analysis of 11 studies of scalp acupuncture treatment in 968 autistic children (some younger than 3 years) found that it may be more effective and faster than typical behavioral and educational interventions in decreasing CARS and ABC scores.[81] A 2011 systematic review of 11 RCTs found mixed evidence of effectiveness.[82]

A significant number of studies included in the systematic reviews above have not reported adverse events. Most available data suggest good tolerability without complications, but infections, bleeding, and injuries from improper use of treatment needles have been reported.

ANIMAL-ASSISTED THERAPIES

There is a recent surge in research studying the efficacy of animal-assisted therapies in children with autism and other disorders. They are often used in hospitalized children and youth. AAT is defined as sessions with therapeutic, health, and wellbeing goals involving the presence of animals.[83] Other forms of Animal-Assisted Intervention (AAI) include animal-assisted activities (animal visits to therapeutic placements) and animal-assisted education. A systematic review of several case studies suggests a general improvement in maladaptive behaviors, classroom participation, self-regulation, and social interactions.[84,85] In a meta-analysis involving 16 studies and 489 school-age autistic children, studies using an active-related comparison arm not involving an animal showed no difference in social interaction and communication skills compared with the animal-assisted intervention. However, the authors could not examine the impact of dosage in this analysis d/t lack of vital information in individual studies.[83]

Because of the popularity of equine therapy, it is prudent to discuss current evidence. Equine therapy can include mounted (hippo therapy and therapeutic horseback riding) and nonmounted equine-focused activities.[87] Hippotherapy (by Occupational Therapists and Physical Therapists) focuses on improving balance and sensory processing skills by using horse movements. Therapeutic horseback riding can focus on riding skills only. Studies have shown the positive impact on social interaction, sensory processing, and severity of autism on teacher-rated scales as long as patients were engaged in the activity.[88]

In a large-scale randomized controlled trial[86], 116 children with ASD aged 6 to 16 yr, were randomized to therapeutic horseback riding (THR) vs barn activity. The study revealed significant improvements in the THR group compared with the control on measures of irritability (primary outcome) (P = .002; d = .50) and hyperactivity (P = .001; d = 0.53), beginning by week 5 of the intervention, based on measures completed by nonblinded caregivers. Significant improvements in the THR group were also observed on a measure of social cognition (P = .05, d = .41) and social communication (P = .003; d = .63), along with the total number of words (P = .01; d = .54) and new words (P = .01; de = .54) spoken during a standardized language sample assessed by blinded speech therapists.[86]

In a systematic review of 15 experimental and quasi-experimental studies involving 294 children and youth with ASD, the authors discussed concerns about the poor methodological quality. Despite these concerns, the results suggested "consistent and reliable positive effects of short-term equine therapy on behavioral skills in autistic children." A current data review highlights the need for larger and longer studies using homogenous samples with strict adherence to treatment fidelity while using subjective and objective measures to assess social communication skills. Evidence of effect on QoL or functional skill is lacking.[87]

ENVIRONMENTAL TOXIN, GLYPHOSATE, AND AUTISM

The results of a systematic review demonstrate an interrelation between Clostridium bacterial colonization of the intestinal tract and autism.[89] Glyphosate is found in an herbicide spread over wheat, soybeans, and other crops. Clostridium, in contrast to many beneficial bacteria, is resistant to the antibiotic effects of glyphosate. Xiong and colleagues compared urinary biomarkers in 62 patients with ASD and 62 non-ASD controls in China, aged 1.5 to 7, and found 3 compounds in higher concentrations in autistic children: 3-(3-hydroxyphenyl)-3-hydroxypropionic acid (HPHPA); 3-hydroxyphenylacetic acid (3HPA); and 3-hydroxyhippuric acid (3HHA) (P < .001).[90] These metabolites are produced by clostridium. After oral vancomycin treatment, urinary excretion of HPHPA (P < .001), 3HPA (P < .005), and 3HHA (P < .001) decreased markedly, which confirmed that these compounds may be from gut Clostridium species. The sensitivity and specificity of HPHPA, 3HPA, and 3HHA were evaluated by receiver-operating characteristic (ROC) analysis. The optimal area under the curve (AUC, 0.962), sensitivity (90.3%), and specificity (98.4%) were obtained by the ROC curve of Prediction probability. Attempting to minimize exposure to toxins, including glyphosate, both in utero and during childhood, passes the SECS criteria, but might require food labeling definitions.

SUMMARY AND CLINICAL CONCLUSIONS

Most families use Complementary and Integrative Treatment of individuals with autism spectrum disorder. It is prudent that practitioners gain knowledge about the benefits and risks of these interventions to have an open, nonjudgmental conversation with families about their role when creating a comprehensive treatment plan. Due to the perceived safety profile of these interventions, families may fail to recognize and report potential adverse effects and drug interactions. In recent years researchers have focused on conducting randomized placebo-controlled studies on these interventions. However, larger and more prolonged-duration studies are needed to establish regular usage.

Additionally, it may be beneficial to examine the impact of these treatments on comorbid physical and psychiatric comorbidities that negatively impact the QoL. Elimination diets (gluten and/casein-free) based on the theories that food allergens trigger autoimmunity as well as "opioid excess" are shown to improve gastrointestinal symptoms in a subset of children with ASD without benefits on the core symptoms of autism. The current review of data points toward the potential benefits of omega-3 fatty acids on hyperactivity, irritability, and social behaviors in a subset of autistic children, with favorable side effect profiles. Vitamin supplementations

Table 1
Strength of evidence and recommendations of biomedical CAM treatment in ASD

Strength of Recommendations based on benefit and safety:

A = Recommend Strongly. There is a high certainty that the net benefit is substantial and safe.

B=Recommend. There is a high certainty that the net benefit is moderate or there is moderate certainty that the net benefit is moderate to substantial and safe.

C=Neutral (offer or provide this service for selected patients depending on individual circumstances, based on professional judgment and patient preferences). There is at least moderate certainty that the net benefit is small.

D = Discourage. There is moderate or high certainty that the service has no net benefit or that the harms outweigh the benefits

I = Insufficient (if the service is offered, patients should understand the uncertainty about the balance of benefits and harms) Current evidence is insufficient to assess the balance of benefits and harms of the service. Evidence is lacking, of poor quality, or conflicting, and the balance of benefits cannot be determined.)

Level of certainty regarding quality:

HIGH Level of Evidence with robust positive data meta-analyses or meta-reviews involving 2 or more RCTs of excellent, robust quality. The available evidence usually includes consistent results from well-designed, well-conducted RCTs in representative child, adolescent or young adult (18–24 year old) populations, assessing the effects on mental health outcomes.

MODERATE Level of Evidence with robust positive data involving 2 or more RCTs of excellent, robust quality. The available evidence usually includes consistent results from well-designed, well- conducted RCTs in representative child, adolescent or young adult (18–24 year old) populations, assessing the effects on mental health outcomes.

LOW Level of evidence with <2 RCTs with good or average quality. The available evidence is insufficient to assess the effects on mental health outcomes.

SECS Criteria:

A guide to clinical decisions is that Interventions that are Safe, Easy, Cheap, and Sensible (SECS) require less evidence to justify individual trials than those that are Risky, Unrealistic, Difficult, or Expensive (RUDE). Because some of the treatments do not have much solid, compelling evidence but would be reasonable to try with a lower bar of evidence, this criterion is also taken into account. Being risky, unrealistic, difficult OR expensive (RUDE) disqualifies from SECS. The bolded conjunctions are essential in applying this guide.

Treatment	Quality of Evidence Grade	Evidence Base in Youth	USPSTF Strength of Recommendations
Melatonin	High	18 trials;5 RCTs	A/Recommend Strongly
Omega 3 Fatty Acids	Moderate	4 Open trials;8 RCTs	B/Recommend
Multivitamin/ Micronutrients	Fair	2 RCTs	B/Recommend
N-Acetyl-Cysteine (NAC)	Moderate	1 RCT with group difference;1 negative 2 RCTs showing benefits of risperidone + NAC	B/Recommend to treat irritability as an augmentation agent to risperidone. Otherwise, C/Neutral.
Methycobalamine	Moderate	2 RCT (both positive, statistically sig positive change in one)	C/Neutral
Immune therapies	Low	None	I/Insufficient data

(continued on next page)

Table 1 (continued)			
Treatment	Quality of Evidence Grade	Evidence Base in Youth	USPSTF Strength of Recommendations
Intravenous Immunoglobulins	Low	None	D/recommend against
Chelation	Low	None	D/Recommend Against
Cannabinoid	Low	1 negative RCT	D/Recommend Against

including B6 + Mg and Vit C have been studied in several randomized controlled trials and have not shown statistically significant improvements in ASD symptomatology. However, Folinic Acid improved stereotypy, attention, and communication in autistic individuals with folate deficiencies. Additionally, multivitamins seem to be reasonably well tolerated and may be beneficial in autistic children with concerns for nutritional deficiencies. Several studies have looked at the role of vitamins, amino acids, and supplements in targeting commonly seen disruptive symptoms such as irritability and sleep-related problems and found limited benefits. One such agent, NAC, can be beneficial in targeting residual irritability and hyperactivity when used in combination with risperidone, with excellent tolerability in autistic children. Dosages of 1800 to 2400 mg/d may be required. Mild gastrointestinal side effects have been reported. NAC can also be beneficial in comorbid impulse control disorders such as excoriation disorder or trichotilomania. The use of exclusion diets continues to be popular in children and youth with autism, but the current data review does not support improvement in core autistic symptoms. There are concerns about nutritional deficiencies arising from some elimination diets in children with Celiac disease.

Insomnia is one of the most common clinical complaints in ASD, which significantly impacts the quality of life of children and caregivers alike. Frequently used sedative-hypnotics and sedative agent studies do not show long-term efficacy and may worsen daytime behaviors. Sleep hygiene techniques and CBT-I are still considered first-line treatments for insomnia in children with ASD. The effectiveness of melatonin in improving sleep efficiency and total sleep duration on both objective and subjective measures has been established in several randomized placebo-controlled trials, in dosages of 3 to 6 mg daily. Melatonin may be effective even in children who fail behavioral interventions for insomnia and is tolerated well with minimal side effects, such as nightmares in a minority of children.[91] Folinic acid seems to be emerging as a potentially safe treatment to target communication and stereotypy but larger sized trials are needed to establish clinical effectiveness and safety. Among other CIM treatments that continue to gain popularity, medical marijuana seems the most controversial. Currently, no double-blinded placed controlled trials studying its impact on either the core symptoms of autism or its comorbid psychiatric symptoms have been completed. Epidiolex, a cannabinoid agent, is FDA approved for complex, severe seizure syndromes associated with ASD. Treatments such as chelation, long-term usage of antibiotics immunoglobulins, secretin, and hyperbaric oxygen therapy have proven to be ineffective. These treatments have been ranked in the table below using the USPSTF scale of evidence-based literature (**Table 1**). In cases whereby specific treatments do not have substantial evidence either way yet, the SECS criteria (safe, easy, cheap, and sensible) have also been used to recommend clinical usage (**Table 2**).

Table 2
Evaluation of evidence of CIG treatment in ASD: authors' personal clinical opinion and application of the SECS criteria (safe, easy, cheap, and sensible) as indicated

Treatment	Strength of REC Based on Benefit/ Safety	Author's Clinical Recommendations
Melatonin	Reasonably Good Studies	Very Useful
Omega −3 fatty acids	Improvement trend noticed	Passes SECS. Trend of improvement in social communication & hyperactivity; small effect. Up to 1.5 g/d. Recommend. Possible side effect of bleeding; overall well tolerated. Studies from premature infants to 18 y old.
Multivitamin/ Micronutrients	Possible benefits	Passes SECS. Routinely Recommend. Significant modest benefits in GI symptoms, insomnia, receptive language, and tantruming. Rare diarrhea SE. Passes SECS at doses within upper tolerable limit. Prenatal MVI prevented offspring ASD
N-Acetyl- Cysteine	Promising	Suggest when targeting residual irritability, hyperactivity, or repetitive behaviors as an augmentation agent. Not to be used in patients with kidney disease. Well tolerated. May need to dose as high as 1800–2400 mg/d. Passes SECS
Methyl cobalamin	Promising for the subgroup of children only	Promising for global ASD in the genetic subgroup. Suggest with caution. Good safety profile. Passes SECS
Probiotics	Possible benefit	Specifically for comorbid gastrointestinal sx in some children. Passes SECS.
Folinic Acid	Possible benefits in individuals with Cerebral Folate Deficiency(CFD)	May benefit stereotypy and communication symptoms in specific individuals with CFD. Passes SECS
Digestive Enzymes	Not good evidence yet	May benefit those with intractable GI sx only. Does not pass SECS
Immune Therapies	No good data	Discourage, does not pass SECS
Intravenous Immunoglobulins	No good evidence	Discourage, does not pass SECS

(continued on next page)

Table 2 (continued)		
Treatment	Strength of REC Based on Benefit/ Safety	Author's Clinical Recommendations
Chelation	No good evidence	Does not pass SECS/Discourage
Medical Marijuana	No good evidence for core autistic sx or comorbid psychopathology	Does not pass SECS except in children with intractable epilepsy.

DISCLOSURE

Dr L.E. Arnold has received research funding from Supernus Pharmaceuticals, Roche/Genentech Pharmaceuticals, Otsuka Pharmaceuticals, Axial Yamo, and Young Living Essential Oils and the National Institutes of Health (USA, R01 MH 100144), has consulted with Pfizer Pharmaceuticals and CHADD, and been on advisory boards for Otsuka and Roche/Genentech. Dr R.L. Hendren has recent research grants from Curemark, Roche, Otsuka, GW LTD, and Axial Biotherapeutics; is on Advisory Boards for BioMarin, Axial Bio Therapeutics, and Janssen. Dr P. Vandana has no financial disclosures. Dr D.R. Simkins has no financial disclosures.

REFERENCES

1. Volkmar F, Siegel M, Woodbury-Smith M, et al. Practice parameters on autism spectrum disorder. J Am Acad Child Adolesc Psychiatry 2014;237–57.
2. Perrin JM, Coury DL, Hyman SL, et al. Complementary and alternative medicine use in a large pediatric sample. Pediatrics 2012;77–82.
3. Valicenti-McDermott M, Burrows B, Bernstein L. Use of complementary and Aolternative medicine in children with autism and other developmental Disabilities: Assocations with ethnicity , Child comorbid symptoms, and parental stress. J Child Neurol 2014;29(3):360–7.
4. Owen-Smith AA, Bent S, Lynch F, et al. Prevalence and predictors of complementary and alternative medicine Use in a large Uninsured sample of children with autism spectrum disorders. Res Autism Sectrum Disord 2015;40–51.
5. Hopf KP, Madren E, Santianni KA. Use and perceived effectiveness of complementary and alternative medicine to treat and manage the symptoms of autism in children: a Survery of parents in a community population. J Complement Med 2016;25–32.
6. Huang A, Seshadri K, Matthews TA, et al. Parental perspectives on use, benefits and physican knowledge of complementary and alternative medicine in children with autistic disorder and attention deficit/hyperactivity disorder. J Altern Complement Med 2013;746–50.
7. Hendren RL, Widjaja F, Lawton B. Complementary and integrative approaches. In: Eric Hollander FR, editor. Autism spectrum disorders. American Psychiatric Association Publishing; 2018. p. 347–70.
8. Rutten BP, Mill J. Epigenetic mediation of environmental Influences in major psychotic disorders. Schizophrenia Bull 2009;1045–56.
9. Buckley AW, Holmes GL. Epilepsy and autism. Cold Spring Harb Perspect Med 2016;6(4):a022749.
10. Giulivi C, Zhang YF, Omanska-Klusek A, et al. Mitochondrial dysfunction in autism. JAMA 2010;304(21):2389–96.

11. Waligóra A, Waligóra S, Kozarska M, et al. Autism spectrum disorder (ASD) - biomarkers of oxidative stress and methylation and transsulfuration cycle. Zaburzenia ze spektrum autyzmu (ASD) – biomarkery stresu oksydacyjnego oraz cyklu metylacji i transsulfuracji. Psychiatr Pol 2019;53(4):771–88.

12. Hagerman R, Hendren R. Overview of Neurodevelopmental Processes and the Assessment of Patients with Neurodevelopmental Disorders in Treatment of Neurodevelopmental Disorders: Targeting Neurobiological Mechanisms. 1st edition Pg 1-21.

13. Goldani AA, Downs SR, Widjaja F, et al. Biomarkers in autism. Front Psychiatry 2014;5:100.

14. Pu D, Shen Y, Wu J. Association between MTHFR gene polymorphisms and the risk of autism spectrum disorders: a meta-analysis. Autism Res 2013;6(5): 384–92.

15. Frye RE, Vassall S, Kaur G, et al. Emerging biomarkers in autism spectrum disorder: a systematic review. Ann Transl Med 2019;7(23):792.

16. Melke J. Abnormal Melatonin synthesis in autism spectrum disorders. Mol Psychiatry 2008;90–8.

17. Pagan C, Delorme R, Goubran-Botros H, et al. The serotonin N-Acetylserotoninmelatonin pathway as a biomarker for autism spectrum disorders. Translational Psychiatry 2014;4(11):e479.

18. Sivertsen B, Posserud M-B, Gillberg C, et al. Sleep problems in children with autism spectrum disorders: a longitudinal population-based study. Autism 2012;139–50.

19. Tordjman S, Najjar I, Bellissant E, et al. Advances in the research of melatonin in autism spectrum disorders: literature review and new perspectives. Int Jounral Mol Sci 2013;14(10):20508–42.

20. Rossignol DA, Frye RE. Melatonin in autism spectrum disorders: a systematic review and meta-analysis. Dev Med Child Neurol 2011;783–92.

21. Maras A, Schroder CM, Malow BA, et al. Long-term efficacy and safety of pediatric prolonged -release melatonin for insomnia in children with autism spectrum disorder. J Child Adole Psychopharm 2018;699–710.

22. Posar A, Visconti P. Omega-3 supplementation in autism spectrum disorders: a still open question? J Pediatr Neurosci 2016;225–7.

23. Freeman MP. Omega- 3 fatty acids : evidence basis for treatment and future research in psychiatry. J Clin Psychiatry 2006;1954–67.

24. Vancassel S, Durand G, Barthelemy C, et al. Plasma fatty acids in autistic children. Prostaglandins Leukot Essent Fatty Acids; 2001. p. 1–7.

25. Parletta N, Niyonsenga T, Duff J. Omega-3 and omega-6 polyunstaured fatty acid levels and Corelations with symptoms in children with ADHD , ASD and typically developing children. PLoS One 2016;11(5):e0156432.

26. Mazahery H, Stonehouse W, Delshad M, et al. Relationship between long chain n-3 polyunsaturated fatty acids and autism spectrum disorder: systematic review and meta-analysis of case-control and randomised controlled trials. Nutrients 2017;9(2):155.

27. Fraguas De. Dietary interventions for autism spectrum disorder: a meta Analyses. Pediatrics 2019;2018–3218.

28. Mazahery H, Conlon CA, Beck KL, et al. A randomised-controlled trial of vitamin D and omega-3 long chain polyunsaturated fatty acids in the treatment of core symptoms of autism spectrum disorder in children. J Autism Dev Disord 2019; 49(5):1778–94.

29. Mazahery H. A randomized controlled trial of vitamin D and omega-3 long chain polyunsaturated fatty acids in the treatment of irritability and hyperactivity among children with autism spectrum disorder. J Steroid Biochem Mol Biol 2019;9–16.

30. Mazahery H, Conlon CA, Beck KL, et al. Inflammation (IL-1β) Modifies the effect of vitamin D and omega-3 long chain polyunsaturated fatty acids on core symptoms of autism spectrum disorder-an exploratory pilot study‡. Nutrients 2020; 12(3):661.

31. Bent S, Hendren R, Zandi T, et al. Internet based , randomized , controlled trial of omega-2 fatty acids for hyperactivity in autism. JAACAP 2014;658–66.

32. Amminger GP, Berger GE, Schäfer MR, et al. Omega-3 fatty acids supplementation in children with autism: a double-blind randomized, placebo-controlled pilot study. Biol Psychiatry 2007;61(4):551–3.

33. Chang JP, Su KP. Nutritional Neuroscience as Mainstream of psychiatry: the evidence- based treatment guidelines for using omega-3 fatty acids as a new treatment for psychiatric disorders in children and adolescents. Clin Psychopharmacol Neurosci 2020;18(4):469–83.

34. Shang T, Liu L, Zhou J, et al. Protective effects of various ratios of DHA/EPA supplementation on high-fat diet-induced liver damage in mice. Lipids Health Dis 2017;16(1):65.

35. Bjørklund G, Meguid NA, El-Bana MA, et al. Oxidative stress in autism spectrum disorder. Mol Neurobiol 2020;57(5):2314–32.

36. Nikoo M, Radnia H, Farokhnia M, et al. N-acetylcysteine as an adjunctive therapy to risperidone for treatment of irritability in autism: a randomized, double-blind, placebo-controlled clinical trial of efficacy and safety. Clin Neuropharmacol 2015;38(1):11–7.

37. Ghanizadeh A, Derakhshan N. N-acetylcysteine for treatment of autism, a case report. J Res Med Sci 2012;985–7.

38. Hardan AY, Fung LK, Libove RA, et al. A randomized controlled pilot trial of oral N-acetylcysteine in children with autism. Biol Psychiatry 2012;956–61.

39. Dean O, Gray K, Villagonzalo K-A. A randomised, double blind, placebo-controlled trial of a fixed dose of N-acetyl cysteine in children with autistic disorder. Aust N Z J Psychiatry 2017;241–9.

40. Wink LK, Ryan A, Zemin W, et al. A randomized placebo-controlled pilot studoy of N-acetylcysteine in youth with autism spectrum disorder. Mol Autism 2016;7:26.

41. James, et al. Metabolic biomarkers of increased oxidative stress and impaired methylation capacity in children with autism. Am J Clin Nutr 2004;1611–7.

42. Bertoglio KJJ. Pilot study of the effect of methyl B12 treatment on behavioral and biomarker measures in children with autism. J Altern Complement Med 2010;555–60.

43. Hendren RL, James SJ, Widjaja F, et al. Randomized, placebo-controlled trial of methyl B12 for children with autism. J Child Adol Psychopharm 2016;774–83.

44. Simkin DR, Arnold LE. The roles of inflammation, oxidative stress and the gut-brain Axis in treatment Refractory Depression in youth: complementary and integrative medicine interventions. OBM Integr Complement Med 2020;5(4):040.

45. Hamza M, Halayem S, Mrad R, et al. Implication de l'épigénétique dans les troubles du spectre autistique: revue de la littérature [Epigenetics' implication in autism spectrum disorders: a review]. Encephale 2017;43(4):374–81.

46. Steluti J, Carvalho AM, Carioca AAF, et al. Genetic Variants involved in one-carbon metabolism: polymorphism Frequencies and differences in homocysteine concentrations in the folic acid Fortification Era. Nutrients 2017;9(6):539.

47. Czeczot H. Kwas foliowy w fizjologii i patologii [Folic acid in physiology and pathology]. Postepy Hig Med Dosw (Online) 2008;62:405–19.

48. Surén P, Roth C, Bresnahan M, et al. Association between maternal use of folic acid supplements and risk of autism spectrum disorders in children. JAMA 2013;309(6):570–7.

49. Ramaekers VT, Sequeira JM, Quadros EV. The basis for folinic acid treatment in neuro-psychiatric disorders. Biochimie 2016;126:79–90.

50. Crabtree MJ, Tatham AL, Hale AB, et al. Critical role for tetrahydrobiopterin recycling by dihydrofolate reductase in regulation of endothelial nitric-oxide synthase coupling: relative importance of the de novo biopterin synthesis versus salvage pathways. J Biol Chem 2009;284(41):28128–36.

51. Batebi N, Moghaddam HS, Hasanzadeh A, et al. Folinic acid as adjunctive therapy in treatment of inappropriate speech in children with autism: a double-blind and placebo-controlled randomized trial. Child Psychiatry Hum Dev 2021;52(5): 928–38.

52. Sadeghiyeh T, Dastgheib SA, Mirzaee-Khoramabadi K, et al. Association of MTHFR 677C>T and 1298A>C polymorphisms with susceptibility to autism: a systematic review and meta-analysis. Asian J Psychiatr 2019;46:54–61.

53. Frye RE, Delhey L, Slattery J, et al. Blocking and binding folate receptor alpha autoantibodies identify Novel autism spectrum disorder subgroups. Front Neurosci 2016;10:80.

54. Frye RE, Slattery J, Delhey L, et al. Folinic acid improves verbal communication in children with autism and language impairment: a randomized double-blind placebo-controlled trial. Mol Psychiatry 2018;23(2):247–56.

55. Vargason T, Kruger U, Roth E, et al. Comparison of three clinical trial treatments for autism spectrum disorder through Multivariate analysis of changes in metabolic profiles and adaptive behavior. Front Cell Neurosci 2018;12:503.

56. Li G, Lee O, Rabitz H. High efficiency classification of children with autism spectrum disorder. PLOS ONE 2018–;13(2):e0192867. Available at: https://doi.org/10. 1371/journal.pone.0192867. Accessed June 5, 2022.

57. Rossignol DA FR. Cerebral folate deficiency, folate receptor alpha autoantibodies and leucovorin (folinic acid) treatment in autism spectrum disorders: a systematic review and meta-analysis. J Personalized Med 2021;11(11):1141.

58. Ramaekers V, Blau N, Sequeira J, et al. Folate receptor autoimmunity and cerebral folate deficiency in low-functioning autism with neurological Deficits. Neuropediatrics 2008;38:276–81.

59. Davies C, Mishra D, Eshraghi RS, et al. Altering the gut microbiome to potentially modulate behavioral manifestations in autism spectrum disorders: a systematic review. Neurosci Biobehav Rev 2021;128:549–57.

60. Arnold LE, Luna RA, Williams K, et al. Probiotics for gastrointestinal symptoms and quality of life in autism: a placebo-controlled pilot trial. J Child Adolesc Psychopharmacol 2019;29(9):659–69.

61. Kang DW, Adams JB, Gregory AC, et al. Microbiota Transfer Therapy alters gut ecosystem and improves gastrointestinal and autism symptoms: an open-label study. Microbiome 2017;5(1):10.

62. Simkin DR. Microbiome and Mental health, specifically as it Relates to adolescents. Curr Psychiatry Rep 2019;21(9):93.

63. Goodwin MS, & Goodwin , T. (1969). In a dark mirror. Ment Hyg, 550-563.

64. McElhanon B, McCracken C, Karpen S, et al. Gastrointestinal symptoms in autism spectrum disorder: a meta-analysis. Pediatrics 2014;872–83.

65. Trivedi MS, Shah JS, Al-Mughairy S, et al. Food-derived opioid peptides inhibit cysteine uptake with redox and epigenetic consequences. J Nutr Biochem 2014;25:1011–8.

66. Croall ID, Hoggard N, Hadjivassiliou M. Autism spectrum disorder and gluten sensitivity. Nutrients 2021.

67. González-Domenech, et al. Influence of a combined gluten-free and casein-free diet on behavior disorders in children and adolescents diagnosed with autism spectrum disorder: a 12-month follow-up clinical trial. J Autism Dev Dis 2020;935–48.

68. Adams J, Holloway C. Pilot study of a moderate dose multivitamin/mineral supplement for children with autistic spectrum disorder. J Altern Complement Med 2004;1033–9.

69. Adams JB, Audhya T, McDonough-Means S, et al. Effect of a vitamin/mineral supplement on children and adults with autism. BMC Pediatr 2011;111(11): 1471–2431. In this issue.

70. Guo BQ, Li HB, Zhai DS, et al. Maternal multivitamin supplementation is associated with a reduced risk of autism spectrum disorder in children: a systematic review and meta-analysis. New York: Nutrition Research; 2019. p. 4–16.

71. Karhson DS, Krasinska KM, Dallaire JA, et al. Plasma anandamide concentrations are lower in children with autism spectrum disorder. Mol Autism 2018.

72. Siniscalco D, Sapone A, Giordano C, et al. Cannabinoid receptor type 2, but not type 1, is up-regulated in peripheral blood mononuclear cells of children affected by autistic disorders. J Autism Dev Disord 2013;2686–95.

73. FDA approves new indication for drug containing an active ingredient derived from cannabis to treat seizures in rare genetic disease. Available at: https://www.fda.gov/news-events/press-announcements/fda-approves-new-indi. https://www.fda.gov/news-events/public-health-focus/fda-regulation-cannabis-and-cannabis-derived-products-including-cannabidiol-cbd#:~:text=FDA%20has %20ap   proved%20Epidiolex%2C%20which,years%20of%20age%20and% 20older. (Accessed February 20, 2023).

74. Aran A, Cassuto H, Lubotzky A, et al. Brief report: cannabidiol-rich cannabis in children with autism spectrum disorder and severe behavioral problems-a retrospective feasibility study. J Autism Sev Disord 2019;1284–8.

75. Sharda, et al. Music improves social communication and auditory-motor connectivity in children with autism. Transl Psychiatry 2018;231.

76. Geretsegger M, Elefant C, Mössler K, et al. Music therapy for people with autism spectrum disorder. Cochrane Database Syst Rev 2014.

77. Ł Bieleninik, Geretsegger M, Mössler K, et al. Effects of improvisational music therapy vs enhanced standard care on symptom severity among children with autism spectrum disorder: the TIME-A randomized clinical trial. JAMA 2017;525–35.

78. Sharda M, Silani G, Specht K, et al. Music therapy for children with autism: investigating social behaviour through music. Lancet Child Adol Health 2019.

79. Wong VCN. Use of complementary and alternative medicine (CAM) in autism spectrum disorder (ASD): comparison of Chinese and Western Culture (Part A). J Autism Dev Disord 2009;454–63.

80. Lee B, Lee J, Cheon JH, et al. The efficacy and safety of acupuncture for the treatment of children with autism spectrum disorder: a systematic review and meta-analysis. Evid Based Complement Alterna Med 2018.

81. Liu C, Li T, Wang Z, et al. ScAlp acupuncture treatment for children's autism spectrum disorders: a systematic review and meta-analysis. Medicine (Baltimore) 2019.

82. Lee MS, Choi TY, Shin BC, et al. Acupuncture for children with autism spectrum disorders: a systematic review of randomized clinical trials. J Autism Dev Disord 2012;1671–83.

83. Dimolareva M, Dunn TJ. Animal-assisted interventions for school-aged children with autism spectrum disorder: a meta-analysis. J Autism Dev Disord 2020.

84. Anderson S, Meints K. Brief report: the effects of equine-assisted activities on the social functioning in children and adolescents with autism spectrum disorder. JADD 2016;3344–52.

85. Kern, et al. Prospective trial of equine-assisted activities in autism spectrum disorder. Altern Ther Health Med 2011;14–20.

86. Gabriels RL, Pan Z, Dechant B, et al. Randomizedcontrolled trial of therapeutic horseback riding in children and adolescents with autism spectrum disorder. J Am Acad Child Adolesc Psychiatry 2015;54:541–9.

87. Srinivasan SM, Cavagnino DT, Bhat AN. Effects of equine therapy on individuals with autism spectrum disorder: a systematic review. Rev J Autism Dev Disord 2018;156–75.

88. Ward SC, Whalon K, Rusnak K, et al. The association between therapeutic horseback riding and the social communication and sensory reactions of children with autism. J Autism Dev Disord 2013;190–8.

89. Argou-Cardozo I, Zeidán-Chuliá F. Clostridium bacteria and autism spectrum conditions: a systematic review and Hypothetical contribution of environmental glyphosate levels. Med Sci (Basel) 2018;6(2):29.

90. Xiong X, Liu D, Wang Y, et al. Urinary 3-(3-Hydroxyphenyl)-3-hydroxypropionic acid, 3-hydroxyphenylacetic acid, and 3-hydroxyhippuric acid are elevated in children with autism spectrum disorders. Biomed Res Int 2016;2016:8.

91. Wasdell, et al. A randomized, placebo-controlled trial of controlled release melatonin treatment of delayed sleep phase syndrome and impaired sleep maintenance in children with neuro. J Pineal Res 2008;57–64.

Moving?

Make sure your subscription moves with you!

To notify us of your new address, find your **Clinics Account Number** (located on your mailing label above your name), and contact customer service at:

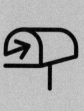

Email: journalscustomerservice-usa@elsevier.com

800-654-2452 (subscribers in the U.S. & Canada)
314-447-8871 (subscribers outside of the U.S. & Canada)

Fax number: 314-447-8029

Elsevier Health Sciences Division
Subscription Customer Service
3251 Riverport Lane
Maryland Heights, MO 63043

*To ensure uninterrupted delivery of your subscription, please notify us at least 4 weeks in advance of move.

Printed and bound by CPI Group (UK) Ltd, Croydon, CR0 4YY

03/10/2024

01040466-0005